For the Sake of the Children

MORALITY AND SOCIETY

A Series Edited by Alan Wolfe

For the Sake of the Children

The Social Organization of Responsibility in the Hospital and the Home

Carol A. Heimer
and
Lisa R. Staffen

The
University
of Chicago
Press

*Chicago &
London*

CAROL HEIMER is professor of sociology at Northwestern University and a research fellow at the American Bar Foundation. She is the author of several books, including *Reactive Risk and Rational Action: Managing Moral Hazard in Insurance Contracts.*
LISA STAFFEN is a Ph.D. candidate in sociology at Northwestern University.

The University of Chicago Press, Chicago 60637
The University of Chicago Press, Ltd., London

Printed in the United States of America

07 06 05 04 03 02 01 00 99 98 5 4 3 2 1

ISBN (cloth): 0-226-32504-0
ISBN (paper): 0-226-32505-9

Library of Congress Cataloging-in-Publication Data

Heimer, Carol Anne, 1951–
For the sake of the children : the social organization of responsibility in the hospital and the home / Carol A. Heimer and Lisa R. Staffen.
p. cm. — (Morality and society)
Includes bibliographical references and index.
ISBN 0-226-32504-0 — ISBN 0-226-32505-9 (pbk.)
1. Neonatal intensive care—Decision making. 2. Neonatal intensive care—Moral and ethical aspects. 3. Neonatal intensive care—Economic aspects. 4. Neonatal intensive care—Social aspects. I. Staffen, Lisa R. II. Title. III. Series.
RJ253.5.H45 1998
362.1′989201—dc21 97-52605
CIP

♾ The paper used in this publication meets the minimum requirements of the American National Standard for Information Sciences—Permanence of Paper for Printed Library Materials, ANSI Z39.48–1992.

To

Ruth Duggins Heimer

and

Diana Marie Staffen

who taught us

our first lessons

about taking

responsibility

CONTENTS

Illustrations

Tables

Figures

ACKNOWLEDGMENTS

IF RESPONSIBILITY IS, as we argue in this book, a social accomplishment, that is no less true for responsible scholarship. Our argument suggests that as those closest to the project, we are the ones who should be held accountable. The norms of the scholarly world concur in this. However, we argue that scholars will be more likely to embrace their responsibilities if, in addition to possessing the requisite resources and skills, they are appropriately supported and encouraged by others. It is for others to judge (we hope responsibly!) whether we had the needed skills and have produced responsible scholarship. Here we wish to acknowledge that, although there were plenty of lonely hours spent at our desks, we received abundant assistance from others.

Although we have many debts, our most important is clearly to the parents we interviewed and to the staff members who allowed us to interview them and watch them go about their work. This book would have been impossible to write without their contribution. But while social scientists often thank their informants for providing data, we wish to express our gratitude to our informants for their analytic contributions as well. The pithy phrases contributed in interviews, wry comments about the other participants in the life of a neonatal intensive care unit, gentle correction when our questions (or, in some instances, our early drafts) indicated that we had misunderstood the situation, all helped us see what direction to go. We have long believed that examples are the keys to good theorizing, and our interviews and field observation provided innumerable rich examples.

We are especially indebted to the social workers who acted as our main informants and sponsors in the two NICUs we studied. It would be difficult to overstate the help they provided—informal discussions, many formal interviews, advice about whom to talk to and how to locate people, introductions to other staff members, space in their offices, comments on our work. Perhaps most important though, their contributions represented an endorsement of the project—a statement that they believed it merited their contributions as well as ours.

If, as we argue in chapter 8, people must function in an organizational world, we would be remiss if we did not mention the organizations that helped (and sometimes hindered) us in working on this book. Three organizations made financial contributions to this work. The National Science Foundation supported Staffen as a graduate student while she combined course work with work on this project. The American Bar Foundation provided salary support for Heimer, a one-year research assistantship for Staffen, and substantial assistance with research expenses (research assistance, transcription, etc.) and provided those resources for more years than may have seemed reasonable. Northwestern University supported the work with a seed grant to Heimer, some support from the Sociology Department in the form of summer support for graduate students involved in co-authoring with faculty, and the "usual" indispensable support for research that we come to take for granted from universities. Both the American Bar Foundation and Northwestern University also contributed immensely to the intellectual development of our work by providing the right mix of solitude and stimulation in a diverse intellectual environment.

Two hospitals, after careful review of our project, permitted us to conduct our research in their neonatal intensive care units. Both hospitals, Northwestern University, and the American Bar Foundation subjected our project to the scrutiny of institutional review boards. While we cannot honestly say that we took pleasure in such reviews, we fully approve of that type of scrutiny. In the spirit of this work, though, we would also add that we have tried to go beyond the formal requirements of those bodies in seeking the consent of our research subjects.

While the hospitals must remain nameless to protect confidentiality, other organizations will remain nameless for a somewhat different reason. In this book we emphasize that people must be adaptable if they are to meet their responsibilities. One of the adaptations we made was to a somewhat leaner budget than would have been optimal in the early days of the project. Universities and other academic bodies put considerable pressure on faculty to apply for grants to defray the cost of research. Such applications take considerable time and are not always successful. We ultimately decided to be responsible scholars and to get the work done (with a higher contribution of our own time and financial resources) rather than to be responsible university citizens and continue to apply for outside funds. We think the book has not suffered for these decisions, although we are probably both somewhat less well known than we might have been had we received funds from the august bodies that declined our proposals or approved them without funding.

We have depended in a variety of ways on the contributions of other individuals. Lorrie Wessel, Zelda Coleman, Carol Nielsen, and Leah Feldman transcribed the bulk of our interviews. As they could testify, interviews done in homes with children and televisions in the background are not easy to transcribe. During their undergraduate years at Northwestern, Debbie Perry, Dan Rost, Amanda Selwyn, and Kim Weber worked on this project, collecting data from hospital medical records, coding and entering them into computer files, checking and rechecking information, compiling bibliographies, and writing us memos about their work. We benefited enormously from their help and were cheered by their interest in the project.

We also received help from graduate students. At various points, Debra Schleef, Sarah Gatson, Elizabeth Lock, and Mitchell Stevens worked on the project, doing many of the same tasks as the undergraduates we employed but also correcting transcripts of interviews, helping administer the project, constructing data files, discussing research strategy with us, commenting on paper and chapter drafts, and sharing the triumphs and setbacks of our work. During the time when we were devoting ourselves to coding data, they provided an indispensable community of people who instantly understood whom we were discussing, why we were chuckling, or what kind of time investment was entailed in some new file-management problem. Mitchell Stevens and Elizabeth Lock were among those who commented on the entire first draft, making suggestions that showed a deep familiarity with the study.

Over the years during which these ideas grew from proposals and papers into a book, we received advice and commentary from many academic colleagues. Among those who commented on paper drafts, chapter drafts, or oral presentations, we would like to thank Bruce Carruthers, the late James S. Coleman, Arlene Daniels, Robert Dingwall, Robert Emerson, Janet Gilboy, Sydney Halpern, Russell Hardin (who ran a wonderful seminar on social and political theory during his years at the University of Chicago), Christopher Jencks, Richard Lempert, Jane Mansbridge, Arthur MacEvoy, Doug McAdam, Mary Jo Neitz, Susan Shapiro, James Short, R. Stephen Warner, and several anonymous reviewers who read and provided commentary as part of publication processes. We owe an enormous debt to those who read and commented on the entire manuscript: John Braithwaite, Daniel Chambliss, Elizabeth Lock, Doug Mitchell, Aldon Morris, Kim Scheppele, Mitchell Stevens, and Alan Wolfe. Alan Wolfe, as editor of the series in which this book appears, indicated interest in the manuscript as it took shape and provided a judicious mix of patience, criticism, and support. Kim Scheppele has followed the project with the biographical insight that only a colleague from graduate school days is likely to have. She provided trenchant comments at the end, but also over the (long) years contributed references, suggestions, and considerable insight about where the project had come from and where it was going. As our editor at the University of Chicago Press, Doug Mitchell helped us through the last stages of writing and rewriting. His enthusiasm and praise alternately made us beam and blush, but he also gave our interactions the right intellectual tone by guiding us to important work in philosophy. Our skilled copy editor, Mark Jacobs, polished our prose and improved the manuscript by making suggestions that showed he was paying careful attention to our argument as well as our grammar.

And then there are those people whose lives are so intertwined with ours that we have asked for and received their help daily, sometimes hourly. Some of this support was given to us individually, some to us as coauthors. Wendy Espeland has probably read the whole manuscript but in two-page segments when we were having trouble with wording, needed advice about whether an argument made sense, or were unsure if we had given a fair rendition of some theorist's argument. Kai and Per Stinchcombe, Heimer's children, helped us understand why it mattered so very much to be responsible parents but also made it important to do the work efficiently. They provided all of the things that wonderful children do—pictures, stories, walks, cuddling, chocolates, tea, endless amusement, some irritation. But they also provided more—some penetrating questions (including one at a seminar), deep pride that their mother was writing a book, and an acceptance that fathers substitute for mothers because mothers have jobs too. Art Stinchcombe has read all of the chapters more than once and read the first draft the weekend it was completed. Because he sometimes doubted our wisdom in investing so much time in a single project (and had to bear some of the costs), we have been especially grateful for his pride in our accomplishment as the project neared completion. In the discipline of sociology he is known for being a reliable producer of incisive comments on others' manuscripts. One of the cleverest parts of our research design was to arrange a family tie with such a person so that we could harness his responsibility to more than just the intellectual parts of the project. We have also been fortunate to have a family tie with Patrick Kerpan, who has occasionally joked about the various ways in which the "Kerpan Foundation" has supported our work. He has been patient and supportive throughout, even when he didn't completely understand how the timetables of academic publishing could be so different from the timetables of software production. Most of the work for this book was completed before Staffen had become a parent, but the birth of her daughter, Elisabeth Staffen Kerpan, helped teach her what it really means to be responsible for another, fragile life—how much work it is (even when a baby is healthy) and how many rewards there are. The copyediting stage undoubtedly went more slowly with one arm occupied by holding the baby, but we wouldn't have had it any other way.

As co-authors, we fully share responsibility for the end product. The project that led to this book has not always been a joint effort. It began as Heimer's project. Staffen joined as a research assistant for a year between undergraduate and graduate school and eventually became a full co-author. Here our accounts diverge somewhat. Heimer believes that it was a stroke of genius to get Staffen signed on as a full participant so that someone else would fully share responsibility for the work. Staffen believes that she was fortunate to join a project that offered unusual opportunities for a graduate student to get full credit for her work. In any case, the evolution of our co-authorship to some degree parallels the evolution of the parents we describe in chapters 5 and 6, with Staffen experiencing an initial period of being an inexpert outsider subject to Heimer's scrutiny and gradually becoming expert herself and fully capable of turning the tables and scrutinizing Heimer's contributions.

The very most responsible friends (and we count our children, husbands, and co-authors among our friends) provide whatever is needed—support, criticism, a sympathetic ear, dinner, written comments, help with child care, and especially a willingness to be put off until we were finished. We are finished now and it is their turn.

ONE

Why We Need a Sociology of Responsibility

"I JUST WANT TO GET TO BE A NORMAL FAMILY," Sue said quietly. "You know, other people get to take their babies here and there or hear them talk. . . . Everybody says just wait, just wait until she starts screaming. I'd be so happy, you know" (1009F, p. 49).[1] Sue and Will had been married for only a few months when Sue became pregnant. It was a planned pregnancy, they both stressed; they didn't think it was right to bring a child into the world inadvertently. They also shared a strong conviction that once a child was born, the parents had an obligation to care for the child, adjusting in whatever way the situation required. As Sue put it, parents "should switch their lives around for the baby," because they "should take care of it no matter what" (1009F, p. 39).

Sue and Will's plans changed abruptly one day sixteen months before our interviews with them, when their daughter was born prematurely. Tiffany spent the next four-and-a-half months in hospitals, overcoming difficulties associated with her prematurity or created by the medical staff's attempts to help her. As many "premies" do, Tiffany had difficulty breathing and was placed on a ventilator. But the fragile tissue of tiny lungs is easily

1. To protect confidentiality, we refer to all people and places by pseudonyms. Throughout this book, we refer to the families we interviewed with case and page numbers from those interviews. The first digit refers to the sample (1 for families from City Hospital, 2 for those from Suburban Hospital), the subsequent three digits to the case number within the sample (we use only numbers 001–040, but kept the leading zero for facility in separating the sample identifier from the case number). We use this four-digit numerical code when we are referring to an infant's case in a general way, but when we refer to a specific interview, we further identify whether it is the female parent (F) or the male parent (M). In a few instances we interviewed the parents together (F&M).

Staff interviews are identified in a parallel fashion, with a four-digit numerical code followed by two letters. The first digit refers to the hospital (1 for City Hospital, 2 for Suburban Hospital), the subsequent three digits identify a specific staff member (again with the leading zero retained for facility in separating the hospital identifier from the code number for a specific staff member), and a letter string identifying the occupation of the staff member (MD for physicians, RN for nurses, DP for discharge planners, OT for occupational therapists, and SW for social workers).

scarred through forced expansion by a ventilator, and infants who spend more than a brief period on a ventilator are likely to suffer permanent damage to their lungs. In addition, their tracheas may be scarred by the endotracheal tube through which air flows from the ventilator into the lungs. Tiffany experienced both problems and as a result had a serious bout of pneumonia, which led to a second hospitalization and numerous surgeries to remove scar tissue and increase the size of her airway. When corrective surgery failed, Tiffany's parents were crushed to learn their daughter would require a tracheostomy. A surgical opening was made in her trachea, and the ventilator was attached to a tracheostomy tube. As a result of these complications, Sue and Will faced great uncertainty about what their daughter's future would be like.

Serious problems such as these often lead to other, more minor problems, which may not be life threatening, but nevertheless wear parents down. For much of her life Tiffany was an extremely reluctant eater. Sue was particularly distressed about this, because it was she who had to organize her day around coaxing her daughter to eat. She also had to explain to physicians and nurses that the problem was not that Tiffany was being held in an uncomfortable position or being fed ineptly or any number of other explanations that they came up with as they laid the blame at Sue's feet.

Over the months of Tiffany's early life, Sue and Will became quite skilled at caring for their child, at training the nurses who were supposed to relieve them for a few hours a day, and at confronting medical staff if they did their jobs ineptly. Sue was particularly galled by incompetence or inattentiveness. Though she was quick to recognize that the hospital staff had skills she lacked, she was infuriated when they failed to recognize that she also had skills and that she was in some ways their supervisor (though she did not describe the problem in quite this way). She complained bitterly that they were unwilling to take her seriously because she was so young. Despite her youth (she was only nineteen when Tiffany was born), she was the one responsible for ensuring that her child received good care.

Sue took her job very seriously, even insisting that Tiffany be transferred from one hospital to another when she became dissatisfied with the quality of care. Sue believed that the nurses did not change the tracheostomy tube that connected Tiffany to the ventilator frequently enough or clean the area around the tube as well as she thought necessary; she also charged them with neglecting to cushion the connection between the tracheostomy tube and the child's skin, failing to tie the tube in place properly to prevent it from becoming dislodged, and leaving soiled diapers on Tiffany so long that she developed severe diaper rash. In addition to arranging for her daughter's transfer, Sue's achievements included successfully resuscitating Tiffany after she stopped breathing one night at home, confronting medical equipment suppliers who brought the wrong parts or who failed to keep machinery in good repair, and detecting signs of illness in Tiffany before the home nurses did (and indeed before the illness could be confirmed by anything other than X rays or ultrasounds).

These young parents had become formidable advocates for their child—they had mastered the intricacies of hospital systems and medical hierarchies, had worked out the arcane details of how to arrange funding through the Katie Beckett program, had figured out how to cope (though unhappily) with a large staff of home nurses, and had reorganized their household by moving in with Will's parents so that they could manage on one working-class salary.[2] And throughout this experience, they retained a sense of what all this effort was for—to raise a child. Sue described her attempts to teach Tiffany to crawl, happily talked about Tiffany blowing kisses to them and clucking her tongue (important evidence that Tiffany was learning the skills necessary for speech even though her tracheostomy prevented her from making much sound), and longed for the day when they would be able to do ordinary things like taking a trip to the zoo, unencumbered by medical equipment.[3]

Sue and Will had risen to the challenges presented by Tiffany's fragile health but nevertheless looked forward to the time when their lives would not be ruled by their daughter's demanding health-care needs. Though neither seemed to have had elaborate plans for his or her own life before Tiffany's birth, they both felt their lives had been put on hold by her prematurity and subsequent medical problems. "We want to go to school, start getting on with our lives, and start doing something" (1009F, p. 17),

2. The Katie Beckett program provides federal funding so that chronically ill or disabled children who would otherwise have to be cared for in a hospital or other institution can instead be cared for at home. The program was signed into law by President Ford, and named after the child whose family had pressed for funding so that they could care for their daughter at home.

3. Will and Sue were fully aware of the importance of these indicators. Will commented on hearing Tiffany's first cry, a particularly welcome sound given the distinct possibility that she might have been stillborn: "It was a real nice first cry because, you know, we didn't expect to hear anything, you know" (1009M, p. 12). He was eager to hear her voice again: "We haven't heard her but make that one noise. That's a little hard, you know, but we're almost to the end, thank God" (1009M, p. 19). The next surgery would remove the "trach," and "she'll be ready to make noise" (p. 36).

Sue said. Quite simply, though, Tiffany's needs had to come first. "Tiffany's my involvement until she gets her 'trach' out," Sue explained (1009F, p. 59). Plans for both parents to go back to school, to buy a house, and to have another child all were deferred. Sue left her job as a sales clerk in a local discount store when she went into labor and was never able to return to work after Tiffany's birth, as she had planned. And Will continued to work as a manual laborer, because they relied on his income, even though he desperately wanted to escape the physically demanding and mind-numbing work. As he put it, though, "The big trauma's over. Now it's just a waiting game" (1009M, p. 36).

As tales of premature births go, this one is not particularly dramatic. But its very mundanity makes it a good starting point for our discussion of what it means to take responsibility. Sue and Will experienced an unexpected event, followed by a long period of considerable uncertainty. The chronicle of their adjustment to Tiffany's birth can be told as a story about a series of unprovoked shocks from the external world or as a tale of a couple's reactions, adjustments, and thoughtful initiatives to improve their daughter's life. Both versions contain a measure of truth, of course—Sue and Will often either had no control over the course of events or only learned about how they might have intervened after the fact. But rather than be passive passengers on a roller-coaster ride (to use a metaphor often invoked by such parents) they had never wished to take, these young parents looked for ways to influence events, to improve the situation even marginally, and to prevent what further disasters they could.

By focusing on what Will and Sue, and others like them, do when confronted with unexpected events with potentially grave consequences, we can learn a great deal about the conditions under which people embrace or reject responsibility. To start with, we learn that there is variability in the people themselves and in the extent to which they accept responsibility. While Will and Sue felt that they had primary responsibility for Tiffany's welfare, not all parents feel that way. Some, for instance, feel that the child only becomes their responsibility after discharge home, and others continue to feel that health professionals have the primary responsibility for some aspects of the child's development. But not all of the variation resides in the people who confront questions about whether to take on responsibilities. Just as a division of labor between professionals and parents may shape parents' sense of what their responsibilities are, so organizational contexts also transform people's views about their responsibilities and their capacity to shoulder them. For those (like physicians and nurses) who are regular participants in an organization, the division of labor may make responsibilities much more manageable. For those who are outsiders (like parents), drawing only briefly on the expertise or resources of organizational members, organizational divisions of labor and boundaries may pose obstacles. Parents who feel, as Will and Sue did, that parental responsibility is not left at the doorstep of the hospital may still have difficulty acting on their views. It may be far from clear how to be a responsible parent on someone else's turf. When contacts with professionals leave some people feeling enlightened and empowered and others demoralized and incompetent, we can be sure that some of the variability is coming from professionals and the organizations in which they work. Some organizations are easy to penetrate, but others are not. Some organizational staff members see outsiders as intruders to be kept at bay while the real work is done by insiders, whereas other staff members see outsiders as potential contributors who must be quickly inducted into the group.

By scrutinizing people's responses to life-altering circumstances, we try to show how responsibility arises and how the acceptance of responsibility can be either undermined or supported by the way that institutions are designed and the way that normative systems (including the informal rules of family life, the rules of professional conduct, the routines and procedures of particular organizations, the administrative regulations of state and federal bureaucracies, and state and federal law) work together. Although we here examine parents' acceptance of responsibility for children, we argue that such an example can tell us much about the general process by which high-quality compliance with norms (what we here call responsibility) comes about.

Situations such as that faced by Sue and Will provide us with the raw materials for studying two fundamental aspects of social life: agency and responsibility. We learn about human agency—the capacity of people to make meaningful choices rather than just do what they have been programmed to do—and what happens when people confront situations for which they have not been prepared either by anticipatory socialization for a particular role or by being supplied with an appropriate "script." It is not that social structure ceases to be important, only that it plays a somewhat different role when extreme uncertainty makes the scripting of activity difficult and when the consequential nature of the events motivates reflection rather than unthinking compliance.

By examining situations like that faced by Will and Sue, we are also able to ask how responsibility arises. Although much of social science is concerned with questions about when people abide by rules rather than violate them, here we instead ask about a different aspect of compliance. We ask how it happens that people actively attempt to figure out what they should do, try to determine which means are most appropriate to the ends, adjust their own behavior and enlist the help of others in a valiant attempt to produce a desired outcome. We turn now to a more formal presentation of the questions that motivated this research and an explanation of why we believe a study of people like Sue and Will is a good way to answer these questions.

Responsibility and Moral Hazard as Concerns of Social Control Systems

Three ubiquitous problems for social systems are how to get people not to violate norms, how to get them to meet minimum standards (e.g., not to shirk on the job), and how to get at least some people to perform at a higher level, providing the flexible adjustment to changing conditions that is the hallmark of responsibility. The first of these problems, the outright violation of norms, or deviance, has been a central concern of sociology since its earliest days (see, e.g., Durkheim's [1982] discussion of the centrality of deviance to the sociological agenda; more recently, see, e.g., Erikson 1966; Gibbs and Erickson 1975; and Merton's brief summary of the history of sociological theorizing about deviant behavior [1987: 8–10]). The second problem, shirking, or moral hazard as it is often called in the social science literature, has received considerable attention in recent years, though until recently most of this attention has come from economists rather than from sociologists (Arrow 1971, 1991; Fama 1980; Fama and Jensen 1983; Heimer 1985; Holmstrøm 1979, 1982). The third problem, which we here call responsibility, has received much less attention.[4] By responsibility, we mean high-quality compliance with norms—thoughtful compliance oriented toward achieving the objective of the norm or meeting one's obligations to others rather than toward avoidance of blame or

4. Two notable exceptions are Selznick (1992) and Wuthnow (1991). Selznick, whose work is cited later in this chapter, discusses both the responsible self and the responsible enterprise, and Wuthnow contributes an empirical study of compassion. Wuthnow argues that the distinction between compassion and corruption is a distinction between two forms of overcommitment (1991: 279–80). Both entail exercising discretion in the application of rules, going beyond a job description, the letter of the law, or the fine print of a contract. But while corruption entails bending the rules for personal benefit, compassion involves going beyond what is required in the opposite direction—overconforming, overperforming for the benefit of others.

superficial conformity. What's crucial here is that people are actively choosing how best to conform to norms, altering their own contributions of labor and other resources as necessary, and monitoring to ensure that the outcomes are what they intended.

Most of the scholarly work on responsibility has asked somewhat different questions from the one we pose here. Our concern is frankly empirical, while the questions posed by others have been more normative. We ask about when people *take* responsibility; others ask either what course of action is the most responsible or when people should be *held* responsible. While we ask especially about empirical regularities and how they arise, other inquiries have focused either on the moral justification of systems of distribution and how to take account of the welfare of others or on the appropriateness of social systems that hold people accountable for some kinds of outcomes (e.g., those over which they have some control) but not for others (e.g., those that are accidental). As we show in the paragraphs that follow, the normative questions posed by philosophers, legal scholars, and economists are closely related to the more empirical questions around which this book is organized.

Notions of what is morally acceptable are key elements of a theory of responsibility. We cannot talk sensibly about when people take responsibility unless we have some consensus about which choices or courses of action are responsible. Although they do not always use a common language and they disagree on the fine points, philosophers and economists do agree that responsibility requires consideration of the welfare of others, a point echoed throughout this book. Kant, for instance, articulates a moral obligation, which he regards as both universally applicable and universally binding, always to treat human beings as ends rather than as means to ends: "So act as to treat humanity, whether in thine own person or in that of any other, in every case as an end withal, never as a means only" (1949:46; see generally 1949, 1965b).

But what does it really mean always to treat other people as ends in themselves? For instance, is it ever responsible to choose one's own welfare over that of someone else? Building on the foundation of Kant's work, other writers have tried to provide guidance about how to think about the inevitable dilemmas that arise in choosing among courses of action that, while respecting the humanity of all, nevertheless lead to inequalities in welfare. The self-interest model of economics contains the rudiments of one theory about the responsible way to take account of the welfare of others. The principle of Pareto optimality, for example, can be seen as articulating a standard for when an action would have the appropriate responsible consequences for the general welfare. In choosing among alternative courses of action, one should choose those actions that improve the welfare of some only if they do not also entail sacrifices in the welfare of others (Cirillo 1979: 42–60).

Some of the modifications of the principle of Pareto optimality offer different views about how people should think about the welfare of others. Rawls (1971), for instance, argues that inequalities are justifiable only when they benefit the most disadvantaged members of a society. We can justify unusually high wages to some occupational group, then, only when the increase in income inequality also improves the welfare of the most-disadvantaged groups, for instance by encouraging the provision of services to them. Although both Pareto and Rawls insist that we must consider the welfare of all members of the society, they diverge in their views on the permissibility of inequality. While Pareto optimality allows any transactions that improve the welfare of some as long as they don't decrease the welfare of others, Rawls's difference principle permits increases in inequality only if the lot of the worst-off members of society is thereby improved.

Such standards for how to balance the welfare of some against the welfare of others include one key component of common conceptions of responsibility—the assertion that it is imperative to take the welfare of others seriously. But they ignore other aspects of responsibility, such as concern with the future as well as the present or the requirement to adjust contributions (of labor or other resources) in order to achieve desired ends. Further, although the principle of Pareto optimality and Rawls's difference principle tell us how people ought to behave—what behavior is morally defensible—they tell us relatively little about when people will in fact conform to such standards or what factors increase or decrease the likelihood that such standards will shape anyone's actions.

Even if questions about what it is morally appropriate to do were resolved, we would still be left with questions about the moral status of actions that people might or might not take to achieve those ends. Here the central issue is the degree to which people have the capacity to choose a course of action and what that capacity to choose implies about how actions should be evaluated by others, for instance in courts of law. When should we hold people responsible, who should hold them responsible, and what consequences should follow when we hold someone responsible? Drawing on Raab (1968), Lempert and Sanders argue that full moral responsibility depends on both agency and intention (1986: 15–41). That is, we can hold people fully responsible only for intentional acts that they had some reasonable way to avoid. If, for instance, a person did not intend to injure someone else or could not avoid the action that led to the injury, we are less likely to hold him or her responsible. Even when we do not feel we should hold someone fully responsible, we may nevertheless continue to pin some of the blame on him or her. Further, legal responsibility need not correspond perfectly with moral responsibility. In some instances, the law (e.g., in strict liability regimes) disregards both agency and intention and holds people responsible for acts they didn't intend and couldn't avoid, on the grounds that such rules of accountability have desirable effects (such as motivating employers to attend to safety or allocating the cost of accidents to those most able to pay for them) (see Scheppele [1991] on tort theory).

Questions about causality are, of course, also important when we move from asking who should be held accountable to asking how we can induce others to take responsibility. McKeon (1957) shows how the word *responsibility,* which only came into use in the late 1700s (he discusses English, French, and German usages), draws on and combines earlier notions of imputation and accountability. Whether we "impute" responsibility to someone, to follow McKeon's usage, is to some degree independent of whether we hold them accountable, he notes. But in distinguishing between imputation and accountability, McKeon sensitizes us to variations in views about where virtue resides (in the nature and will of individuals vs. in the mores and laws of communities), who makes evaluations (other community members forming their opinions as individuals vs. a community body making a more formal assessment), and what is being evaluated (the actions and choices that are the causes of an act vs. the consequences of the act). The imputation of responsibility, he argues, entails both assessing causal efficacy and praising or blaming others for making choices and taking actions that are judged to be either particularly good or particularly evil. The imputation of responsibility is a statement about what we think we can expect from others in the future and about whether we can expect them to be sensitive to questions of principle and to the relation between means and ends. Accountability, in contrast, is about the relationship between private interests and the common good, McKeon suggests. Communities mete out rewards and punishments as a way of holding people accountable for the good or evil consequences of actions, regardless of whether anyone intended the consequences.

Both streams of discourse also recognize that independent moral evaluations may conflict with common opinion and community rules and that it may sometimes be responsible to buck popular opinion or violate a law: "The hero in fact and in fiction is either the man who conforms in the highest degree to the standards of estimation and praise or the man who ignores common opinion to pursue what is praiseworthy" (McKeon 1957: 10). To be responsible, then, entails making an independent assessment of whether the situation requires one to follow the rules or break them, and McKeon here recognizes that responsibility entails considerably more than perfunctory compliance with obligations. At the end of his essay on the concept of responsibility, McKeon moves beyond his concern with questions of how we assess behavior as responsible or not to ask explicitly about the link between holding people responsible and encouraging them to take responsibility. "The basic elements of responsibility are accountability and imputation," he comments, "but the moral problem of responsibility is to find the means to use them in discussion and common action so as to increase the probability that responsible action will develop moral character and rational perceptiveness" (1990: 85). It is these questions about how imputation, accountability, and other causal mechanisms increase the likelihood of responsibility that we pursue in this book.

Although a few scholars have conducted empirical investigations about the causal mechanisms that increase the likelihood of responsible behavior, they have rarely identified the problem in a way that highlights the underlying dimension of compliance with obligation or shows the relation of responsibility to deviance and shirking. Moreover, these researchers have been concerned with such diverse empirical settings and have categorized the work in sufficiently disparate ways that little theoretical progress has been made. For instance, much of the work on regulation could be conceived to be about the ways that regulators try to induce responsible behavior in those they regulate. From this perspective, Bardach and Kagan (1982), Braithwaite (1985), Stone (1975), Vaughan (1996), and many of the authors whose work is collected in Hawkins (1992) could be conceived as studying responsibility, though only Bardach and Kagan explicitly discuss the difference between responsibility and other levels of compliance with obligations. This book is explicitly concerned then with how normative systems foster responsibility. We argue that Will and Sue's reaction to their daughter's plight can only be understood when we analyze it as an attempt to take responsibility—to comply thoughtfully and wholeheartedly with their normative obligations to Tiffany.

Though responsibility has received scant attention from social scientists, it has become a buzzword in politics and public discourse on issues ranging from the decline of the American family to the escalation of corporate greed. Legislators often debate how welfare recipients can be induced to take responsibility for their own lives rather than rely on the public purse (although scholars like Luker [1996] point out that such discussions are plagued by deep misconceptions about teenage pregnancy and unwed motherhood and their relation to poverty). At the same time, given that children now make up a larger percentage of the nation's poor than at any time since we began keeping statistics (Coltrane 1996: 124), legislative debate about welfare cannot completely ignore questions about societal as well as parental responsibilities for children. Juvenile crime has also been a focus of national concern, and questions about responsibility have been raised in that discussion as well. If parents would take more responsibility for their children, some suggest, juvenile crime rates would fall. Concerns about responsibility are pervasive. Teachers are accused of failing to take responsibility for their students' learning. Corporate managers, we are told, have conceived themselves as beholden only to shareholders and have neglected their responsibilities to other stakeholders. Responsibility was also the rallying cry of the controversial and closely watched Million Man March, of African-American men, in Washington, D.C., in 1995. The refrains are familiar: If individuals, groups, and large organizations took more responsibility, the world would be a better place. But what exactly does it mean to take more responsibility? Who should take responsibility? How is responsibility encouraged? And alternately, how is it undermined?

Responsibility, as it is commonly understood, has a multiplicity of meanings. But whether they are onerous obligations or rewards for past achievements, and whether they are individual or collective ones, responsibilities carry with them an obligation to achieve some desired, but perhaps ambiguously defined, objective. In analyzing responsibilities, we need to make understanding the nature of the obligation our first task. Here we are interested in how widely shared the obligation is, asking whether it falls on the shoulders of one person or is shared with others. We are also interested in how compulsory the obligation is and ask whether one is drafted or volunteers. In addition, we are interested in how the desired outcome is defined, whether by those who must meet it or by other authorities, in how closely compliance is monitored, and in how rewards and punishments are distributed for meeting, exceeding, or falling short of expectations. Responsibility implies some social group. We must therefore ask: Responsible to whom? For what? And with what consequences?

In using the word *responsibility*, we wish to emphasize our agnosticism about motivations that lead to responsible behavior, the goals that are being pursued, and the settings in which responsible behavior occurs. One may pursue the goals of an organization, a profession, a family, or world peace using reason and calculation, and the pursuit of such goals would ordinarily be called responsible. Though responsibility is clearly a moral issue as well as an empirical one, here we treat it empirically. This is not because we are unwilling to take a stance on such moral questions as whether responsibilities should be met or who should meet them, but instead because many of the deepest questions can only be answered through empirical investigations. For instance, although one can say in the abstract that it is responsible to take account of others' welfare, to add content to that statement requires empirical investigation to determine what others' interests are. The customary split between normative and descriptive (or "positive") work is overdrawn. Moral and empirical approaches work together. Sensible moral prescriptions require an empirical foundation, and empirical investigations often lead us to see more clearly what is morally acceptable and what is not. Before philosophical principles can be translated into practical prescriptions, for instance about how to balance the welfare of one against the welfare of another, they must be combined with information about the needs and interests of various parties, current levels of welfare, the costs and benefits of supplying the goods and services most needed or desired, the unanticipated costs and benefits of altering levels of inequality, and the causal processes entailed in building empathy, planning courses of actions, and fostering the cooperation necessary for complex activities. Rather than prescribe what families ought to be doing, we instead ask what families are in fact doing when they are confronted with unexpected burdens. Our purpose here is not to condemn some parents while praising others but to explore the variation among parents in how they conceive their obligations to their children and ultimately how some parents come to have a very narrow conception of their role, while others define it much more broadly.

Here we make the case for why social scientists should be interested in responsibility. Sociologists have been accused of believing that social structure and norms are so determinative of human action that there is little room for human agency (e.g., Wrong 1961; Giddens 1979; Sewell 1992). Clearly people do make choices, as Sue and Will did, and real choices at that. Our premise is that many such choices are oriented to the welfare of others, of social groups, or of values. Choices and agency are "responsible" only when they are social. But how much people really *choose* varies from one situation to another; we have knee-jerk responses in some situations, while in others we think long and hard before deciding what to do or how to do it. To develop sociological theories that incorporate human agency, we need to examine situations that require agency—situations in which people must use their human capacities to reflect, strategize, and choose. Variations between situations or roles that require responsibility and those that do not supply raw materials for constructing theories that incorporate a more sophisticated understanding of human agency.[5] Human agency that takes account of others we call "responsibility" since that is the core meaning of the word as it is usually used. As Selznick puts it, the responsible self is "both genuinely other-regarding and constructively self-regarding" (1992: 227). For example, when people point to variations in levels of responsibility as a justification for variations in wages (Jaques 1972; Soltan 1987), they apparently mean that occupants of positions requiring more responsibility have to think, strategize, and choose on behalf of a complicated system of social values.

The most important parts of social structure cannot be created or managed without agency, and responsibility is the core of what we try to achieve through incentive systems, the design of the legal system, the instruction of our children in values, and similar devices to get others to take a larger view or to consider the relation between an action and a complicated set of purposes. This requires social arrangements that make people look beyond themselves to consider the needs and interests of the organizations, families, friendship groups, or societies in which they are embedded. When we try to get someone to "take responsibility," for instance by assigning a task or mandating some behavior, we are disappointed if we

5. Although much of the work on the capacity of people to make meaningful choices focuses on structural constraints that limit and shape choice, more recent work has also looked at the extent to which people's capacity to make choices is limited or expanded in other ways. For instance, the essays in Loewenstein and Elster (1992) examine how problems of choice and constraint are altered when we look at them over time, and Sanchez (1997) shows that people continue to experience themselves as agents making meaningful choices even when they are relatively powerless. Sewell (1992) argues that social structures do not always constrain actors; instead they empower some actors while disempowering others. While we will be looking at some of the kinds of constraints examined by other authors—difficulties with choice over time, bureaucratic impediments to choice, variations in power—we will be especially interested in how people's sense of their own agency is affected by the importance of the stakes.

get legalism rather than thoughtful compliance. In giving their children chores, parents hope to instill a sense of obligation for the collective welfare and to teach that many rules are guidelines for coordinating the activities of a group of people. Even if the work gets done, parents are disappointed when their child repeatedly chooses the easiest jobs or fails to notice when a task needs to be done, insisting that no rule specifies when it has to be done. Responsibility is about a moral competence that goes beyond accountability and legalism; it entails moral agency based on an "inner commitment to moral restraint and aspiration" (Selznick 1992: 345) rather than simple conformity to an external standard.

Responsibility is also fundamental to caring.[6] Gilligan (1982) argues that moral development can proceed along two different paths, one guided by the ethic of justice, the other by the ethic of care.[7] A person can either reason deductively from principles of justice or attempt to decipher and balance the needs of various parties. Gilligan suggests that those guided by the ethic of care are more likely to feel responsible for finding a solution that works well for everyone. At the highest level of development, though, the ethic of justice and the ethic of care tend to converge. Paying attention to the spirit as well as the letter of the law and attending to the rights as well as the needs of concrete people would, by our argument, often lead to the same outcome.

This connection between responsibility and caring is especially strong when responsibilities are fates rather than opportunities, as we explain below. Gender differences in distributions of caring work encumber women with responsibilities not easily shifted to others, leaving men freer to invest in responsibilities that are both more likely to lead to rewards and easier to escape should they become burdensome.[8] For men, responsibilities are

6. In presenting her argument for a more political notion of the ethic of care, Tronto (1993) discusses the relationship between care and responsibility, which she regards as a central moral category. See esp. her comments on the elements of an ethic of care (1993: 127–37). Interestingly, Tronto also is concerned about the association of care with women (as we are below, for a somewhat different reason) and how to move the ethic of care into the moral and political mainstream. See Menkel-Meadow (1996) for a skeptical assessment of the wisdom and practicality of weakening the tie between gender and the ethic of care.

7. Gilligan's book stimulated a cottage industry of scholarly work debating the link between gender and the ethics of justice and care, discussing the adequacy of Kohlberg's (1981) and Gilligan's research, extending the analysis to include variations by ethnicity and social class as well as gender, and noting applications of Gilligan's ideas to other settings. Tronto provides an overview of much of this work (1993: 61–97).

8. It is important to keep in mind that there are also intragender differences in the constraints of family roles. Childless women will usually be less constrained by family roles than other women. But sometimes being childless or unmarried only means that other fam-

more likely to be taken on as strategic opportunities or investments, while for women responsibilities are more likely to be fates that limit their capacity to strategize and to invest outside the family (Heimer 1996b). Any empirical study of the social organization of responsibility will thus need to address questions about how responsibilities come to be assigned to one group of people rather than another and why there is more choice about the acceptance of some kinds of responsibilities than others.

Responsibilities as Fates or Opportunities

We can distinguish between two different ways that people come to have particular responsibilities and their correspondingly different experiences with them. Briefly, responsibilities can be either opportunities or fates; they can be more strongly associated with positions or with persons. People may come to have particular responsibilities because they choose them, for instance by volunteering for one task rather than another at work, or by deciding on a line of employment. The physicians who cared for Tiffany during her hospitalization acquired a responsibility for her (and other patients) when they chose to become neonatologists; one or more of her nurses might have requested to care for her in particular and to act as her "primary nurse." In choosing one responsibility rather than another, a person might be driven by the chance to do an interesting task, to get credit for a job well done, to avoid an onerous alternative task, or to win the opportunity to undertake an especially attractive job later. Reactions to this first type of responsibility are tapped by survey questions that ask whether respondents would like to take more responsibility at work or whether they already have as much responsibility as they want. Evidence from surveys suggests that people like their jobs better when those jobs carry more responsibility.[9]

But not all responsibilities are so freely chosen. Some responsibilities are received as accidents of fate and experienced as burdens rather than opportunities, though a person may still be able to refuse a responsibility or to limit his or her obligations. A premature birth, such as Tiffany's, or

ily members will assume that the unmarried sister is the obvious caretaker for their aging mother.

9. These surveys do not usually measure actual responsibility. Instead they ask about numbers of superiors and subordinates, ownership of the business, frequency of supervision, and sometimes whether the respondent is happy with current responsibilities or would like to have more or fewer. As one example, Jencks, Perman, and Rainwater's (1988) index of job desirability includes some items that could be construed as measures of responsibility.

the illness of an aging parent does not lead to fantasies of credit for a job well done or of future opportunities to care for disabled relatives.[10] Instead people worry about how to balance the new responsibility with preexisting commitments and how to husband their resources or find new ones. Rather than seek rewards, people strive to avoid guilt and blame. The best they can hope for is credit for having "done their duty" despite the unfairness of being dealt a hand of inescapable obligations.

Though in some senses a responsibility is a "fate" whenever one does not freely choose the responsibility and cannot escape it (and so exercises agency more in deciding how to meet the obligation rather than in whether to meet it), the potential disproportion between obligations and resources is fundamental to the consequential character of fatelike responsibilities. When a responsibility is a fate, one must dip into or even deplete one's own resources even though others do not pitch in. A responsibility is a fate, then, whenever one might be stuck in a permanently losing situation, in which a responsibility can be discharged only by exhausting one's resources. It is even more a fate if such a permanently losing position does not leave one with sufficient resources to discharge the responsibility adequately. But fatelike responsibilities are not limited to personal life. One is confronted with property ownership as a fate when one's business goes bankrupt with unlimited liability, especially if one then feels an obligation to pay all the creditors even after the bankruptcy. And in social systems, such as caste systems, in which occupations are ascriptively assigned (on the basis of such immutable traits as gender, race, and ethnicity), occupational responsibilities are more likely to be experienced as fates.

Two aspects of responsibility—the inescapability of the obligations and the relation between resources and obligations—predict being stuck in a situation similar to bankruptcy. When resources do vary with the magnitude of an obligation, and when one can escape burdens that have become intolerable or just unattractive in comparison with other responsibilities one might shoulder, a person retains the flexibility to strategize about

10. Although people do not think of "opportunities" to care for sick or disabled relatives or to take on other similar fates as "investments," they may nevertheless subsequently choose to make use of the skills and knowledge acquired in the course of meeting such obligations. People might, for instance, be called on to offer advice and solace to others experiencing similar events. Sue and Will's decision to build on their experiences with Tiffany by enrolling in a nursing curriculum, and so to use their new empathy and skills in a professional capacity, is rather unusual. We suspect that the likelihood of treating the new knowledge and skills as "human capital" is greater when people experience these crises before having made major decisions about careers.

which package of obligations to accept. In contrast, when resources cannot be adjusted in response to contingencies, and when one retains responsibility "come hell or high water," one's capacity to maneuver is decreased, and previous obligations act as rigid constraints on one's ability to respond to other opportunities that might arise. It is this constraining aspect of fatelike responsibility that so deeply shapes women's experience of responsibility. As we discuss below, women and men are not equally exposed to the burdens of fatelike responsibilities. There is a central irony here: though fate implies inevitability, fatelike responsibilities are more inevitable for women than for men. Fate, in short, is quite an elaborate social achievement.

In this book, we explore the various mechanisms that bind people, sometimes loosely, sometimes tightly, to their responsibilities and the mechanisms that are only sometimes available to adjust resources to obligations. Gender predicts how fateful the responsibility is, and we will discuss this first. But other characteristics of people also play an important role in shaping how they view their obligations and in determining whether they have the room to maneuver to meet those obligations, and we will return to those, as well, in our examination of how parents view their obligations to their children.

Gender: A Strategic Resource

Because responsibilities carry contingent obligations, assuming one responsibility tends to limit one's capacity to accept others. The conflict is more acute for responsibilities that are fates than for those that are opportunities, because fates cannot as easily be shed or reduced to accommodate new possibilities and because they are more likely to be associated with the shallower pockets of families than the deeper pockets of organizations. Characteristics that are associated with taking on fatelike responsibilities are therefore key subjects in an empirical study of responsibility. We argue that women are disproportionately likely to shoulder such fatelike responsibilities as the care of children and the elderly and that this gender inequality is a deep and abiding constraint on the capacity of women to seek or accept more highly rewarded responsibilities. While gender is clearly not the only variable that affects the likelihood that a person will take on such responsibilities, we believe that we cannot understand either how acceptance of responsibility affects gender stratification or how responsibilities are allocated without taking a close look at this piece of the puzzle. In this book our concern is more with how such gender inequalities come about than with the consequences of such inequalities. But because inequalities tend to reproduce themselves, we will necessarily focus on both causes and consequences.

We need not dig very deep to find evidence that women disproportionately shoulder the burdens of caring for small children or aged, ailing, or disabled family members. Clearly, maternal responsibilities are less often shed than paternal ones.[11] In 1995, 23% of children under eighteen lived with their mother only, 69% with both parents, 4% with their father only, and 4% with neither parent (U.S. Bureau of the Census 1996: 65; people under eighteen who maintained their own households or family groups were excluded). Indeed, McMahon (1995) argues that shirking parental responsibilities is almost unthinkable for women, because motherhood is so central to their identities. In consonance with our argument that some responsibilities come to be associated more with the person rather than with a position, McMahon finds that for mothers "the feeling of responsibility for their children is more than the expectation of a social role; it becomes constitutive of the self, making the denial of such responsibility almost unthinkable. Thus for a woman to be remiss in feeling responsible for her child would implicate her whole moral character. Being responsible for her child is about being moral as a person . . . motherhood [is] associated with female morality" (270).

Over the life course, women's ties with kin are stronger than men's, and their sense of normative obligation to kin is also stronger (Rossi and Rossi 1990). Women spend more hours per day on child care and household work whether or not they are employed, and women with children at home have fewer hours of leisure than men. Daughters are more likely than sons to assist aging parents (Spitze and Logan 1990). Women also do the kin-work of maintaining ties across households (DiLeonardo 1987). And women shoulder obligations to others even when it hurts—Simmons, Klein, and Simmons (1977) found that, controlling for the type of relationship (parenthood, sibling, etc.), women are more likely than men to donate kidneys.

To understand apparent gender differences in the extent to which responsibilities are inescapable and constraining personal obligations, we need to look at three sets of conditions. First, concerning how responsibili-

11. It may be somewhat easier to give up motherhood by refusing the role at the start, for instance by relinquishing a child for adoption or having an abortion. Still, the lore about "birth mothers" (but not "birth fathers") needing to compensate for having given up babies or worrying about how their children have fared, and about the lingering guilt felt by women years after having abortions, suggests some residual sense of personal obligation.

ties are assigned, we need to ask whether women are more likely than men to define obligations as theirs rather than as someone else's. We also must ask whether others see obligations as belonging to particular women but not to particular men. Second, concerning the conditions under which obligations are incurred, we need to ask whether women are more likely than men to believe that a relationship is at stake and that they might jeopardize the relationship if they failed to take responsibility. Do gender differences in expressivity (e.g., awareness and discussion of their own and others' feelings) shape the sense of obligation? Are women more likely than men to be embedded in ongoing exchange relations, and do these relations create different obligations for the two sexes? Third, concerning whether other resources give relief from obligation, we need to ask whether men and women differ in their access to resources such as money with which to meet obligations. When are substitutions, for instance money for one's own labor, acceptable? Are others (e.g., neighbors or the state) more likely to provide assistance to men than to women, so that familial obligations can be met without substantial changes in a care provider's life. Although questions about how responsibilities are assigned to individuals, about the extent to which obligations are incurred in the context of ongoing relationships, and about how other resources substitute for contributions of one's own labor are analytically separable, they are not empirically independent. In particular, often it is through relationships that obligations come to feel and be defined as personal, and relationships arise and are sustained through repeated exchange.

To say that women are disproportionately saddled with the burdens of fatelike responsibilities says little about how these "personal" responsibilities shape men's and women's capacities to take on responsibilities outside the home. Pleck (1977) long ago suggested that the boundary between work and home was asymmetrically permeable for men and women—that for men work intruded into the time and space allocated to family life, while for women family life intruded on work time and space. Men then use the resources of the home to provide the flexibility needed to make a go of their careers—working weekends when necessary, entertaining a customer or colleague for the evening, working an extra shift because a co-worker is ill. In contrast, women are more likely to use whatever flexibility can be wrung from a job to handle the uncertainties of family life—they make deals with bosses about making up hours so they can stay home with a sick child, rank potential jobs by how tolerant the supervisor is of obligations to children, and refuse offers of extra hours or chances to enter-tain business associates because such tasks are incompatible with household obligations (Freeman 1982). Working men tend to work longer hours than working women, and men are more likely to be employed in the sorts of occupations that require them to work especially long hours. But even when both spouses are employed, women spend more time than men on housework and child care (Hochschild 1989; Szalai 1972; Robinson 1977).[12]

For both men and women these statistical differences in hours spent on household versus employment obligations are produced by processes that are often uncomfortably constraining. Although both sexes are constrained, we must not overlook the differences both in how behavior is shaped and in the long-term consequences of these patterns. For men and women, hours of labor very likely go up in response to increases in the demand for their labor. For both sexes, increases in hours are at least partly an attempt to reduce costs—for instance by providing more attention for a troubled child at home or by placating an angry supervisor at work. But when men placate angry supervisors or put in extra hours because of a bulge in the flow of work, they anticipate that such investments will yield returns in stability of employment, increases in wages, or opportunities for advancement. Women have no similar expectations about changes in returns at home, although they may expect some gratitude (and Hochschild [1989] discusses the family economy of gratitude) and hope that their children will benefit from the attention.[13] Because some family obligations are accepted almost unconditionally, the economy of family life does not require as close a tie between investment and return.

As one rises in an organization, whether it be a firm, political party, religious group, or voluntary association, the variability of demands increases. People who have other responsibilities are less able to adapt quickly to new demands unless a staff of assistants can carry much of the load.

12. Bielby and Bielby find that "compared with men with similar household responsibilities, market human capital, earnings, promotion opportunities, and job responsibilities, women allocate substantially more effort to work activities" (1988: 1055). Although this says that women work harder than equally situated men, it ignores other important issues such as gender differences in labor-force participation (esp. during the months after childbirth), in likelihood of working part-time, in hours worked, and even in decisions about what kinds of jobs to accept. Household and family obligations do not make women shirk once they accept paid employment, but they make them more reluctant to take on employment obligations that they would be unable to meet.

13. Research, however, suggests that mothers' expectations of gratitude may not be fulfilled. Because children expect their mothers to care for them, they are not grateful to their mothers for providing care, but only to their fathers (Maccoby and Mnookin 1992: 36).

But fatelike responsibilities typically must be met with resources from the flexibility of small groups of people and the shallow pockets of families and friends rather than the large staffs and deep pockets of organizations. Further, family work is more constraining than many commitments at work. Family life is more variable in its demands—only really exceptional employment situations call for round-the-clock work, as sick children occasionally do in every family—and therefore calls for more adaptability than most other occupations. Anyone assigned the primary responsibility for a home and family will have little capacity to take on responsibilities in other settings. As long as such responsibilities are perceived as *personal* and women lack the resources to decrease the burden, they will be unable to invest equally with men in the world of positional responsibilities. The fateful consequence of being the gender that shoulders fatelike responsibilities is that women are less able to invest strategically in responsibilities that are also opportunities.

The facts are not new, and indeed they have been pithily presented before: wives provide their husbands with continuous flexibility (Hertz 1986); the boundary between work and family life is asymmetrically permeable for men and women (Pleck 1977); because of gender differences in the "second shift," employed women with children in effect work an extra month of twenty-four hour days (Hochschild 1989); women are more likely than men to be assigned the high-periodicity household tasks that preclude their joining the councils of state or business (Douglas and Isherwood 1978). As Hochschild (1989, 1997), Hertz (1986), and Gerson (1985) argue, changes in the workplace have outstripped changes in the home.[14] Women continue to do more than their share at home despite participation in the labor force, and this inequality in both labor and responsibility stunts or distorts women's careers. The link between the domestic sphere and the public sphere, between the more complete revolution at work and the stalled one at home (Hochschild 1989), continues to pose a puzzle.

We argue (esp. in chapter 3) that in whatever setting they occur, roles that carry a lot of responsibility differ from other roles in requiring a person to look out for the interests and needs of others, to define obligations diffusely, to think about both long- and short-term consequences, to use

14. Coltrane (1996) presents evidence that over the last three decades fathers in intact families have become more involved in family work, although he concedes that most men still avoid doing routine child care and housework. Although this increased involvement by some men is good news, we must keep in mind that it is evidence about intact families and that a lower proportion of families are "intact" than in the past.

discretion in adapting to contingencies, and to accept the consequences "come hell or high water." But when responsibilities are tied to persons (as family obligations are especially tied to mothers, daughters, wives, and sisters) rather than to positions (as responsibilities at work often are), it is difficult to escape responsibilities that have become losing propositions.[15] Further, one is more likely to have to meet personal obligations with one's own time, skill, and money. Because one must meet whatever obligations life brings from one's own reserves and because the responsibilities of family life are quite variable compared with the demands imposed by the world of paid work, women cannot as easily invest their reserves in high-powered careers. Neither family life nor high-powered careers come packaged in limited-liability, forty-hour weeks with specified tasks. But having a wife makes family life more like a "job" for men; the bulk of the uncertainty is absorbed by a woman, leaving the man free to make strategic investments in his career. The complaint that husbands are willing to "help out" at home but don't accept responsibility is then not a petty gripe but a key element of the persistence of gender inequality.

Gender is, in short, not just a variable, but a resource for men, and we treat it as such in our analysis. Though we wish to acknowledge women's agency in their decisions about taking responsibility, we also cannot deny that people face constraints that vary with gender. Women lack some of the resources that allow men to escape some of the most burdensome familial responsibilities. Gender is thus important for understanding the variation between parents in their acceptance of the responsibilities of caring for a sick child, but there are other important variables as well. There are no simple explanations as we try to account for variations among families in their willingness and ability to shoulder a burdensome responsibility. But richer families can more easily accommodate the additional burden by hiring extra help and seeking the opinions of experts. Likewise, parents with more education can more easily understand the arcane medical details, master the necessary care routines, arrange complicated schedules, and coordinate the efforts of many participants. However, we

15. In arguing that responsibilities associated with persons are different from those associated with positions, we do not wish to minimize the importance of variations among families and among jobs. How much familial responsibilities are personal rather than positional varies with family structure and with one's position in the family. And the work-related obligations of professionals sometimes become associated with the person, particularly when the professional possesses rare expertise or has special information about interaction partners, as occurs in the relationship between faculty and long-term student, physician and chronically ill patient, lawyer and client, or therapist and patient.

must emphasize that wealth and education do not necessarily produce responsibility and are certainly not the only routes to a desired outcome. Gender works somewhat differently from these other resources, then. It determines whether one will be expected (both by others and by oneself) to shoulder a burdensome responsibility. These other resources help to lighten the load.

Of course, noting that women are disproportionately likely to shoulder burdensome familial responsibilities or that parents with more money and more education may have an easier time of it is nothing new. However, when we recast these all-too-familiar facts in a new light, we learn something new about responsibility. When we look closely, as we do in this book, we see variations among parents and among families that elucidate the process by which incumbents of roles come to define their obligations so differently. We begin to see how it is that some parents come to embrace an onerous responsibility and others reject it. By then comparing this case with other settings, we begin to understand the general process through which responsibility is produced or undermined well beyond the infant intensive care units where we begin our investigation.

Neonatal Intensive Care: A Strategic Site for the Study of Responsibility

To answer some of these questions about the social organization of responsibility, we studied the allocation and acceptance of responsibility for infants who spent the first part of their lives in an infant intensive care unit. Neonatal intensive care units (NICUs) provide care for premature babies, those with congenital anomalies or serious genetic abnormalities and those who suffered traumatic births.[16] Babies may stay for only a day or two, or may be hospitalized for many months. They may need only to "feed and grow," or they may need ventilatory support, special feeding regimens, complex surgeries, drug therapies, and the like.

16. A newborn is called a "neonate" during its first twenty-eight days. Neonatology, focusing on the treatment of critically ill newborns, evolved as a specialty during the 1960s. Probably the best sources of general information on neonatal intensive care are by sociologists Guillemin and Holmstrom (1986) and by journalist Lyon (1985). Other, somewhat less general social scientific treatments are provided by Anspach (1993) and Frohock (1986). Mehren (1991) and Stinson and Stinson (1979, 1983) present parents' perspectives on NICU experiences, and Harrison's (1983) and Lieberman and Sheagren's (1984) discussions are intended to provide guidance for parents of premature or critically ill newborns. Medical information is available in sources such as Rathi (1989) and Cloherty and Stark (1991).

Neonatal intensive care units are also sometimes called infant intensive care units, infant special care units, or newborn intensive care units.

In choosing a site for our empirical work, we sought a case that had a variety of features that would make it both theoretically interesting and practical. We wanted a case in which there was some ambiguity about how to meet obligations, the obligations were consequential, the assignment of obligation was to some degree contested, the enforcement of obligations was the concern of a variety of social control systems and their agents, and at least some of the negotiations about obligations were directly observable. We also believed that because of its importance to our understanding of both responsibility and the persistence of gender inequality, it was necessary to focus on some type of fatelike responsibility that to some degree "belonged" to both a man and a woman. We also believed that we should investigate some unexpected obligation that arose relatively early in the life cycle so that we would not simply be investigating a process by which inequalities created during people's early adult years were perpetuated in their middle and later years.

The focus of activity in the NICU is on the lives, health, and development of infants, and good outcomes depend on coordinated contributions from doctors, nurses, administrators, therapists, social workers, and, of course, parents. Though a wide variety of people are involved directly in the care of infants, overall responsibility lies mainly with parents and physicians—parents because they are the ones who take the infants home and must make many choices on their behalf, and physicians because they are at the top of the medical hierarchy, with the capacity to direct or veto others' actions. It is vitally important to the welfare of the infants that physicians, ancillary health-care workers, and parents take their obligations to the infants seriously and comply with them in a flexible and thoughtful manner. With such precarious newborns, "good-enough parenting" and "good-enough doctoring" are not sufficient. But how are devoted and attentive parenting and doctoring motivated and supported? The high stakes of NICU care call forth unusually thoughtful responses from the participants. Parents and physicians both worry, though to different degrees, about saving the child's life and about how damaged the child is likely to be. The NICU is, for this reason, a good site to study how normative systems encourage and sustain performances that exceed those that are more routinely expected. When failures to meet obligations have very real consequences, participants are likely to be especially concerned about how to produce such exemplary performances regularly, and we are therefore more likely to be able to learn what works and what doesn't.

In the neonatal intensive care unit, then, questions about full and flexible compliance with obligations—what we call responsibility—are particularly compelling because what is at stake is the life and death of tiny, fragile newborns. If hospital staff members or parents meet their obligations in a perfunctory or ill-informed way, their small charges suffer the consequences—pain, severely compromised lives, prolonged dying, or death. Though the vast majority of the adult participants in these dramas are well intentioned, competent, and caring, differences of opinion about what is technically possible, wise, or moral can lead to tense conflicts, as occurred more than once in Tiffany's case. Such conflicts may undermine commitment or degrade performance.

Parenting a child who has been critically ill differs from parenting a healthy child by degree, not kind. Most parents worry about their children's well-being, feel the pressures of caring for someone so dependent, plan for their children's futures, and otherwise attempt to provide what their children will need as they grow and develop. However, parenting ordinarily goes on in private, without any particular instruction in how it ought to be carried out. Wide variations in parenting are usually tolerated as long as parents do not fall below the state-specified minimum standard for abuse or neglect (a standard that is sometimes dangerously low). In the NICU, in contrast, the negotiations about what each child needs are relatively public and the standards, as we have already noted, are higher. Processes that are usually hidden from the researcher's view are brought into an institutional setting, the hospital, where they can be observed, recorded, and analyzed. Even though the time spent in the NICU is only the beginning of many years of parenting, it is here where consequential decisions are made whose effects may be felt for years to come, where the standards for the health and well-being of the child are set, and where parents struggle to master the skills necessary to meet their obligations. Even when these obligations are not particularly onerous, parents who have weathered this initial crisis still have much to teach us about responsibility. The long-term burdens faced by parents whose infants are discharged home from the NICU vary quite a bit. Some children, like Tiffany, have demanding health-care needs long after discharge, while others go home essentially normal. This variation allows us to examine how changes in the magnitude of the obligation affect the parents' acceptance of responsibility.

All of the parents in our study accept some degree of responsibility for their children. Our purpose here is not to focus on the small number of parents at the extreme end of the continuum who relinquish their parental rights or grossly neglect their children, but instead to explore the subtler differences among parents in how they conceive their obligations to their children. These subtle differences nevertheless have profound effects and are the key to understanding how high-quality compliance is produced. Of course parents take responsibility for their children, the skeptic may argue. And indeed, most parents do. However, the dichotomy between those few who clearly neglect or abuse their children and everybody else masks quite a lot of variation. This book explores this variation within the category of "responsible" parent and teaches us something not only about parenting but also about responsibility more generally.

Of course, no research site is ideal. Along the way, we encountered some difficulties that limited our research, but we also made some unexpected discoveries. Though, as we noted above, we never intended to focus our research on parental deviance (why some parents relinquished custody of their children or had them taken away), we were nevertheless discouraged by the difficulty we had locating some parents and getting them to agree to an interview. Young, single fathers were especially difficult to locate and interview. Though we were more successful when these fathers were still involved with the mothers of their infants, we were disappointed by the small number of interviews we managed to complete with unmarried fathers. As we discovered, the father's tie to his child is often mediated by his tie to the child's mother, and when the fathers were no longer involved with the mothers, they were often no longer involved with their children. The fathers who were the most difficult to interview, then, often represented the low end on our responsibility scale. We know from the mothers' interviews that they assumed very little responsibility, but because we interviewed very few of them ourselves, we could only rarely uncover how such fathers thought about their obligations to their children and how they became detached from a responsibility to care for them. The variation among the parents we interviewed is, in this limited sense, less than we would have liked.

The flexibility of our research plan, however, proved to be a boon. Because we entered the NICU with only educated guesses about what would be important to parents, we made lengthy observations in the unit before beginning our interviews. During our observations, we discovered an elaborate social control system aimed at shaping parental behavior in the NICU and ensuring that parents are taught to care for their infants at discharge. As we describe in chapters 5 and 6, parents exercise a good deal of agency, defining what their roles should be, and becoming at various times both the objects and agents of social control.[17] Parents exercise agency in the NICU but are not free simply to do as they please. They meet a formidable social control system that is tethered to the laws of the state and helps define minimum standards of parental competence. Some parents must be prodded by the NICU staff to meet even the most minimal standards, but others must be restrained from attempting to impose standards of their own. The intricacies of the social control system in the NICU could not have been anticipated, and we benefited greatly from a flexible research strategy that allowed us to make the necessary adjustments as our knowledge accumulated. We pursued a similar strategy as we carried out our interviews, using a flexible research guide rather than a rigid interview format. This technique allowed the respondents' stories to take shape in a way that reflected what was important to them, not just what was important to us. As we read the interviews and laboriously coded them for various chapters of this book, we often cursed ourselves for choosing this method, but we believe the interviews are far stronger because of it. In this way, we made discoveries that we never could have anticipated, and some of these discoveries became cornerstones of the arguments in this book.

Overview of the Book

Understanding when and how responsible compliance with obligations—be they legal or moral—is produced and sustained requires an examination of the main normative systems (medical, familial, and legal) that govern the activity in the NICU and of the roles of participants as agents and objects of social control who encourage, cajole, or coerce each other to take responsibility. We must also ask about the infrastructure, well developed in some social locations but completely absent in others, that provides a template for the division of tasks and coordination of activities. And we must

17. In this book we use the word *agency* in two distinct ways. In chapter 1, we discuss agency primarily as the capacity to make and implement choices. We argue that responsible action necessarily entails strategizing and making choices and so presupposes a conception of human actors as agents whose actions are not completely constrained by social structures, conventions, preexisting scripts, or cultural definitions of objects and persons. In chapter 6, we draw on agency theory (from economics) to help us understand parents' relationships to their babies and to the hospital staff, arguing that parents see hospital staff members as agents who need to be induced to act on behalf of the infants and their families. Although both are standard usages, it is crucial to recognize that discussions of agency can refer to two quite different social science traditions, one concerned with the extent to which people are autonomous individuals who can make meaningful choices, and the other with effective methods for the selection, motivation, and control of others who act on our behalf.

ask what mechanisms people employ when rigid boundaries between organizations and between positions in organizations make coordinated activity difficult. Finally we must inquire about how people come to define particular obligations as belonging especially to them and what differentiates those with more expansive notions of their obligations and more flexible approaches to fulfilling them from others with narrower definitions of their responsibilities or more restricted repertoires.

Before returning to a more detailed discussion of just what we mean by *responsibility,* we first take a guided tour through the NICU in chapter 2, supplying readers with basic information about how an NICU is organized, who the main participants are, what kinds of tasks they are assigned, and what kinds of medical problems bring newborns to NICUs. We begin with the "insider's" view of the NICU, describing how the organization looks to those who work there (and to some others, like researchers and parents, who come to share this view after spending a great deal of time in the unit). We then describe our research sites, "City" and "Suburban" Hospitals, and the kinds of data we collected, including extensive observations at both NICUs, formal interviews with twenty-two staff members and eighty-six parents, and data from 951 infants' medical records. And finally, we take a second look at the NICU, this time from the point of view of the "outsider." Though the NICU is a well-ordered place with a meticulously arranged division of labor, it is nevertheless quite confusing to new participants. Parents are novices in neonatal intensive care and are often overwhelmed by the admission of an infant. While many parents are quick studies, mastering both the medical and organizational details, many others remain mystified by the complexity of their child's illness and never manage to make sense of unit policies and protocols or the division of labor among staff in the NICU.

In chapter 3, we return to the core theoretical concerns of the book. We describe several dimensions of responsibility and illustrate the variation between roles that require considerable responsibility and those that require less by drawing on examples from our study as well as from other settings. Roles vary in how much responsibility they require, but occupants of roles also vary in the extent to which they accept the associated responsibilities. In this chapter, we explore this second type of variation by analyzing our interviews with NICU parents.

We group parents according to how needy their child was at the time of our interviews: Was the child essentially normal, or did the child require extensive medical care? After assessing the nature of the obligation, we then used our elaborated definition of the dimensions that distinguish more responsible from less responsible behavior to ask how adequately the parents in our study shouldered the responsibility of caring for the child. Did the parents embrace the responsibility, as Will and Sue did, planning for the future, taking the child's welfare seriously, defining their obligations as parents broadly, setting goals and strategizing about how to achieve them, and postponing some of their own plans or making other accommodations to meet the child's needs? Or did the parents reject the responsibility, going on with their lives as if their child had no special needs or as if the needs of siblings or of the parents themselves should always take priority? Did the parents think about the future, or was planning beyond next week simply not possible given the uncertainty about the child's condition or the resource constraints with which the family lived? Did they follow routines that might be appropriate for other children but were not appropriate for this child? Did they simply not see that their child needed to be taught skills that other children might learn "naturally," did they believe that such therapeutic interventions were unlikely to be effective, or did they believe these tasks belong to specialists rather than to parents? Did they conceive of parenthood as a dyadic relationship with their child, or did they believe that parental responsibilities extend well beyond the boundaries of the home?

The task of this chapter, classifying parents by their level of responsibility, is both intellectually challenging and morally loaded. Although we sympathize with the concerns of those who argue that we should be extremely cautious about evaluating parents, we believe that there is meaningful variation among parents and that the only way to understand what factors encourage an occupant of a role either to embrace a responsibility or to reject it is to address that variation squarely.[18] The definitions, illus-

18. Opposition to evaluating parents and classifying them as "good" or "bad" is grounded in three concerns: (1) evaluations of "parents" in fact end up being evaluations of mothers rather than of both parents, (2) evaluations of parents are too much based on a white, middle-class understanding of what children need and are intolerant of the parenting styles of other groups such as ethnic or racial minorities or single mothers, and (3) evaluations of mothers too often are simply thinly veiled attempts to pin the blame for bad outcomes (e.g., delinquency or poor performance in school) on mothers whether or not their parenting has anything to do with those outcomes. For discussion of these points, see Campion (1995), Luker (1996), Ribbens (1994), and Stacey (1996). Further, Seligman and Darling argue that the parents of disabled children should not be treated differently than the

trations, and categorizations we provide in this chapter lay the foundation for the rest of the book, where we ask how the variations we observe arise and are manifested.

In chapter 4, we begin the work of explaining how variations among parents arise by examining the three main groups that define responsibilities to critically ill infants and oversee the efforts of those charged with caring for them. Our task is to give an overview of the jurisdiction and perspective of the legal, medical, and familial institutional systems that influence the care of infants in the NICU and after discharge. Responsibility for the care of a critically ill infant belongs jointly to the family into which the baby is born and to which it is eventually discharged, to the staff members who care for it during the period of hospitalization, and to the state, which often pays for the care and sets and enforces standards both for medical care and for parenting. Each of these parties has a distinctive view of what responsibility entails and a stake in ensuring that critically ill infants are well cared for and that other parties live up to their obligations (as it construes them). In this chapter, we ask how responsibility for a critically ill infant is divided among these groups, how that division affects the capacity of each to do its job, and how each helps to shore up, or undermine, the commitment of the others. We give special attention to the role of the law, asking about legal definitions of the obligations of the medical staff and the parents. We show how these legally defined standards help shape parents' and medical staff's views of their own obligations while simultaneously supplying them with tools to reshape the behavior of others.

---

parents of other children; they believe that it is unfair to subject parents to additional scrutiny or to require them to demonstrate mastery of a standardized set of parenting skills just because their children happen to be disabled (1989: 247).

In assessing parental responsibility, we take account of these concerns by evaluating both mothers and fathers; noting variations in parenting style associated with social class, ethnicity, and family configuration; evaluating the actions and orientations of parents rather than the outcomes; and assessing the responsibility of other care providers, such as hospital staff members, who often evaluate parents but are less often themselves subject to evaluation. We also have been careful to listen to those who do the bulk of the child care—the parents themselves—and in fact base much of the book on an analysis of our interviews with parents.

After all is said and done, though, it is important to acknowledge that we are in fact categorizing parents as more and less responsible. While we do believe that there is a strong ideological component to contemporary understandings of what children need, as Hays (1996) argues, we also believe that children have fundamental biological and developmental needs that must be met by the adults in their lives if they are to thrive. That does not mean that children cannot develop properly without educational toys or infant swimming lessons, of course, but it also does not mean that children have no objective needs.

Underlying the legal regulation of medicine in the NICU and the legal attention to parenting is a common concern with how to get people to take responsibility. In the hospital itself, the objective is to get physicians and the other members of a health-care team to juggle a variety of obligations to patients, the hospital, and other team members while providing the best possible care; for parents, the dual objective of the law is to ensure that parents' rights to raise their children as they see fit are protected at the same time that parental obligations to provide minimally adequate care are enforced. In both cases, the law must be articulated with other, suppler normative systems to achieve higher-than-minimal compliance. Put bluntly, for both hospitals and parents, the object is not just to reduce neonatal mortality or to decrease the chance of producing a "defective" child but also to increase the chance that the child will grow to a healthy, productive, and happy adulthood. The challenge is perhaps posed especially starkly in neonatal intensive care, but this is hardly the only setting in which there is tension in legal and normative systems between avoiding disasters, or punishing those responsible for them, and motivating the high-quality compliance that will achieve the goals of the legal or normative system. A fundamental theoretical question is how social control systems induce people to take responsibility by shaping incentive systems, setting standards, and shaping our sense of the social world we inhabit, and this question is addressed in subsequent chapters.

In chapter 5, we focus on how supervision and social control by NICU staff members contribute to parental responsibility. As a baby approaches discharge from the NICU, staff members become increasingly concerned about whether the baby's family is willing and able to assume full responsibility for the child. Staff members are concerned about the commitment of the parents to reorganizing their lives to meet the needs of an unusually demanding newborn. Do the parents visit often enough to learn their baby's schedule? Have they arranged for time off from work when the baby comes home from the unit? NICU personnel are also concerned about whether the parents (and especially the mothers) have the skills to provide rudimentary therapies, to administer routinely required medications, to discern when the baby needs more expert medical care, and to evaluate the care provided by experts. Do the parents know how to thread a nasogastric tube through the nose, throat, and esophagus into the stomach if that is how their baby is fed? Are parents able to work with staff members? Will parents jeopardize their child's health by developing irrational attachments or antagonisms to particular health-care providers? One physician, for instance, questioned Sue's assessment that Tiffany would receive poor care at a particular hospital and warned her about the dangers of having Tiffany treated at an alternate facility whose staff would be unfamiliar with her case.

Much of the social control machinery of the NICU is thus designed to determine which parents are "appropriate" (in the parlance of the NICU staff) and which are not, to bring "inappropriate" parents up to a minimal level of competence and commitment whenever possible, and to draw on the authority of the state to make other arrangements for the baby's discharge (e.g., adoption, foster care, or placement in a shelter) if parents' behavior cannot be reshaped. Though the hospital staff members are the main social control agents in this case, the legitimacy of their intervention into family life depends on the family's relation to the legal system. State laws establish minimum standards of acceptable parental behavior (below which parents can be charged with neglect or abuse) and specify when particularly inadequate parents must be referred to child-welfare agencies. NICU routines for the social control of parents are built on this legal foundation. But because of the deep interdependence between the hospital and families, the system has a reintegrative character that is somewhat unusual for social control systems. The hospital unit needs to discharge its patients, but it cannot easily accomplish this without the cooperation of parents. Unlike other social control systems, then, the NICU has a strong incentive to reform rather than expel deviant participants.

Just as staff members may be worried about whether parents will perform adequately, so parents are worried about the performance of hospital staff members, and chapter 6 reexamines the problem of social control in the NICU, this time looking at the parents as the agents, rather than the objects, of social control. Though not all parents conceive it as their responsibility to monitor their infant's care in the NICU, most parents feel some obligation to "test" staff competence and concern in the early phases of the baby's hospitalization, and some parents become increasingly attentive overseers if they conclude that staff routines are lax or that not all staff members are equally qualified. But which parents conceive of themselves as overseers of hospital staff members? Which parents will cease to believe that doctors are essentially interchangeable because "they are all perfect," as Sue once did (1009F, p. 35)? And what can parents do to protect their child's interests in a setting in which they themselves are novices?

Although each tries to control and shape the other's behavior, parents and hospital staff members are hardly identical as agents of social control.

How such social control efforts are carried out varies with the resources of individuals and the infrastructural support provided by organizations, and we should not expect parents and staff members to carry out the tasks of monitoring and correcting each other's actions in the same ways. Staff members are trained experts and are regular participants in the NICU; parents are novices and are unfamiliar with the setting. Staff members have strong ties with other participants; parents do not. Staff members have the infrastructure of organizational routines, including routines for the social control of parents, but parents have no corresponding "social control machinery" to shape staff behavior. Most parents must start from scratch, defining for themselves what their roles should be, learning enough about NICUs to intervene intelligently, and finding allies in the NICU itself or in the legal system.

And just as the social control tools that work for the staff do not work well for the parents, so the theoretical tools that help explain social control by staff members work less well to explain social control by parents. While a labeling theory explanation of how one group (here, the staff) evaluates and labels members of another group (the parents) works well to account for the collective social control of parents by staff members, agency theory—with its focus on how principals (here, the parents) hire and motivate agents (medical care providers) to act on their behalf—better accounts for the much more individualistic social control strategies used by parents.

In these two chapters on social control we emphasize the relationship between social control and responsibility. Taking responsibility often requires a person to act as an agent of social control. When people cannot meet their own obligations without the cooperation of others, they must continually assess whether others have done their jobs adequately, substitute their own effort or the effort of someone with the requisite skills to compensate for inadequacies, and attempt to prevent subpar performances in the future by showing clearly what kind of contribution is required. In situations where those who accept responsibility cannot meet their obligations by their isolated efforts—and this includes virtually all of social life—accepting responsibility necessarily brings with it the obligation to monitor and correct the behavior of others.

Once an infant leaves the intensive-care nursery, the roles of the family, the state, and hospital staff members shift dramatically. Unlike the other parties that share responsibility for critically ill infants, parents have a continuous and long-term obligation. The state may intervene episodically if child-welfare workers become convinced that parents are not meeting their obligations in even a minimal way, and for some infants a continuing relationship with a variety of medical specialists is necessary. In many families, though, after the initial hospitalization parents are left to shoulder most of the responsibility by themselves.

Although the child needs many of the same things whether it is being cared for in the hospital or in the home, taking responsibility for a child is quite a different matter when one is a member of a health-care team from when one is a parent. Parents take their newborns home to an organization that is much more primitive than an NICU. Homes lack emergency medical equipment, obviously, but they also lack the infrastructure of a complex division of labor with provision for supervision and quality control, interchangeable staff members to fill positions around the clock, procedure and medication protocols that provide guidance about what to do under a wide variety of circumstances, and schedules and forms to coordinate the activities of numerous care providers. Such infrastructure is important in ensuring the consistency and quality of care in an infant intensive care unit. In the absence of elaborate organizational infrastructure, the care provided by parents after they take their newborns home is much more variable than the care provided in NICUs. Some parents provide more attentive care than could be provided in an NICU, but other parents hardly notice that their recently discharged infant has special needs.

In chapter 7, we take another look at the variation among parents that we first described in chapter 3. Here we ask about variations among families and parents in how they conceive their responsibilities, where ideas about how children should be raised come from, how the parents' relationship with the child shapes feelings of obligation, and what parents do to try to meet obligations to their children. We know that parents' ideas about what children need are shaped by social class, education, gender, ethnicity, race, and age. For instance, mothers are more likely than fathers to conceive that their presence in the hospital is essential to the child's well-being; they are also more likely to believe that they have special contributions to make to the baby's development once it comes home. Parents with professional occupations are less likely than others to believe that they should accept the authority of hospital staff members and completely entrust the infant to these people during the baby's hospitalization, and they are correspondingly less likely to bow to medical opinion once the baby comes home.

In addition to shaping conceptions of what parental obligations are, however, these characteristics also shape a parent's capacity to meet obligations. For instance, richer people can more easily hire help; better-educated people are likely to have more information about child development and what kinds of interventions might help avert some of the sequelae of prematurity; women are more likely than men to have read books about pregnancy, childbirth, and infant development; and people with steady middle-class jobs are more likely to be able to negotiate time off to take a child to a physician, to stay home to recover from a difficult pregnancy, or to spend time with the baby after its release from the hospital. And parents differ in the extent to which others expect them to shoulder the burdens of caring for a sick or disabled child and in the variety of excuses that might enable them to escape child-care tasks.

In some senses chapter 7 assesses whether all of the social control machinery of the state, the hospital, and the extended family have been adequate to the task and have fostered in parents a willingness to take seriously the burden of caring for a child who may (or may not) continue to suffer the effects of a rocky start. As we will demonstrate in this chapter, there is more than one route to responsibility. Resources like money and education provide flexibility and a cognitive framework for thinking about what children need, but they do not predict perfectly who will embrace a particularly burdensome responsibility. Although some of our most responsible parents had the fewest resources, on the average wealthier and better-educated parents took more responsibility for their infants, and they were especially advantaged in being skilled organizational participants able to work effectively across organizational boundaries.

In chapter 8, we return to a topic that has been a subordinate theme throughout the book: the organizational worlds in which individuals must meet their responsibilities. The parents who are the main focus of this study begin caring for their infants in NICUs under the watchful and somewhat critical gaze of health-care providers. As parents, they are initially bit players in a drama directed by hospital staff members. Gradually their roles are enlarged and they often begin to feel that they should have some say even on matters closer to the medical core. When the baby leaves the NICU, the organizational infrastructure largely disappears, and parents must learn what it means to care for their infant without the infrastructure that was present and seemed necessary in the hospital. Even though households bear little resemblance to NICUs, they to some degree resemble NICUs in the permeability of their borders. NICU staff rely on labor inputs from personnel outside the NICU, and parents similarly must seek assistance outside the home in the offices of pediatricians, in the emergency rooms of community hospitals, in zero-to-three programs for children with special needs, and in their contacts with low-level bureaucrats who manage insurance claims or administer aid programs. In bringing the organizational backdrop into the foreground of our analysis, we show that being a skilled organizational participant is now a key part of taking responsibility. We also show that some of the important variation is among organizations rather than among individuals. Individuals may vary in the extent to which they conceive it to be their job to bridge organizational boundaries and in their skill as organizational participants, particularly in organizations where they are interlopers. But organizations also vary in the kinds of impediments they pose to those who must work in the boundary regions. Some organizations are welcoming, providing guidance about routines, the jobs of those who are regular participants, and the like; others are essentially impenetrable, with cultures that justify making clients wait, shifting scut work to clients whenever possible, and protecting core routines and personnel from clients even when they have legitimate reasons for intruding. When organizations are brought into the foreground, it becomes clear that if we wish to encourage people to take responsibility, we must redesign not only normative systems but also organizations.

The focus on organizations also allows us to move beyond the world of infant intensive care to address more theoretical questions about the production of responsibility, to assess the causes and consequences of gender inequalities in acceptance of fatelike responsibilities, to show how responsibilities to individuals and to groups are reconciled, to examine how routinization and moral agency work together, and to suggest how normative systems grounded in different spheres jointly support responsible behavior.

TWO

Life in Two Neonatal Intensive Care Units

THE MOST ADVANCED MEDICAL CARE for newborns is delivered in neonatal intensive care units, where human expertise and high technology combine forces. The NICU is filled with a constant flurry of activity and the disquieting sound of alarms—some serious, most not, but all demanding immediate attention. The pace of activity, the noise, and the bright lights all violate common notions of what a nursery should look like.[1] But, of course, this is not a regular nursery. The patients treated in the NICU have a wide range of serious medical problems, including prematurity and the respiratory problems that often result, various congenital anomalies, and problems resulting from the injuries of birth or the accidents of genetics.[2] The care of these critically ill infants requires the precise orchestration of the skills of a large number of health-care providers, including attending physicians, fellows, and residents, along with consulting physicians from various medical specialties, nurses, therapists, and technicians. Rounding out the cast are social workers, discharge planners, and administrative staff, who provide crucial services, if not direct patient care. Along with these organizational members, parents are important participants in the NICU. As one might expect, however, the parents and the medical staff regard the infant's hospitalization quite differently. To borrow from sociologist Everett Hughes (1971), the emergencies of laypersons are transformed into the routines of professionals in the NICU.

Parents are often overwhelmed by the admission of a newborn to the NICU. Not only are they faced with complex medical information, but they must also negotiate their way through a complex system of care. On admission, parents are given thick packets of information to orient them to unit rules and introduce them to innumerable staff members. They are

1. Indeed, research has suggested that the stress of this noisy, bright environment may contribute to neonatal morbidity (Zylke 1990).

2. See Table 2.2 for a summary of the primary diagnoses of the infants admitted to the two NICUs we studied.

told who will care for their babies, when they may visit, when and whether other family members may visit, which phones they may use, and where they may talk with other NICU parents. Even routine baby care is not routine in the NICU. Parents receive instruction on feeding, bathing, and clothing their babies. In the most critical cases, parents may be restricted from holding or even touching their infants. Additional instructions are prominently displayed throughout the unit. Signs, for instance, instruct all visitors to check in with the unit secretary, and to don hospital gowns and scrub arms and hands before going to the bedside. These organizational rules and routines are designed simultaneously to protect the patients from harm, to protect the unit from disruptions in the smooth delivery of intensive medical care, and to comply with the specifications of accrediting bodies and insurers. The care of these critically ill infants, then, also requires the careful orchestration of the role of parents.

The purpose of this chapter is to provide an orientation to this complex world of neonatal intensive care from two different points of view. We will describe how the organization of the NICU looks to those who are "native" to the setting and to those, like parents, who are entering the NICU for the first time—in short, insiders and outsiders. Descriptions of complex organizations, like hospitals or other critical care units, often rely heavily on the insider's view. When one begins research, much of the early time is typically spent getting oriented to the setting, learning who is responsible for what, how the obligations of one position relate to those of another, and the like. After some time in the setting (if all goes well), the researcher begins to develop a rich understanding of the organization and ceases to be an organizational novice. One of the researcher's goals, in fact, is to learn how the organizational participants view the organization. However, one of the key organizational participants in our setting is not an insider. The parents of the infants are often overwhelmed and confused about how the organization works, reactions we understood from our own bewilderment in our first days in the NICU. Only gradually did we realize that our initial bewilderment about the NICU world was as important data as our subsequent understanding. Our descriptions of the roles and responsibilities of various NICU medical personnel are essential to providing a full understanding of the organizational setting. Equally essential, however, is the parents' view. Although we began our analyses with what the insiders and outsiders themselves experience, our job is to explain how those differences arise, and this necessarily requires us to uncover facts that would not be available to members of either group and to make comparisons that they would be unlikely to make.

We begin the chapter with a brief description of neonatal intensive care medicine, including the main categories of participants who provide care to the patients in the NICU, their roles and responsibilities, and the main problems that lead to the hospitalization of newborns. We describe our two research sites, "City Hospital" and "Suburban Hospital," in some detail and then turn to a more detailed description of our research methods, including how we gathered data from medical records, observations in the NICU, and detailed interviews with NICU staff and parents, and how parents were selected for interviews. Although the NICU is a well-ordered place with a meticulously designed division of labor, it is nevertheless quite confusing to anyone who is not a regular participant. We conclude by taking a second look at the NICU, this time from the point of view of the parents. Here we highlight the difficulties of mastering the organizational details of the NICU—collecting information, determining which expert is responsible for what part of their child's care, having a question answered, or lodging a complaint. We also describe the visitation patterns of parents in the NICU. As organizational participants, parents are quite distinctive. Their turnover rates are higher than those of other participants, and their participation is often rather unpredictable even during their tenure in the organization. This pattern of rapid turnover and episodic participation makes it difficult to incorporate parents fully into organizational routines and is crucial in helping explain parents' feelings of dislocation. Further, parents enter the NICU with a wide array of different circumstances. We therefore have nearly as many "outsider" views of the organization as we have parents. The importance of the asymmetry between the experts and the parents cannot be overstated, and we will revisit this issue in much more detail in later chapters. In chapter 5, we will describe how the organization attempts to shape the roles of the parents, and in chapter 6, we will turn the tables to explore variation in how the parents view their roles in the organization. But these arguments first require an introduction to the organizational setting of this research, the neonatal intensive care unit.

Neonatal Intensive Care: The Insider's View

A Brief History of Triumphs and Controversies

Neonatology is a relatively new medical specialty, evolving as a separate discipline in the 1960s. The limits of viability have been continually redefined, as new breakthroughs in technology and treatment have followed one after another since its inception—an exciting field for those who can keep up. During the course of our research, infants just twenty-five weeks' gestation and weighing as little as 500 grams were considered viable.[3] More recent treatment advances have pushed the edge of viability even further, so that infants as premature as twenty-three and twenty-four weeks' gestation are now being treated.[4] In addition, infants with congenital anomalies like spina bifida or hypoplastic left heart, and those with severe necrotizing enterocolitis (NEC), who were not considered viable only a relatively short time ago (Frohock 1986), have also become candidates for aggressive treatment.[5] Studies indicate that regional intensive-care facilities for newborns have contributed to a significant decline in infant death rates.[6] By this mea-

3. An infant who is at least thirty-eight weeks gestation is considered full-term. An average full-term infant weighs about 3,300 grams, or 7 pounds, 4 ounces (Stubblefield 1984).

4. These advances are largely due to the development of surfactant replacement therapy. The FDA approval of synthetic forms of surfactant has led to some important changes in how respiratory problems of premature infants are treated. Surfactant coats the lungs of the full-term infant, allowing them to remain elastic while expanding and contracting. Without the coating of surfactant that mature lungs have, the lungs of premature infants have too little surface tension, often collapse, and are difficult to reinflate. While surfactant therapy was new while we were doing our research, many premature infants with hyaline membrane disease (a respiratory disease of unknown cause that occurs in newborn premature infants and is characterized by deficiency of the surfactant coating the inner surface of the lungs, by failure of the lungs to expand and contract properly during breathing, with resulting collapse, and by the accumulation of a protein-containing film lining the alveoli and their ducts) are now treated routinely with surfactant. The administration of surfactant has been shown to be associated with an increase in lung volume (see, e.g., Cotton 1994), and has had a "significant impact" on infant mortality and on some complications of prematurity (Kliegman 1995). It is now much more common to see small premature infants breathing without respirators.

5. Spina bifida is a congenital cleft of the spinal column with hernial protrusion of the membranes that envelop the spinal cord and sometimes the spinal cord itself, and may result in paralysis and severe brain damage. Hypoplastic left heart is a congenital malformation of the heart in which the left side is underdeveloped, resulting in insufficient blood flow. Until fairly recent surgical innovations, it was considered fatal. Necrotizing enterocolitis is a condition that results in the death of intestinal tissue. It often requires emergency surgery to remove the damaged tissue, and may still be fatal if there is too little healthy tissue remaining.

6. For the fifteen years from 1967 to 1982, neonatal mortality declined about 4% per year, a rate of decline almost entirely attributable to advances in neonatal intensive care (Paneth 1990:791). Survival rates for the extremely-low-birth-weight infants (weighing less than 1,000 grams, or 2 lbs., 3 oz.) increased dramatically during the late 1970s and early 1980s. By 1985, expected survival rates with neonatal intensive care were over 80% for infants weighing 750 grams (1 lb., 10 oz.) to 1,000 grams and 50% for infants as small as 700 grams (1 lb., 9 oz.) to 750 grams (Hodgman 1990:2657).

sure, the brief history of neonatology is a history of great triumphs. But these triumphs have also sparked controversy and debate: When these very premature and sick infants survive, what kind of future awaits? Because neonatology is a young and rapidly changing discipline, the future is often murky. Any time the limit of viability is redefined, the survivors are too few to determine the future with any certainty.[7] Quite simply, the future has yet to unfold. Of course, this uncertainty is felt especially acutely by parents, who are intensely aware that their infants will be the inheritors of this uncertain future.

Prematurity is the most common reason for admission to an NICU.[8] The lungs of preterm infants are not fully developed, and these patients often suffer from respiratory distress syndrome and require mechanical ventilation.[9] In extremely premature infants, other complications often follow: difficulty feeding, difficulty weaning from the ventilator, ongoing respiratory difficulties, and intracranial hemorrhages. The second most common diagnostic category in the NICU is congenital anomalies, including heart defects like patent ductus arteriosus or defects of the digestive system like an imperforate anus, many of which require immediate surgery. Other diagnostic categories include genetic syndromes, such as Down's syndrome; gestational accidents, such as amniotic banding or malformations that occur because of maternal illness or injury at key points

---

However, for the tiniest infants, there is some evidence that neonatology simply prolongs the inevitable. Hodgman reports that the decline in the neonatal infant mortality rate encouraged physicians to treat ever-smaller infants. Summarizing a stream of research on outcomes for low-birth-weight infants, Hodgman says: "Length of gestation is a significant determinant of outcome in these tiny infants. A gestation of 28 weeks was accompanied by a good prognosis for survival. At 26 weeks, the survival rates were significant although long-term morbidity was increased, while an infant of 24 weeks' gestation or less rarely survived. In a recent study that compared results of intensive care for infants with a birth weight less than 750 g in 1982 to 1985 with 1985 to 1988, mortality and long-term morbidity were not improved. The only significant difference in the two periods, an increase of mean age at death from 73 hours to 880 hours [or 37 days], raises a serious question as to whether routine intensive care can be justified for the very immature infant" (1990:2657).

7. The American Academy of Pediatrics Committee on Fetus and Newborn recently issued a statement arguing that while the survival rate for infants at the threshold of viability is improving, still too little is known about the costs of care and the long-term outcomes of survivors (1995:974–76).

8. Although neonatal mortality rates improved at an unprecedented rate from 1967 to 1982, the proportion of infants who were born preterm and with low birth weights remained virtually unchanged (Paneth 1990:791).

9. Respiratory distress syndrome is also called hyaline membrane disease. For an explanation of this, and recent advances in its treatment, see n. 4.

in fetal development; and birth injuries, such as meconium aspiration and asphyxia.[10] Nearly 9% of patients at Suburban and 15% at City did not survive their initial hospitalizations. Many of the infants who leave the unit are discharged with demanding health-care needs and a great deal of uncertainty about long-term outcomes.[11] Although no pregnancy can be perfectly safeguarded from the accidents of genetics and the tragedy of preterm labor, some pregnancies carry more risk than others. Both poverty and maternal age are risk factors for preterm delivery and genetic defects, and NICU patients are disproportionately likely to be born to older mothers and to very young, poor mothers. Both groups have special difficulties accepting unusually heavy child-care obligations: older mothers because they are especially likely to face competing demands on their time (either from other children or from established careers), and young mothers because they have fewer resources.

In spite of general agreement about the impact of neonatal intensive care medicine on infant mortality rates, there has been considerable debate

10. Patent ductus arteriosus (PDA) is an abnormal heart condition in which the ductus arteriosus (a short broad vessel in the fetus that connects the pulmonary artery with the aorta and conducts most of the blood directly from the right ventricle to the aorta, bypassing the lungs) fails to close after birth. An imperforate anus is one that is lacking the usual or normal opening and so does not allow the normal passage of feces. Down's syndrome (also called Trisomy 21) is a genetic disorder caused by an extra chromosome on the twenty-first pair, characterized by moderate to severe mental retardation, slanting eyes, and other distinctive features. Amniotic banding is a band of fibrous tissue extending between the embryo and the amniotic sac, and is often associated with faulty development of the fetus. Meconium aspiration causes severe respiratory difficulties and results when the fetus passes the meconium plug (a dark greenish mass of sloughed cells, mucus, and bile that accumulates in the bowel of a fetus and is normally discharged shortly after birth) before birth and inhales the meconium-tainted amniotic fluid.

11. A recurrent concern regarding neonatal intensive care is the health status of the survivors. In a survey of research on outcomes of former patients of neonatal intensive care units, McCormick (1989:1767) reports that the proportion of very-low-birth-weight infants (less than 1,500 grams, or 3 lbs., 5 oz.) that survive with moderate to severe handicap has remained relatively small and stable—between about 4% and 10%. Although McCormick acknowledges that these stable figures are encouraging, she raises three concerns: (1) the failure to assess accurately survival rates at the current frontier of survival (which is much less than 1,500 g), (2) a stable rate of handicap that hides an inflation in the absolute numbers of infants who survive with handicaps, and (3) the limited generalizability of the follow-up data that are reported by individual institutions and so affected by their referral patterns. Harrison (1986) raises additional questions about studies of the health status of survivors, noting that often the data are collected too early for major disabilities to be evident; some children classified as "normal" may later turn out to be very far from normal. Although there is little consensus in the scientific community about outcomes for former NICU patients, there is widespread agreement about the need for more research (see, e.g., McCormick 1989; Paneth 1990; Hodgman 1990; and Strandjord and Hodson 1992).

about the long-term effects of that care.[12] Research suggests that decisions about viability are often made without adequate regard for the quality of life of the infants and their families (Anspach 1993). Low-birth-weight infants are often at risk for serious, long-term disabilities, some of which may result from the very therapy they receive as neonatal patients. For example, the oxygen therapy that keeps preterm infants alive may cause blindness (Silverman 1980) and chronic lung disease (Strandjord and Hodson 1992). Many patients also suffer intracranial bleeds that may—depending on the size of the bleed and its placement—result in serious neurological impairments. In the NICU, there is a delicate balance between the tragedy of overtreatment and the horror of undertreatment, a balance that has received quite a lot of scholarly attention. The now-famous Baby Doe cases drew the public's attention to the possibility of undertreatment in NICUs (as we'll describe next), but critics have argued that intensive-care medicine errs on the side of aggressive intervention rather than undertreatment. Many scholars have written about the ethics of intensive care medicine, asking such difficult questions as how to balance the patient's right to life with the quality of life and when to discontinue treatment. Other scholars have asked whether the cost of intensive care can be justified in a system where many poor women have no access to adequate prenatal care.[13]

Neonatology has captured the public's attention as well, as both the tragedies and the miracles have been chronicled in the press and paraded across prime-time television news magazines. The debate about ethics in neonatology reached a national audience when the Reagan administration initiated what came to be called the "Baby Doe" regulations. Briefly, the Baby Doe case involved an infant in Indiana who was born with Down's syndrome, not fatal in itself, but who also had a throat obstruction that would be fatal if left untreated. The parents refused treatment and took the case all the way to the Indiana Supreme Court to assert their right. The controversy produced perhaps the most famous legal drama in the field of neonatal medicine and drew the nation's attention to the delicate balance between the parents' rights to refuse treatment and the infant's right to receive treatment. The Baby Doe regulations followed, forbidding nurser-

12. See n. 6. These debates are, of course, not unique to neonatal intensive care. For comparisons, see, e.g., Zussman (1992) on adult intensive care, and Bosk (1992) and Rothman (1986) on genetic counseling and prenatal screening.

13. The bioethics literature is extensive. Readers may wish to consult Anspach (1993) for an excellent review of the bioethics debates in neonatal intensive care.

ies from withholding food, water, or medical treatment from disabled newborns, but the regulations were eventually struck down by the U.S. Supreme Court. The horrors of undertreatment exposed, a 1985 federal law mandated state child-welfare agencies to investigate cases of "medical neglect," defined as withholding medically indicated treatment from critically ill infants.[14]

The horrors of overtreatment have also been chronicled for mass consumption. Perhaps the most widely read example is a moving *Atlantic Monthly* article and book written by the parents of an infant who eventually died in an NICU (Stinson and Stinson 1979, 1983). *The Long Dying of Baby Andrew* describes these parents' journey from hope to the grim reality that their son either would not survive or would be seriously impaired. While their story portrays the devastation and pain of overtreatment in the NICU, stories of triumph have also captured the public's attention. One such triumphant story involves six premature babies, conceived with fertility treatment, successfully treated in an NICU and eventually discharged home to their parents. Dubbed the "Dilley six-pack," their story was aired on national television and even published in a book (Dilley and Dilley 1995) before they were superceded in 1997 by the McCaughey septuplets.

In short, the great triumphs and equally great tragedies have received a disproportionate share of both scholarly and public attention. The social science and ethics literatures on neonatal intensive care are focused quite heavily on the most dramatic cases, especially the drama of life-and-death decisions. Most of life in the NICU, however, is much more mundane than the popular or academic literature would lead one to believe. More of the medical staff's time is spent making routine decisions and following established protocols than in making explicit life-and-death decisions or consulting lawyers about treating a patient against the parents' wishes. Our focus in this book, then, is not limited to the part of the NICU that interests ethicists most or that has most troubled the public and fascinated academic researchers. Instead, we look at the mundane, everyday decisions, including such matters as whether infants are warm enough, whether they should be bottle-fed or nursed, whether they should be dressed in attractive clothing that pleases parents but may hinder quick medical access, whether their oxygen levels should be adjusted or the respirations increased on a ventilator, and so on. Most treatment decisions in the NICU

14. See chapter 4 for a more detailed discussion of the Baby Doe Regulations and related references.

are incremental and so are very different from the consequential single decision about whether to operate that faced the parents of Baby Doe.

Although questions about the ethics and distribution of care are both timely and important, our purpose here is somewhat different. Rather than ask whether neonatal intensive care is ethical or effective, we ask how the obligation to care for an infant, whose long-term outcome may be uncertain and whose care may be burdensome, is constructed and maintained. That is, we are interested in the roles and responsibilities of the participants in the NICU not only as they consider life-and-death decisions but more commonly as they carry out the routine business of caring for patients and getting them home. Our task, then, is to show how the responsibility for a critically ill infant is shared by the family to whom it will eventually go home, by the hospital staff members who succor it through the dangerous first days, weeks, or months, and by the state, which often pays for the baby's care and which sets and enforces standards both for health care and for parenting. Because the first phase of this allocation of responsibility is worked out in the intensive care unit, our explanation of variations among parents in their conceptions of what they owe their child must include an account of how responsibility is constructed and assigned in the NICU and who the main actors are in that setting.

The Insiders

Neonatal intensive care demands the best of the best. Hospitals must be specially equipped to care for critically ill infants, and the staff must be specially trained. The hours are long, the work demanding, but rarely dull. Research activities are combined with patient care. Clinical trials test new technologies, procedures, and drugs as the age of viability is lowered. Many who work here do so because, in pediatrics, this is where the "action" is. Although many patients die (sometimes grim deaths), many more survive. This is the business of saving lives—but not just any lives, babies' lives. Few jobs are more rewarding, or more demanding. If success is measured by how many years may be added to a patient's life, then never is more at stake than in neonatal intensive care.

Although neonatal intensive care is first and foremost the business of saving infant lives, its mission extends well beyond that. Patient care is combined with research and the education of future generations of physicians. NICUs are, in addition, involved in educating parents. Though evaluating the skills of fellows and residents is part of the main function of the organization, evaluating parents and teaching them new skills are necessary tasks that follow from treating such young patients. NICUs are not simply responsible for treating the clinical problems of their infant patients but must also be concerned with whether these patients will be discharged to homes where they will be cared for adequately.

NICUs draw their patients from large geographic regions and are organized in regional referral networks. Medical care facilities for newborns are designated as Level 1, 2, or 3 nurseries: The most-advanced care is delivered in NICUs, or Level 3 tertiary care centers, while Level 2 nurseries offer an intermediate level of care, and Level 1 nurseries care for only the healthiest newborns. Level 3 nurseries are linked to Level 1 and 2 nurseries through regional referral contracts and are usually found in major medical centers that also function as teaching hospitals. Most Level 3 nurseries receive a large number of their patients from hospitals that are not equipped to care for critically ill or extremely premature infants. Some NICUs are located in pediatric hospitals without labor and delivery wards, so all of the patients in the NICU must be transported from the hospitals where they were born. Others receive a large proportion of their patients from their own hospital's labor and delivery ward while continuing to accept referrals from outside. Patients in the NICU may be transported many miles from where they were born and, in some cases, may even cross state lines to receive potentially life-saving treatment.

Attending physicians sit at the top of the hierarchy in the NICU. These physicians rotate on- and off-service, splitting their time between patient care and research. During each rotation in the nursery, the attending physician is responsible for ensuring not only that each patient receives appropriate care but also that each fellow and resident receives appropriate training. Under the direction of the attending physician, fellows and residents are responsible for most of the routine diagnostic and treatment decisions in the NICU, but the attending remains formally and legally responsible for those decisions. The neonatology fellows are the next most senior physicians. Fellows have completed their training in pediatrics and are receiving specialized training in neonatology. They share responsibility for teaching the less-advanced residents and in the attending physician's absence are in charge of the unit and the medical decisions. Groups of "green" residents rotate through the nursery every six weeks or so as part of their training in pediatrics and are an important source of physician labor in the NICU.

In addition to the efforts of physicians, the NICU depends on large numbers of highly skilled nurses. Nurses in the NICU are responsible in large part for carrying out the essential work of monitoring the patients' medical conditions. In the NICU, patients can deteriorate rapidly, and nurses are often the first to notice a critical change. While the physicians are formally responsible for diagnostic and treatment decisions, nurses provide much of the hands-on care. For instance, they respond to monitor alarms, make minor adjustments in ventilator rates and oxygen concentrations, administer medications, and start and change IVs, in addition to feeding, rocking, bathing, and changing the infants. The nurse-to-patient ratio ranges from 2:1 for the most intensive medical care to 1:4 for those patients who are the healthiest. With the rotation of physicians through the unit, the system of primary nursing adds some measure of continuity to the care. Primary nurses choose their "primaries" soon after admission, and some patients also have additional nurses who sign on as associates. Primary nurses are then responsible for managing the care plan for their "primary" and are assigned to that infant whenever on duty. Primary nurses often become quite attached to their primaries over the course of the infant's hospitalization, decorating the infant's bedside, dressing the infant attractively, and otherwise acting as a surrogate parent.

Patients in the NICU often require additional services from specialists and therapists. Consultations are frequently sought from such pediatric specialists as cardiologists, neurologists, surgeons, gastroenterologists, ear-nose-throat specialists, and nutritionists. In addition, the services of physical, occupational, and respiratory therapists, phlebotomists, X-ray and ultrasound technicians, lactation consultants, social workers, and discharge planners are often required as well.

Though NICUs have a fairly rigid division of labor, coordinating that division of labor is a never-ending task. Several organizational routines help coordinate the efforts of this vast array of health-care professionals. On daily morning rounds, the head nurse, residents, fellows, and attending physician on duty gather to discuss each patient. As they move through the unit, the resident in charge of each patient's care gives an oral report to the others at the bedside. This report serves to update the others on the patient's progress and provides an opportunity for the attending physician to assess both the patient's progress and the resident's training.[15] Daily progress reports are recorded in the patient's medical chart by the physicians, along with any changes in the patient's status or course of treatment

15. For an excellent analysis of the training of surgical residents, see Bosk 1979.

and reports from any consulting physicians. As residents finish their rotations in the NICU, they write more lengthy off-service notes to brief the incoming residents on the patient's hospital course. Nurses also keep detailed written records. The nursing chart is kept at the patient's bedside, where the nurse records observations of the patient's status throughout the shift. When a nurse's shift comes to an end, an oral summary of the patient's status ("report") is given to the nurse on the next shift. In addition to these formal organizational routines, nurses and physicians communicate regularly about their patients. As a patient's condition changes or as diagnostic test results are returned, there is much informal communication between and among physicians and nurses throughout the day and into the night.

Because the flow of patients is unpredictable, the management of admissions and discharges is an ongoing problem (see Devers 1994). Every effort is made to restrict admissions so that the census does not exceed the number of patients the unit is authorized to treat. However, there is a competing pressure to keep the beds full. The attending physician has formal authority to admit or refuse patients. According to the referral contract, the unit cannot refuse to accept the transfer of a patient who is critically ill. If the unit is full, then the attending must either try to make room by transferring patients who are well enough to continue their treatment in Level 2 nurseries or by finding another Level 3 nursery that will accept the critically ill infant. Discharge planning begins the day a patient is admitted because of the pressure to ensure that some beds will be open for the never-ending flow of new patients. The head nurse spends most of her day tracking the progress of patients and adjusting the nursing staff assignments as needed. Elaborate contingency plans are continually updated so that if bed space is needed, some patients can be moved from one room to another, and others can be discharged either home or to a lower-level nursery. These contingency plans depend not only on the medical status of the patients but also on the preparedness of their parents to take their babies home.

Other organizational business takes place in meeting rooms outside the unit rather than at the bedside. In many NICUs, weekly meetings are held to discuss discharge plans and any problems the families may be having that will affect their ability to take care of their infants at discharge. There is some variation from hospital to hospital, but these meetings (variously referred to as "social service rounds," "discharge planning rounds," or "interdisciplinary rounds") usually include some combination of physicians, nurses, social workers, discharge planners, and therapists. Other communication between discharge planners, social workers, and medical staff takes place more episodically as it is needed. Other meetings may also be held regularly to discuss the organizational business of the NICU. In these meetings, physicians and nurses have the opportunity to discuss any problems of coordinating work on the unit and to propose solutions. Topics may include such matters as the development of new protocols, preparations for accreditation reviews, discharge instructions to parents, and nursing complaints about physicians and residents (and vice versa). Additional meetings are convened, some on a regular schedule, some as the need arises, to review mortality and morbidity statistics, to sift through the evidence on troublesome cases, or to spread the good news about an important breakthrough. Some of these meetings are strictly internal affairs, though others bring in outsiders such as quality assurance specialists, ethicists, or visiting neonatologists.

While communication between staff members is highly regularized, communication between staff members and parents is much more episodic. Parents are expected to visit the unit or to telephone the unit if they cannot visit. Communication is not routinely initiated by the staff unless there is a medical emergency or the parents have failed to phone or visit for a long time. The rules of informed consent require that staff initiate at least some contact with the parents, but many medical procedures do not require informed consent, so this organizational routine enforces only episodic contact, at best. Instead, more regular contact with the NICU remains the parents' responsibility. Here we find that organizational position has a direct bearing on the amount and kind of interaction staff members have with parents and that frequency of contact tends to be inversely related to the staff member's position in the status hierarchy.

Nurses, who are on the bottom of the medical status hierarchy, are on the front line of communication with parents. Phone calls from parents are directed to them, and visiting parents spend a great deal of time at the bedside with the nurses assigned to care for their babies. Nurses have considerable responsibility for teaching parents both normal baby care and any special care that will be needed at discharge, and they are also responsible for documenting parents' behavior. Visits and phone calls from parents are recorded by the nurses in their notes, which later become part of the medical record, and nurses also document which medical skills parents have acquired and which still need to be mastered before the patient can be discharged home.

Among physicians, residents are on the bottom of the status hierarchy. They provide much of the day-to-day patient care and have the most regular contact with parents. Because residents are on the unit more hours of the day than other physicians, they are more likely to be nearby when parents call or visit. Attending physicians and fellows are often not on the unit for parent visits and rarely linger at the bedside except during rounds. Parents are most likely to have contact with them during formal meetings that take place outside the unit (although some savvy parents schedule their visits to coincide with rounds). These meetings may be requested by the parents or called by the physicians but are nonetheless most likely to occur during a time of crisis. Although nurses give parents many progress reports, they typically shy away from revealing poor prognoses. Bad news is almost universally delivered by physicians (or sometimes it is not delivered at all).

Social workers also play a key role in relations with parents. Whereas nurses and physicians treat patients first and families second, social workers have primary responsibility for identifying and resolving the social problems that complicate the practice of pure medicine (Heimer and Stevens 1997). Social workers engage parents in private conversations and counseling sessions both at the patient's bedside and in private, closed-door meetings. They listen sympathetically to devastated parents and phone absent ones. They encourage visits and help parents plan for the future. They assess how the parents are coping with the crisis and whether they will be able to manage both the emotional and physical work of parenting. They record contacts with parents and their evaluations of parents in the patient's medical record alongside physicians' evaluations and notations about the patient's medical condition. Social workers' assessments are also shared with other staff members at weekly interdisciplinary meetings where each patient's discharge status is discussed and plans are developed to avert potential discharge problems.

The staff of the NICU spends much of its time evaluating: whether the patient is improving, the care plan needs adjustment, and the like. But, as we have already hinted, the staff also evaluates the parents, focusing attention on the capacity of the parents to manage the patient's care at discharge. When infants are healthy, parents take them home with very little instruction and even less scrutiny of how they will be cared for. As long as the children are not placed in danger, parenting is largely a private matter. But when infants are critically ill, the issue of how child care ought to be carried out cannot be left to the parents alone. Because the hospital depends on parents to take their infants home and because they can be held responsible if patients are sent to unprepared parents or inadequate homes, the evaluation of parents plays a prominent role in the organizational business of the NICU.[16] As a patient approaches discharge from the NICU, then, staff members become increasingly concerned about whether the family is willing and able to provide rudimentary therapies, to administer medications, to discern when more expert medical care is needed, and somehow or other to get it all paid for. As we will argue in more detail in chapter 5, the social control machinery of the NICU is designed to determine which parents are "appropriate" and which are not, to bring "inappropriate" parents up to a minimum level of competence and commitment whenever possible, and to draw on the authority of the state to make other arrangements for the baby's discharge if the parents' behavior cannot be reshaped.

The NICU is an organization, then, where the emergencies of new parents are transformed into routine organizational business. There is a routine for nearly every problem, whether it be medical or interpersonal. Though one might expect a somber mood in a unit filled with critically ill infants, the transformation of troubles into routine business means that the mood in the NICU is often as buoyant as in any other workplace. When parents are absent (and even sometimes less discreetly in their presence), the air is often filled with jokes and laughter. Nurses chat about their weekends and their families, gossip about co-workers, and replay the mistakes and tragedies of patient care in the NICU with "black humor." Some days are slow, and the nurses and physicians long for some "action" to make it interesting. Other days are too full of action: a transport team is sent out for twins born very prematurely at the same time that another patient is admitted and immediately placed on a heart-lung bypass machine (called ECMO, an acronym for extra-corporeal membrane oxygenation) in a last-ditch effort to save its life. The staff and the patients must be juggled as new patients require beds and old patients must be discharged, or transferred, to make room.

This brief "insider's" view provides a general portrait of the organization of the NICU and the main categories of participants, their roles, and responsibilities. But as we will describe below, parents navigate the NICU without the benefit of a detailed map like the one we have just constructed. As researchers, we had the luxury of constructing our map over the course

16. At Suburban Hospital, we were told of one family who wanted their son discharged to them even though they were living in their car.

of several years, combining our own extensive observations and interviews with staff members in two NICUs with a review of the academic and popular literature on neonatal medicine. What is quite orderly—and even mundane—from the inside appears quite different indeed when viewed from the outside. But before we turn our attention to the parents' view of the NICU, we will first describe our research design, give profiles of City and Suburban Hospitals' NICUs, and explain how we collected our data.

The Research Design

The arguments in this book rely on data from several different sources. We made extensive observations at two different NICUs beginning in the late 1980s and ending in the early 1990s. Both are located in teaching hospitals in a major metropolitan area, one within the city limits, "City Hospital," and the other in a nearby suburb, "Suburban Hospital." Our own observations are combined with documentary evidence from patients' medical records and scores of interviews with staff members and parents from each unit. This approach yielded volumes of evidence for analysis: hundreds of pages of field notes, file drawers full of interview transcripts, and nearly a thousand file folders of information collected from patients' medical records. Many different kinds of evidence can then be used to answer our research questions: not just interview data, but also data from observations and from organizational documents. By studying two different NICUs, we gain further confidence that our conclusions are not based on the practices of a single NICU. Next, we introduce readers to the NICUs at City and Suburban Hospitals before we return to a more detailed description of our data.

City Hospital

City Hospital is a nationally renowned pediatric center that is nestled among brick brownstones and storefronts and close to public transportation. The NICU occupies one-half of an upper floor of the hospital. When visitors step off the elevators, they are greeted by a large, cheery mural that softens the sterile environment and serves as a reminder that this is a place for children. Large double doors mark the entrance to the nursery. A sign instructs visitors to check in with the unit secretary. Although parents may visit the unit any time, day or night, access by others is limited, and visitation policies are strictly enforced. Through the double doors is a long corridor with several doors on each side. Patients are treated in three rooms, where they are grouped according to severity of illness. These rooms have glass windows shielded by white horizontal blinds. In spite of the blinds, a few of the patients and their caretakers can be glimpsed from the corridor. The other doors in the corridor hide conference rooms, offices, a staff lounge, and a storage room for medical supplies. On one wall, a corkboard displays a crowd of pictures of former patients—the successes—and letters of thanks from their parents. The "front desk" where the unit secretary works is not really a desk at all, but a small three-walled room that serves as a hub of activity. Separated from the corridor by a chest-high partition, the unit secretary busily tracks incoming and outgoing patients, transfers calls, pages physicians, greets visitors, and otherwise keeps track of the ever-changing patient population of the NICU. As visitors approach the unit secretary's desk, they are often met by the backs of residents and other physicians busily making notations in patients' charts. A few computers are visible as well. Although the notes in the patients' records are written by hand, during the course of our research computers were being introduced to track some aspects of patient care.

A white board on the wall of the corridor displays important unit information. Each patient's last name is listed under the room where the patient is being treated. Next to the patient's name is written the name of the resident who is assigned primary responsibility for the patient's care. Nursing assignments are recorded at the front desk. The unit has the capacity to treat twenty-four patients, but the patient census often dips below this number and occasionally exceeds it. Because City Hospital does not have a labor and delivery ward, all of the patients in the NICU are born outside the hospital and must be transported to the unit. This NICU, like all others, receives patients from a regional referral network, as well.

Before patients are discharged, they usually spend some time in the room designated for "feeders and growers." The patients in the annex, as this room is called, are the healthiest in the NICU. Although all of the patients here are connected to cardiorespiratory monitors, none of them are on ventilators. Since these patients are less seriously ill, they require less intensive nursing, and each nurse cares for three or four patients. Most patients in the annex have graduated from isolettes (or incubators) to open cribs and are being bottle-fed at least part of the time. Several rocking chairs are scattered around the room, and babies are often taken out of their beds to be fed and rocked by nurses, parents, and an occasional volunteer. Though the patients in the annex are not yet well enough to be discharged home, they seem quite well when compared with the other patients in the unit.

Although the two rooms in the main part of the NICU are larger than the annex, the additional equipment and personnel make them, even with the same number of patients, more crowded. And although the nurses have fewer patients to care for, they are more pressed for time. As the patients are sicker, the mood here is decidedly more intense and serious than in the annex. The patients in the main part of the NICU often require far more technological support than those in the annex. Many of them require ventilators and oxygen and depend on IVs to deliver vital fluids, medications, and nutrition. These patients lie either in open beds with warmers above or in isolettes, and they often cannot be removed from their beds to be rocked or bottle-fed. The open beds allow quick access to the patients and are often used for the most critically ill, while the isolettes are enclosed and provide precise temperature regulation. A low-tech accommodation is made for some of the tiniest of the ventilated patients: They are placed in open beds and covered in ordinary household plastic wrap to protect their delicate skin and prevent dehydration.

A fourth room, called the parent room, is adjacent to the annex and is primarily used by parents who are ready to take their infants home. In the days just before discharge, some parents take care of their infants there, demonstrating that they have mastered the necessary skills, routines, and procedures. A nurse occasionally checks in with the parents and is available to assist or answer questions, but most of the care is performed by the parents. The parent room is also used for private time between parents and their infants. Some of these infants are well enough to be moved from the annex to the parent room for breast-feeding. Others are so sick that they are taken there to be held and comforted by their parents as they die. The parent room offers a measure of privacy in this very crowded place.

Among the nurses who care for patients at City's NICU are regular staff nurses, "float" nurses, and agency nurses. Because of the unpredictability of staffing needs, the unit often compensates for staffing shortages with the use of float nurses, who are employed by the hospital and rotate to different units as needed, and agency nurses, who are employed by a nursing agency that has a contract with the hospital and are referred to the hospital as needed. Hospital floating nurses and agency nurses are often assigned to the annex. The use of such temporary personnel allows the unit the flexibility it needs to adjust to changes in the demand for nursing services. But these temporary personnel are often unfamiliar with the patients and unit policies and procedures. Thus, flexibility has its price. The unit manages this price by employing the same agency personnel whenever possible. In-

Table 2.1 Profiles of two NICU patient populations: City Hospital and Suburban Hospital, circa 1990

	City Hospital (N = 379)	Suburban Hospital (N = 566)
Race of infant (percentage)		
White	50.9	85.5
African-American	26.6	4.1
Hispanic	11.6	6.5
Other	7.9	3.7
Unknown	2.9	0.2
Method of payment (percentage)		
Insurance	59.1	82.3
Public aid/uninsured/ method of payment unknown	40.9	17.7
Parents' marital status (percentage)		
Married	59.9	83.4
Unmarried/unknown	40.1	16.6
Mean length of hospitalization (in days)	24.0	22.6

deed, some agency personnel work at the unit often enough to be assigned to more critically ill patients, but primary nursing responsibilities are reserved for regular staff nurses.

In addition to the nurses, the staff of City's NICU includes three attending physicians, two fellows, and a social worker assigned half-time to the unit. Scores of residents also rotate through the unit in small groups about every six weeks. The patient population served by City Hospital is drawn from a large region and is racially and ethnically diverse. As Table 2.1 shows, about half of the patients treated at City's NICU are nonwhite, and some 41% of their parents are on public aid or have no insurance at the time of hospitalization. In addition, a substantial portion of the parents are not married.

The patients who are admitted to City's NICU have quite a wide range of medical problems. The majority are admitted because of prematurity and its associated complications. Table 2.2 illustrates the range of primary diagnoses of patients admitted during a twelve-month period. In addition to prematurity, many infants were admitted because of heart, gastrointestinal, neurological, and other problems. Others were admitted because of

TABLE 2.2 Primary diagnoses of two NICU patient populations: City Hospital and Suburban Hospital, circa 1990 (in percentages)

Diagnoses	City Hospital (N = 379)	Suburban Hospital (N = 566)
Prematurity	29.0	59.2
Respiratory disorders	35.6	43.5
Respiratory Distress Syndrome (RDS)	18.7	28.1
Diaphragmatic hernia[a]	2.9	0.9
Gastrointestinal/Genitourinary disorders	26.6	9.9
Imperforate anus[a]	4.8	0.4
Nectrotizing enterocolitis (NEC)[a]	2.9	3.2
Heart disorders	22.7	14.7
Patent Ductus Arteriosus (PDA)[a]	5.3	8.1
Multiple heart defects	4.2	1.1
Neurological disorders	10.8	6.5
Myelomeningocele[a]	2.4	1.1
Intraventricular Hemorrhage (IVH)[a]	1.8	2.1
Genetic/Other Syndromes	10.3	3.4
Multiple congenital anomalies	3.2	1.4
Down's syndrome	2.6	0.5
Meconium aspiration[a]	5.3	6.2
Sepsis[a]	2.7	11.0
Amniotic fluid aspiration	0	7.4
Other	11.6	28.6

Note: Percentages do not sum to 100. Data for this table were collected from patients' medical records. The mean number of primary diagnoses is 1.6 at City and 2.0 at Suburban. The diagnoses listed under the general category are the two most common.

[a]*Diaphragmatic hernia*—a hole in the diaphragm that allows the intestines to invade the chest cavity. *Imperforate anus*—an anus that does not open to allow the normal passage of feces. *NEC*—a condition that causes the bowel tissue to die. *PDA*—a heart defect where the bloodflow bypasses the lungs. *Myelomeningocele*—a form of spina bifida where the neural tissue and the membranes that envelop the spine protrude from the spinal column forming a sac under the skin. *IVH*—a hemorrhage in the ventricles of the brain. *Meconium aspiration*—causes severe respiratory difficulties and results when the fetus inhales meconium-tainted amniotic fluid. *Sepsis*—a serious systemic infection of the blood.

the accidents of birth, like meconium aspiration and asphyxia, and still others were admitted because of the accidents of genetics.

Suburban Hospital

Located in the same metropolitan area but in a nearby suburb, Suburban Hospital serves a more affluent and less racially and ethnically diverse population than City Hospital. As shown in Table 2.1, about 85% of the patients treated in Suburban's NICU are white, and approximately 83% of the parents are married and have some form of medical insurance. As is illustrated in Table 2.2, the infants in the NICU at Suburban Hospital were by and large admitted for the same kinds of medical problems as those at City, although a higher proportion of patients were simply very premature, often because they were the products of twin or triplet gestations.[17]

Suburban's NICU is larger than City's and has a ward layout with bed spaces for thirty-six infants. Although Suburban accepts transfers from other regional hospitals, many of the patients in the NICU are born at Suburban and admitted directly to the NICU. Suburban Hospital specializes in obstetrical care for high-risk pregnancies, and many of these pregnancies result in admissions to the NICU. In fact, physicians from the NICU are often present in the delivery room. Neonatologists are requested to be present in cases where a need for immediate critical care for the newborn (or newborns) is anticipated. In these cases, treatment decisions can begin just moments after birth.

Suburban Hospital is a sprawling medical complex that rises impressively above its suburban surroundings. A newer structure has been attached to the main hospital building, where construction is continuing in order to improve the facilities that make up the core of the hospital. During our research, the construction plans for the hospital included increasing the size of the NICU to accommodate more patients. Neonatal intensive care is a growth business. As the noise of construction one floor above invaded the NICU, the unit seemed even less like a nursery for newborn babies. Exhausted by the struggle to survive, however, the babies seemed oblivious to the din of construction.

All thirty-six beds in the NICU are located in one large, rectangular room that is divided into four quadrants of roughly equal size. Patients are

17. Twins and triplets are less likely to be carried to term than single fetuses and are therefore likely to be overrepresented in NICUs. Furthermore, the use of fertility drugs, which increase the odds of a multiple birth, is more common among Suburban parents than among City parents.

assigned to quadrants on the basis of severity of illness. The most critically ill patients are treated in quadrants one and two, and the less seriously ill in quadrants three and four. Visitors enter the unit after walking down a long corridor, passing the attending physicians' offices, the social work office, and the parent lounge. While the doors to these offices are often closed, the door to the parent lounge is almost always open and a television can frequently be heard from the hall. The lounge is cozy, has room for several people to be seated, and is often scattered with children's toys and books. At the end of the corridor and just before the entrance to the unit is a large mural of photos of previous patients. The successes are displayed prominently here, as well. Just outside the door to the unit sits a small table that holds a visitor's book. A small note asks visitors to sign their names before entering the unit. Some parents do; most do not. The first door to the unit opens into a small scrub area. Large signs instruct visitors to "gown" and scrub before entering a second door that opens into the NICU.

The front desk is located just to the left of the main entrance to the unit. This front desk is very much like the one at City Hospital: the unit clerk pages physicians, answers phones, screens visitors, and carries out administrative support tasks; physicians write orders and make entries in patients' charts; and the head nurse tracks existing patients and plans for incoming patients. Just beyond the front desk is the first quadrant. Each quadrant is long and narrow with a path defined by the space between the beds on either side. The second quadrant is behind the first and extends to the back of the room. The third quadrant is adjacent to the second, and the fourth quadrant is directly in front of the main entrance to the unit and next to the first quadrant. The quadrants are separated not by walls but by functional barriers. The two long sides of the quadrants are defined by shoulder-high partitions several inches thick, which have several electrical outlets and a source for oxygen and another for suction at each of the numbered bed spaces. On top of the partition is a counter where monitors and other equipment can be placed while in use. The quadrants in the front of the room (one and four) are separated from the quadrants in the back of the room by a long counter with supply cabinets above and below. At the very back of quadrant two is a long table with several chairs. This table is sometimes used by nurses and physicians as a gathering place. A small room at the very front of the unit offers a measure of privacy for administrative meetings and meetings between families and staff, for breast-feeding mothers, and for parents saying good-bye to their dying infants.

A row of windows lines the outside wall shared by quadrants three and four. These windows look onto the hallway outside the unit—or, perhaps more important, the hallway outside looks into quadrants three and four. Quadrants three and four are noticeably wider than quadrants one and two, and this design was intended to provide more space for the additional equipment often required by the more critically ill patients: IVs, ventilators, and the like. However, the more critically ill patients are not treated in these more spacious quadrants because, as a nurse explained to one of us during fieldwork, "We aren't running a freak show." Rather than a "freak show," interested onlookers can view rows of babies sleeping in open cribs and isolettes, while others are being rocked and fed by parents or nurses. As in City's NICU, the sickest patients in quadrants one and two are often lying in open beds with warmers above. Though parents are undoubtedly grateful not to have onlookers gawk at their infants, the more cramped quarters of the first two quadrants make it more difficult for parents to find room to sit at their infants' bedsides. Many of them perch on stools, switching sides of the bed as needed to get out of the way.

The nurses in the NICU at Suburban are all employed by the hospital. Unlike City's NICU, this NICU does not employ agency nurses to provide flexibility. Instead, it tries to maintain a stable patient census.[18] During the course of our research, the census hovered close to full capacity. When more flexibility is needed, nurses who work part-time are often asked to increase or decrease their hours. At other times, the head nurse fills in the gaps by caring for patients while carrying out her other responsibilities. This system provides less flexibility than the system at City Hospital but increases continuity. All of the nurses at Suburban's NICU are familiar with the policies and protocols of the unit. The differences between City and Suburban should not be overstated, however. Both units use the system of primary nursing, where the primary nurse is routinely assigned to care for her patient.

Because the number of patients treated at Suburban is larger than at City, the staff is also larger. Suburban's NICU has five attending physicians and two social workers (who alternate spending half-time in the perinatal unit) on staff. In contrast to City Hospital, these attending physicians continue to follow their patients, even meeting with parents, after they have

18. This policy is an accommodation reached after a long period of tension. Before the implementation of this policy of limiting the patient census, nurses had been very angry at physicians' willingness to stretch nursing resources to the limit by frequently operating above capacity.

rotated off-service. They are, therefore, more likely to be seen in the unit when they are off-service. The attending physicians are not always in the hospital, however. They also rotate to the referring hospitals, where they combine patient treatment with physician education. This program was initiated to improve the quality of treatment of the patients before they were transferred to Suburban. In addition to the attending physicians at Suburban, several fellows and a handful of residents share responsibility for treating patients.

The Data

We began our research at City Hospital, which is widely thought to set the standard of care for NICUs in its geographic region. On the one hand, this means City's NICU is not typical. Because of its reputation for excellence, some of the worst cases are transported to City for treatment. On the other hand, in such a setting we would be quite likely to find a concentration of the burdensome responsibilities we were interested in studying. As already described, City Hospital serves a racially and ethnically diverse population and treats many patients who are on public aid or have no insurance. City Hospital thus provides us with some important sources of variation within the patient population: married parents as well as unmarried, rich parents as well as poor, black and Hispanic parents as well as white ones.

Suburban Hospital was chosen as the second research site to provide a contrast to City Hospital. Whereas City Hospital treats a racially and ethnically diverse population, Suburban treats a more affluent and more homogeneous population. Among the other NICUs in the region, Suburban offers perhaps the greatest contrast to City on this dimension. But the contrast between City and Suburban serves another important purpose as well. A second research site is an important check on any tendency to overgeneralize from evidence from a single setting and gives some sense of variations in practices. The sociological research on NICUs tends to suggest that NICUs have much in common with one another—Guillemin and Holmstrom (1986), Frohock (1986), and Anspach (1993) describe events and practices from other locations and earlier periods that are strikingly similar to what we observed. However, the extent to which NICUs with different resources and very different patient populations would share similar organizational features and practices was an empirical question for us. In order to facilitate comparisons between the two hospitals, we followed the same research design as faithfully as possible in the two settings, completing our research at City before beginning at Suburban.

Our first contacts at both NICUs were negotiated largely through the social workers, who turned out to be receptive to our research and irreplaceable allies throughout the research period. They oriented us to each unit, introduced us to key personnel, helped us negotiate the details of access to medical records (once we had official permission to use them), and in other ways smoothed our path. We began our research by doing fieldwork and making extensive field notes on our observations. The fieldwork had two main purposes. First, if we planned to interview families about their experiences and the responsibilities they had shouldered, we needed to know enough about what NICUs were like to be able to interpret their comments. In addition, we believed that the NICU staff did more than just provide medical care. But we needed to observe the full round of activities in the NICU to uncover the relationship between parents and staff and to learn how this relationship might shape the commitments and reactions of parents.

We tried as much as possible to observe comparable activities in the two units and were largely successful in this.[19] We spent about one year doing fieldwork in each NICU and made a concerted effort to observe the full round of NICU activities. Although we were initially introduced to some key NICU personnel by the social workers, we were quite quickly on our own. We spent countless hours at the infants' bedsides, simply "hanging out" and watching the activities in the NICU. Here, we witnessed the routines of organizational life in the NICU: from admission to discharge and everything in between. We talked to nurses about their jobs, their patients, and their patients' families. We asked questions about procedures and protocols. We observed interactions between staff members and parents at the bedside. We visited the NICU during the day, the evening, and even overnight. We also tagged along occasionally on rounds, sat in parent and staff lounges, and otherwise made every effort to understand the complex world of the NICU.

We had an advantage conducting fieldwork in the NICU, because researchers can remain relatively inconspicuous in the crowd of people in the nursery—including therapists, nurses, parents, grandparents, attending physicians, residents, chaplains, social workers, phlebotomists, volunteers, janitors, and even other researchers. At times, we used the crowds to our advantage to make observations like the proverbial "fly on the wall," and

19. Those who would like to learn more about our data collection and methods may wish to consult the methods appendix, where we discuss some of the trials, tribulations, and triumphs of our research project.

at other times we quite actively pursued people with our questions. Though we would have often liked to dig deeper, we exercised considerable restraint with the parents whose infants were hospitalized in the NICU while we were making observations. We made observations and talked with many parents informally but did not attempt to interview any of them more formally during the crises of their infants' hospitalizations. We kept a respectful distance during the hospitalization, but we pursued them with great determination after their infants were discharged home (as we'll describe in more detail below).

From the beginning of our fieldwork in the NICUs, we also attended staff meetings at which patients' families were discussed. We believed these discussions about evaluations of parent performance and strategies to reshape parents' behavior would be important for our purposes. At these meetings, individual staff members' evaluations of parents are compared and reconsidered. Social work and nursing attention to reforming parents depends largely on the assessments made in these meetings. And what we learned at these meetings, combined with our insights from observations and staff interviews, makes up the core of our argument about the social control of parents in the NICU.

We later concluded that meetings between families and staff members were especially important in shaping parents' understanding of their obligations, and we arranged to attend many of these meetings as well.[20] In these meetings staff members comment on whether the parents are learning the skills, showing appropriate concern, and visiting frequently enough. Family members and medical personnel also discuss their disagreements about proposed treatments. During these meetings, we observed several protracted discussions about whether to continue to treat critically ill babies, a tense day-long discussion about whether the daughter of Jehovah's Witnesses would receive blood products, and several negotiations about whether a mother was going to give up custody of her child and about the conditions under which other parents would be permitted to take their children home.

These observations were supplemented by formal interviews with a variety of staff, including neonatologists, nurses, physical therapists, social workers, discharge planners, and staff associated with the hospital's follow-up program. Our aim in selecting staff members for interviews was mainly to get a variety of perspectives so that we would have a clear sense of what

20. Heimer (1992b) discusses these meetings between parents and staff members.

role each type of worker played in the complex division of labor and in ensuring high-quality medical and parental performances. In these interviews, we asked staff members to describe the kinds of interactions they had with patients' families and to explain the division of labor among different categories of workers (e.g., who would be responsible for talking to parents about a child's impending death). We also asked staff members how they dealt with a variety of common troubles—ranging from disputes between parents and staff members over treatment to difficulties getting parents to learn to care for their infants—and whether there were any particular types of parents with whom they had special difficulties. Though we conducted formal interviews with the social workers, we also interviewed them informally on other occasions. As key informants, social workers in both hospitals provided considerable information about hospital policy.

In addition to direct observational data, we collected information from the medical records of former patients as well. During the first year of our research at City Hospital, we collected data from the medical records of 379 former patients who had been hospitalized in City's NICU during one twelve-month period.[21] At Suburban Hospital, we collected a corresponding set of data from one twelve-month period, or 566 admissions. The information contained in the medical records focuses, of course, on medical matters, many of which are tangential to our research interests. In addition to this medical information, though, the record includes information about the age, marital status, race, and employment status of parents. We were also able to record the patient's primary diagnoses, a brief summary of the patient's medical course, and verbatim transcripts of notes written by physicians, social workers, discharge planners, and nurses detailing their interactions with and assessments of the patient's parents.

Especially useful for our purposes is the information from the record that documents the visitation patterns of the parents and staff reactions to parental behavior. These data provide crude indicators of the level of compliance with some of the most basic obligations of parenthood and allow us to study how compliance varies with other parental characteristics. The notes of social workers and discharge planners provide systematic evidence on reports to child-welfare agencies about, for example, maternal

21. The unit admitted 389 patients during this time period, but ten records were unavailable: one had been subpoenaed, and another nine either could not be located in the medical records department or were unavailable because the infant had been subsequently rehospitalized.

drug use, plans to relinquish a child for adoption, or failure to visit. Nursing notes include evaluations of parental competence in routine baby care and rudimentary medical care. These data supply valuable information about parental compliance with obligations (as conceived by the hospital) and about staff attempts to shape parental behavior (through meetings, teaching sessions, and, much more rarely, formal contracts with the parents and involvement of the state child-welfare agency).[22] Although an important part of the evaluation of parents is done orally and continues to exist only in the oral tradition of the unit, these written records supplement our observations nicely and allow us to make some systematic comparisons across a large number of cases.

Interviews with the parents of former patients round out our picture of how the rights and obligations of parenthood are understood, defined, and carried out by the parents themselves. Interviews with them were intended to provide information about how mothers and fathers conceived their obligations, how those conceptions had changed over time (particularly as they adjusted their views to take account of new information about the seriousness of the baby's condition), what kinds of pressure others had applied to parents to get them to take on onerous obligations, and how they balanced obligations to the hospitalized infant with other obligations. In order to allow the parents to discuss the issues that were salient to them and to their experience, the interviews were based on an interview guide (which we pretested with personal contacts and with members of parent-support groups) rather than standardized questions. The interviews were wide-ranging and included a more or less chronological account of the child's hospitalization, as well as questions about parents' roles during and after the hospitalization, the division of child-care labor (both between parents and between parents and other care providers), and how they conceived their obligations to the child. Information about the length of the hospitalization, the age and marital status of parents, the educational and occupational history of parents, family income, religious beliefs and affiliation, and childbearing history was collected from all parents, but the bulk of an interview focused on the child's hospitalization, its current condition, the family's adjustment to the child's needs, attempts by hospital staff members and others to shape parents' behavior, accounts of disputes be-

22. A formal contract might specify when and for long the parent would visit, what child-care tasks the parent would perform during the visit, when the parent should have mastered important skills, and what consequences would follow (e.g., placement of the child in a long-term care facility) should the parent not abide by the contract.

tween staff members and the parents, parents' assessments of the competence of the staff (and plans to bring malpractice suits in some instances), discussions of resources available to the family, accounts of the process of learning to care for the child, reactions to the division of effort between father and mother and their different levels of commitment, and comments on the costs and pleasures of having that particular child.

We began interviews with a sample of parents of former patients at City Hospital, which we drew from the list of patients whose medical records we had viewed. Because our research focuses on the burdensome obligations that result from having a sick child, we first excluded all patients who were known to have died in the NICU or a subsequent hospitalization.[23] We then selected a simple random sample of forty former patients from this shorter list. Because we expected that hospital staff members (and other people as well) would treat mothers and fathers differently, and because parents often share the burden of caring for a critically ill baby, we attempted to conduct separate interviews with both parents.[24] Though it was relatively easy to arrange to interview both parents when they were married, it was often difficult to make contact with fathers who were not married to the mothers of the infants. In spite of the difficulties we encountered, we successfully completed forty-four interviews with the parents of twenty-eight former patients at City Hospital. At Suburban Hospital, we altered our sampling strategy slightly. We began, as before, with the list of NICU admissions from a twelve-month period, but this time we drew a simple random sample of infants who had been hospitalized for longer than twenty-eight days and had survived. The sampling strategy was modified for the second hospital because we wanted to increase the proportion of respondents who were facing a long-term rather than a short-term crisis. If a child's hospitalization is relatively brief, the odds that he or she will go home requiring little more than ordinary newborn care are quite good. And although the experience may have been traumatic, adaptations to normal parenthood do not speak as clearly to the core theoretical issues of this

23. Issues of death and dying are certainly salient to this research project. In fact, many of the parents we interviewed had to face the grim, but very real possibility, that their child might die. And the child of at least one couple we interviewed did in fact die following our interview. However, we reasoned that those parents who lost their infants shortly after birth, in most cases without ever taking them home, would have less to say about the core issues of this book.

24. While many current books on motherhood rely on interviews only with mothers (e.g., Ribbens 1994; McMahon 1995; Hays 1996), Coltrane's (1996) book on fatherhood is notable in that he interviewed both mothers and fathers, as we did for this study.

book. With this modified strategy, we successfully completed thirty-nine interviews with the parents of twenty-one former patients at Suburban Hospital.

Taken together, these data yield a comprehensive picture of how obligations to critically ill newborns come to be defined and assigned to various parties and how performances are evaluated and rewarded or reshaped. Different data sources speak to different theoretical and empirical questions, and by combining them we are able to piece together a picture of the complex process of taking responsibility. Recognizing that different participants will often see the same events quite differently, we collected data that allow us to capture a range of perspectives. Given the importance of the divide between parents and staff members, we now take a second look at the organization of the NICU, this time from the parents' point of view.

A Second Look at Neonatal Intensive Care: The Outsider's View

One is struck, when first entering the NICU, by the dramatic contrast between the size of the patients and the mass of medical machinery that surrounds them. Respirators help infants breathe, ultraviolet lights for curing jaundice glow over beds, cardiorespiratory monitors track heart rate and respirations, blood-gas monitors check oxygen-saturation levels, IVs slowly administer medications and fluids for calories and nutrition, isolettes encircle patients to keep them warm, and portable X-ray machines and ultrasound units are wheeled in and out of the NICU as needed. Although parents are encouraged to visit the NICU—and most want to visit as soon as possible—few are prepared for what they will confront. One couple poignantly described the helplessness of their tiny infant and how different he looked from a normal, healthy newborn. The mother was unprepared for the sight of her very premature baby, who was "just laying, not moving" and seemed more like a "vegetable" to her than a robust newborn (2022F, p. 10); the father compared him to a piece of meat (2022M, p. 2). When planning for parenthood, the overwhelming majority of parents we interviewed had not even discussed the possibility of something going wrong. And then suddenly, with little or no warning, everything seems to have gone wrong. Their baby is critically ill.

Danny was born full term, but with a diaphragmatic hernia, a condition that allows the intestines to invade the chest cavity, preventing the lungs from developing normally and resulting in severe respiratory distress. Just a few months before his birth, his mother had turned twenty-one, and she had married Danny's father, Jack. The pregnancy was unexpected, but the difficulties following Danny's birth were even more unexpected. Indira gave birth to Danny, and he was whisked away to Suburban's NICU for treatment before she had even seen him. She was given a polaroid snapshot of her son, and she clung to it during the long week she was separated from him. During that week, he had surgery to correct the diaphragmatic hernia and was placed on ECMO (a heart-lung bypass machine). Indira was unfamiliar with her son's condition, had never heard of ECMO, and couldn't see for herself what was going on. When she was finally able to visit, Danny's condition had worsened. He required a second surgery for a complication from the ECMO treatment: "They said it [the surgery] was going to be two or three hours, but it ended up being five and we were just sitting there waiting and waiting. We were like, 'Is there any news? Is there any news?' you know. We're in this little lounge over there waiting and waiting and waiting, and I was going out of my mind. I was like, 'Oh, God, oh, God, help.' We went, we went to the chapel, and we were praying for him, and my mother-in-law and father-in-law were there. We were all crying. We didn't know what to do" (2002F, p. 28). Parents often feel overwhelmed during the initial stages of their infant's illness, unable to imagine how they will cope with the crisis.

Fathers are often the first to see their infants in the NICU. And they, too, tell heart-wrenching tales of their shock and grief after discovering how sick their newborns are. One father describes the first time he saw his son in the NICU. The pregnancy of his wife, Jean, had been perfectly normal until her water broke unexpectedly at just twenty-nine weeks' gestation. When Nick went to visit Tom, who was born eleven weeks premature, in the NICU, he describes how difficult it was to see his son attached to all sorts of medical equipment: "It was scary. The kid looked so small and he was, you see the IVs, all these monitors attached and then you see these tubes going through his nose to feed the baby. So it was very tough. And his heart wasn't fully developed. . . . Obviously, you have the worst possible scenarios you can think of. The first couple of days, the first few days, I was very worried that he was not going to make it, but after two, three, four days, I knew he was going to make it" (2033M, p. 3). When asked how he knew his son would survive, Nick describes how a lifeless body started to look more like a baby: "The first two, three days, he was absolutely, he had no life in him, it seemed like. He had no movement. He opened his eyes once in awhile, and it was as if he had no life in him. But after two or three days, he started moving, he was moving around" (2033M, p. 3). Before Tom's birth, Nick had some limited knowledge of neonatal intensive care but thought: "The NICU exists for sick babies or for premature babies. I don't really pay too much attention, because not my baby. My baby won't be there. He'll be full term. He'll be healthy" (2033M, p. 4).

No parent plans to have a sick baby. This simple observation underscores the asymmetry between the parents and the hospital staff. Although the critical illness of an infant is what brings both the parents and the staff to the NICU, they have very different relationships to this central fact. Quite simply, parents are novices in critical care medicine, and they are novices on somebody else's turf. Collecting information about how their infants are doing, evaluating that information, exploring treatment options, evaluating the quality of care, and the like all pose challenges to parents in the NICU (as we will describe in more detail in chapter 6). At the same time, NICU parents cannot do what they had planned to do—care for and get acquainted with a healthy newborn.

As members of the baby's team, parents face formidable impediments. Though they may have planned to be parents, and some even "trained" for the job, they did not plan to join an intensive-care-nursery health-care team. Although only a few of the parents talk about NICU parenting as a "job," our point here is to show how the insertion of parents into what is for others an employment situation leads to considerable discomfort as the disconcertingly different orientations of parents and staff members are juxtaposed. Insofar as parents have a job to do in the NICU, it is a very unusual one, which fits only awkwardly into the unit's life. Aside from the emotional trauma of having a critically ill baby, this substantial shift in the job of parenting is very confusing, even more confusing than the first weeks of employment in a new position. New employees are not usually assigned to high-stakes projects, nor are they usually so desperately committed to ensuring a good outcome. And new employees usually are assigned tasks and told when to be at work. Parents are told that they play a vital role but are not assigned any work. They are expected to be in the NICU, though they are not told how often they should be present or for how long. Little attempt is made to incorporate them into the NICU division of labor, and parents therefore receive little information about what roles others play. In fairness, staff members do not wish to overwhelm already distraught parents with irrelevant details. And for a variety of reasons, staff members cannot incorporate parents into the regular round of work—even if hospital accrediting organizations would tolerate increased parent participation, parents vary too much in skill level, the regularity of their presence in the NICU, and squeamishness about medical work. Parents then play a largely peripheral, often ceremonial role. They name the baby but do not care for it; they must be consulted about treatment, but if for some reason they are unable or unwilling to give consent in some emergency situations, the baby may be treated anyway.

The result of this partial incorporation into the NICU work routine, though, is that the elaborate division of labor that we described earlier in this chapter is largely lost on parents. Rather than the refined map of the NICU world that staff members possess, parents have only crude maps. In their versions, physicians are distinguished from nurses, but residents, fellows, attendings, and consultants all are lumped together into a single category. Only a few parents could correctly categorize ancillary staff members. Though they sometimes noted the presence of these workers, parents described them by gender and sometimes by task. A social worker might be "that nice lady who always asked me how I was doing," and a respiratory therapist could be "the man who always pounded the baby on the back." Such a crude category system does not capture the detail that makes NICU life predictable. If residents are not distinguished from attendings, for instance, the different work schedules of the two groups appear as "noise" rather than as two different, but orderly and predictable, patterns. Similarly, without an understanding of how therapists, X-ray technicians, nutritionists, or social workers fit into the hospital division of labor, and what schedules they follow, any regularity is lost and parents instead see a disordered flow of personnel through the NICU.

Of course the patterns of parent presence and participation in the NICU are also hard to describe. But just as nurses' shifts and physicians' rotations are key aspects of the experience of these staff members, so too parents' visitation patterns (hard as they are to uncover and describe) are an important feature of the experience of being the parent of a critically ill baby. As a category, parents are more variable than health-care workers (a point to which we return later in the book). Some parents visit several times a day, others come to the hospital once a week or even less frequently; some parents stay for several hours when they come, others stay for only a few minutes. Because parents' knowledge of NICU routines and familiarity with their infants' care providers are shaped by the frequency and duration of their visits, big variations in the amount of time parents spend on the unit lead to substantial differences in how much parents know about the unit and about their child's medical condition. In addition, though the effects of variability among staff members are reduced by the discipline of schedules and bureaucratic routines, the effects of parental variability are not similarly contained by any schedule of required visits. The loose articulation between the work of staff and the work of parents in the NICU thus arises partly from each group's inability to discern the pattern that underlies the other group's schedules and activities.

Just as parents (and researchers, we might add) gradually learn how to categorize the numerous staff members they encounter and ferret out information about NICU staff schedules, so staff members gradually gain some capacity to predict the comings and goings of parents. In both cases, though, local knowledge is more common than general knowledge. Parents learn about the schedules of *their* nurses, doctors, and therapists, and staff members (especially nurses) learn enough about the lives of *their* patients' parents to predict whether they will come in the morning, in the afternoon, or in the middle of the night, how long they will stay, and whether they will visit daily, once a week, or only when they are asked to come in and sign consent forms.

Because parent visitation is not much governed by bureaucratic rules, the patterns that exist cannot be uncovered by describing the rules for participation. For the most part NICU rules about visitation are rules that permit, but do not mandate, visiting. This is not to say that there are no observable patterns to parent visitation (or other forms of participation), but only that most of the constraint that produces the patterns comes from outside the NICU itself. To complete our portrait of the NICU, then, we describe the patterns of parent visitation, the rudimentary form of participation which typically undergirds other forms of participation, and explain the main pressures that shape parent visiting. Some of these pressures arise from the rules of other organizations (e.g., employers) with which the parents are involved, while others arise from other features of the parents' lives.

Perhaps the most important barrier to parent visitation can be summed up quite simply: distance. The physical distance that separates the sick infant from its parents has a different effect on mothers than on fathers. Mothers are disproportionately affected by the barrier of distance in the first few days following the infant's admission to the NICU. During this early period, many mothers are unable to visit their infants in the NICU because of the need to recover from the labor and delivery, a recovery that frequently takes place in another hospital. However, in the long run, distance often presents more of an obstacle to fathers, who are more likely to return to work while the infant is being treated. In the early period, the crisis often warrants time off work. But when the crisis goes on for weeks and months, extended leaves are often not feasible. So the physical distance between the infant and the parents has a more pronounced effect on the mother's ability to visit in the early stages of the hospitalization and a more pronounced effect on the father's ability to visit for the duration.

As we show in Table 2.3, parents vary quite a bit in how frequently they visit the NICU. When we control for variations in the lengths of the infants' hospitalizations by dividing the number of parent visits by the length of the hospitalization, we find that mothers visit a bit more often than fathers. Table 2.3 shows that at City Hospital, mothers have a visit recorded in their infants' charts on about 29% of the days their infants were hospitalized, while fathers have a visit recorded on about 23% of those days. Mothers of Suburban babies have a visit recorded on about 26% of the days their child is in the NICU, while fathers have a visit recorded on about 21% of those days. This table also shows that unmarried and uninsured mothers have far fewer visits recorded than their married and insured counterparts. And perhaps not surprising, unmarried fathers are the least likely of all to visit, with visits recorded on only about 9% of the days their infants are hospitalized.

The data on parent visitation patterns are taken from the medical records of their infants. At City Hospital, nurses record all contact with parents on a form titled "Nurse-Parent Communication Record," where notations are made about the duration and content (e.g., parents' comments and questions, child-care tasks performed by them, instructions given to them) of any visits, along with the content of any phone conversations with the parents. At Suburban Hospital, contact with the parents is simply recorded in the nursing notes along with the rest of the nurses' notations about their patients: patients' vital signs, IV settings, medications, tests, feedings, urine and bowel output, and the like. Because these data are produced for organizational purposes (and not for social science purposes), we must first understand how they are used by the organization before interpreting them with any confidence.

Certainly not every visit by a parent is recorded in the medical record. Nurses are often very busy and are primarily concerned with recording medical information about their patients. However, as we noted earlier, NICUs are not just in the business of treating patients, they are also in the business of ensuring those patients are discharged to places where they will receive adequate care. Contact with the parents is recorded in the medical

TABLE 2.3 Mean percentage of days a parent visited the NICU during the infant's hospitalization (N in parentheses)

	City Hospital	Suburban Hospital
All mothers	28.8 (374)	25.5 (524)
White	35.4 (192)	26.1 (449)
Black	18.9 (100)	20.3 (20)
Hispanic	28.7 (44)	19.2 (34)
Other, unknown	21.9 (38)	27.1 (21)
Married	34.2 (226)	26.9 (446)
Unmarried, unknown	20.5 (148)	17.5 (78)
Insured	35.7 (221)	26.7 (436)
Uninsured, public aid, unknown	18.9 (153)	19.5 (88)
Older	29.0 (320)	25.9 (487)
Younger (< 20)	17.9 (38)	20.8 (35)
All fathers	23.2 (374)	21.2 (524)
White	29.9 (192)	21.8 (449)
Black	8.6 (100)	16.5 (20)
Hispanic	27.0 (44)	17.6 (34)
Other, unknown	23.6 (38)	18.9 (21)
Married	32.1 (226)	23.3 (446)
Unmarried, unknown	9.7 (148)	9.1 (78)
Insured	31.4 (221)	22.7 (436)
Uninsured, public aid, unknown	11.4 (153)	13.8 (88)
Older[a]	28.6 (89)	21.4 (364)
Younger (< 20)[a]	13.4 (9)	9.9 (11)

Note: Number of visits by each parent, as recorded in the infant's medical record, divided by the length of the infant's hospitalization, yielding the proportion of days on which the parent visited the infant in the NICU. No visits would be 0%; a visit every day would be 100%. Ns are lower than the total number of medical records reviewed (379 at City and 566 at Suburban), because in some cases information on parents' visits was missing from the infant's medical record. At City, this would mean that the form for recording parents' visits was missing from the record; at Suburban, this would mean that the nurses' notes could not be located in the medical records department or for other reasons were not available for review.

[a]Ns are much lower for fathers than for mothers, because the mother's age was routinely recorded in the medical record, but the father's age was not.

record, then, as a way of building a case about the adequacy of the parents as caretakers of the infant. Here we are concerned only with the number of visits (or, more precisely, the proportion of days of the infant's hospitalization when a parent visit was recorded in the medical record). Other written notations in the medical record by nurses, physicians, and social workers at both hospitals also address what takes place during the visit: whether the parents are "appropriately concerned," whether they ask "appropriate questions," and seem to have an "appropriate understanding" of the infant's diagnosis and prognosis. We will return to these evaluative statements and the role they play in the NICU social control system in chapter 5. Here, the content of the evaluations is less important than understanding that because these notations are part of the NICU social control system, we would expect more scrutiny of some parents than of others. Parents who may be expected to have difficulty coping with the critical illness of a newborn, such as the young, poor, and unmarried, are more likely to receive close scrutiny than parents who are married and middle-class. Because such parents have fewer resources, visitation may be difficult, and the staff needs to determine whether this is an indication of resource constraints or of detachment that may compromise the infant's chances for good health and survival after discharge. If there is any systematic bias in the medical record, then, we would expect the visits of young, poor, and unmarried parents to receive more attention than the visits of older, richer, married parents. So although parental visits are likely to be understated overall (that is, not every visit is recorded), the visits of the young, poor, and unmarried are, if anything, overstated relative to the visits of other parents. In short, the gap between these groups is likely larger, not smaller, than what is represented in the medical records. Furthermore, the slightly higher rates of visitation at City than at Suburban must also be interpreted in the light of how these visits are recorded at the two units. Because City has a special form on which contact with parents is recorded and Suburban does not, the visitation of Suburban's parents is likely understated relative to City's.

The gap between different categories of parents is even more dramatic when we examine Table 2.4, which shows the percentage of parents who had no visits recorded in their infants' medical charts. Although mothers are less likely than fathers to have no visits recorded, mothers and fathers at City Hospital are about twice as likely as their Suburban Hospital counterparts to have no visits. Only 8.4% of mothers at Suburban Hospital have no visits, while the proportion more than doubles at City to 17.6%; and

TABLE 2.4 Percentage of parents with no visits during the infant's hospitalization (N in parentheses)

	City Hospital		Suburban Hospital	
All mothers	17.6	(374)	8.4	(524)
White	13.0	(192)	7.8	(449)
Black	22.0	(100)	25.0	(20)
Hispanic	15.9	(44)	2.9	(34)
Other, unknown	31.6	(38)	14.3	(21)
Married	14.6	(226)	7.4	(446)
Unmarried, unknown	22.3	(148)	14.1	(78)
Insured	13.6	(221)	7.6	(436)
Uninsured, public aid, unknown	23.5	(153)	12.5	(88)
Older	17.2	(320)	8.4	(487)
Younger (< 20)	23.7	(38)	5.7	(35)
Mean length of infant's hospitalization (days)	6.6	(66)	8.3	(44)
All fathers	28.1	(374)	14.9	(524)
White	20.3	(192)	14.2	(449)
Black	48.0	(100)	35.0	(20)
Hispanic	20.4	(44)	8.8	(34)
Other, unknown	23.7	(38)	14.3	(21)
Married	12.8	(226)	9.2	(446)
Unmarried, unknown	51.4	(148)	47.4	(78)
Insured	15.4	(221)	11.2	(436)
Uninsured, public aid, unknown	46.4	(153)	33.0	(88)
Older[a]	18.0	(89)	10.7	(364)
Younger (< 20)[a]	33.3	(9)	36.4	(11)
Mean length of infant's hospitalization (days)	15.1	(105)	15.8	(78)

Note: Data for this table were collected from the infant's medical record. Ns are lower than the total number of medical records reviewed (379 at City and 566 at Suburban), because in some cases information on parents' visits was missing from the infant's medical record. At City, this would mean that the form for recording parents' visits was missing from the record; at Suburban, this would mean that the nurses' notes could not be located in the medical records department or for other reasons were not available for review.

[a]Ns are much lower for fathers than for mothers, because the mother's age was routinely recorded in the medical record, but the father's age was not.

14.9% of fathers at Suburban have no visits, while the proportion nearly doubles to 28.1% at City. The difference between mothers at Suburban and City may be explained by the fact that all of the NICU patients at City are transported there from the hospitals where they were born. The mothers at City, then, may simply be recovering from labor and delivery in another hospital and may therefore be physically unable to visit. Indeed, the mean length of the infant's hospitalization for those mothers who never visited shows that the infants were only in the NICU for about a week on average. Many of the mothers at Suburban Hospital, on the other hand, delivered their infants at that hospital and only had to travel a few floors to see their infants rather than a number of miles. Fathers do not have to recover from the physical trauma of labor and delivery, so this is no help in fashioning an explanation for their failure to visit. Brief hospitalizations are not the key. Indeed, the infants of fathers who failed to visit were hospitalized on average about two weeks, twice as long as the infants of mothers who failed to visit. Marriage, however, does seem to be a key. Approximately half of all unmarried fathers have no indication in the record that they ever visited.

These admittedly crude data about visitation patterns are only the tip of the iceberg, of course, because they tell us little about what parents actually do during their visits. Some parents discover that they are entitled to read their child's medical record and regularly do so; other parents are either unaware of the existence of the medical record, too intimidated by the setting to inquire about their right to see the record, or sufficiently respectful of medical authority that they wish to leave such matters to the authorities.[25] Some parents know their child's team members by name and are aware of nursing shifts and vacation schedules and physician rotations; other parents refer to their child's team members only by category labels ("nurse" and "doctor") and seemed to feel that NICU health-care providers were organizationally interchangeable and that there was nothing parents could do about the rapid turnover of these highly skilled workers. Just as one wouldn't expect to become acquainted with the pilot of a plane but would simply entrust one's fate to him (or her), so one had to entrust one's child to the care of skilled, but anonymous, health-care providers.

From the inside, then, the NICU may appear to be a well-ordered organization with carefully choreographed routines for saving lives. But from the perspective of outsiders, the NICU often seems bewildering, the infant's progress full of uncertainty, the staff innumerable, anonymous, and

25. This right varies by state. In the state where we conducted this research, people have the right to view and even copy their own medical records and those of their minor children.

inaccessible. As frightened parents face what is often the biggest crisis of their lives, there is no one in sight willing to give firm answers. For most parents, the NICU remains a frightening place. For some parents bewilderment is gradually replaced by a sense of familiarity and even occasionally mastery. But for most others, the NICU is nearly as bewildering on the day their child leaves as on the day they first walked through the doors.

In describing the parents' experience of the NICU, we have tried to show that even very carefully ordered environments can be difficult to negotiate if one does not know the categories and principles by which the order is generated. Foreigners to any culture have difficulty discerning the rules of interaction, and parents entering the NICU are certainly entering a foreign culture. But they arrive with a mission. Because their child is in the custody of "foreigners," parents are unusually motivated to learn enough about the culture to ensure the safety of their child and to maximize the chance that they will finally gain physical custody of the baby. Some view the foreign culture as benign, others view it as hostile. But nearly all regard the NICU as foreign and feel that they cannot do their job as parents unless they successfully negotiate the cultural barrier. To see the NICU only from the insiders' perspective is grossly to misunderstand the task facing NICU parents.

THREE

What Do We Mean by Responsibility?

RESPONSIBILITY IS FUNDAMENTAL to the social world we inhabit yet is curiously undertheorized. We have a common understanding of what responsibility entails, believe we know it when we see it, and bemoan its absence when we don't. Responsibility is a virtue. Those who "take responsibility"—whether they are individuals or organizations—are heralded. Those who shirk are vilified. This, then, might be read as a story of heroes and villains. Our approach, however, is somewhat different. Rather than treat responsibility as an issue of character, morals, or ethics, we instead ask how responsibility is socially produced and sustained. Rather than treat responsibility as a personal attribute, we instead ask what conditions increase the likelihood that people will care about the welfare of others or choose the common good over their own welfare. Rather than simply chronicle personal triumphs and failings, we instead illustrate how human agency and social institutions are jointly required to produce outcomes that are oriented to the welfare of others.

Human agency that is flexibly oriented to the welfare of others is at the core of our definition of responsibility. In this chapter, we define responsibility more precisely along five dimensions. We argue that those who take responsibility differ from others in taking the interests and needs of others seriously, focusing on both present actions and future outcomes, defining obligations broadly (even following them across organizational boundaries), using discretion to meet unforeseen contingencies, and accepting whatever costs and benefits are entailed. To illustrate these dimensions, we draw on examples from an array of settings, including the NICU. Our purpose here is to lay the foundation for our analysis in the rest of the book.

Two types of variation are of interest to sociologists studying responsibility: variation among roles and among individual occupants of the same role. That is, some roles require or permit incumbents to assume more responsibility than others, and some occupants of a role take more responsibility than others even though the role ostensibly requires the same level of responsibility from all. In both cases we want to know what kinds of social arrangements facilitate the acceptance of responsibility and increase the chance that people will be able to meet the obligations that they have accepted. This book is primarily about variations among incumbents of a single role—parenthood—although the tools that we use to differentiate parents who take a lot of responsibility from parents who take only a little also can be (and are) used to distinguish among disparate roles.

The first task of this chapter is to define what we mean by responsibility by describing and discussing its five dimensions. This theoretical apparatus, once constructed, allows us much greater precision in discussing variations in the amount and kind of responsibility various people assume. This conception of responsibility is meant as a general theoretical formulation and therefore applies just as well to other settings as it does to parents of NICU graduates. Here, however, we are interested primarily in explaining the variation among parents, and we turn to this analytical task next. We begin our empirical analysis with portraits of seven children and their parents to illustrate the rich variation among the families we interviewed. All parents ostensibly share the same role—parent of former NICU patient—but we find a great deal of variation. We translate the five dimensions developed in the first half of the chapter into coding categories to analyze our interviews with parents and discuss our results.

In effect, we ask how much responsibility each of the parents we interviewed actually assumes. Does the parent assume a great deal of responsibility, taking the child's welfare seriously, planning for the future, defining obligations broadly, using discretion, and accepting contingencies? Or does the parent assume only a limited responsibility? But individuals did not face identical situations, and we take account of this by further classifying parents according to the magnitude of the burden they faced. Is the child essentially normal, or does the child require extensive medical care? In this chapter we explain how we made assessments both of the magnitude of the burden that parents faced and of the extent to which they shouldered those burdens. We also present our evidence about how parents stacked up on these matters—how large their burdens actually were and how much responsibility they in fact accepted.

Our interviews with parents contain a great deal of variation, and describing that variation systematically proved to be one of the most challenging tasks of writing this book. Though our aim was to transform "taking responsibility" into an empirical question, it nonetheless remains morally loaded. Taking responsibility, alas, is a virtue, and there is no way to make either the acceptance of responsibility or the refusal to take responsibility morally neutral.

Defining Responsibility: Two Types of Variation along Five Dimensions

A theory of responsibility, if it is to be useful in understanding variation in the empirical world, must have the kind of precision that allows us to make systematic comparisons.[1] How do we know responsibility when we see it? Our gut may tell us, but this is simply not enough. Here we continue the theoretical discussion of responsibility we began in chapter 1 by adding the kind of precision that allows researchers to begin to make such systematic comparisons.

We are primarily interested in why some parents act more responsibly than others, and to explain these variations we look at how exactly parenthood is arranged, how motherhood differs from fatherhood, how people conceive the obligations of parenthood, and what resources and constraints shape the experiences of particular parents. Individual parents differ in such matters as the details of recent biography, including childbirth classes or other experiences that might shape their orientations to parenthood, access to the kinds of resources that might allow them to adjust to their child's unusual needs, whether their kin networks include anyone with medical expertise or anyone who will help with child care, and whether their employers are stingy with time off for family medical emergencies.

To shed light on parenthood, we also compare parenthood with other roles, noting for instance how positions in an organization are configured and what kinds of incentive systems motivate planning for the future or the use of discretion. We turn often to examples from hospital settings. Such examples serve, first, as comparison points for parenthood. Doctors, nurses, and social workers also vary in the extent to which they accept responsibility and for some of the same reasons. But medical examples also allow us to show how the activities of people in nearby roles shape and constrain parenthood. During the baby's NICU stay, what parents do depends a great deal on what hospital staff allow and encourage them to do.

1. Some of the material presented in this section has been adapted from Heimer (1996b).

Since our primary interest here is in parents, our argument is framed initially as one about variations among individuals who occupy the same role. But, as we show, variation between roles may be described and explained in the same fashion as variation between incumbents of a single role, and we thus generalize the argument from incumbents to roles. Just as those occupants of a role who accept more responsibility can be distinguished from those accepting less by comparing them along the five dimensions we discuss below, similarly roles requiring substantial responsibility can be distinguished from those requiring less responsibility along the same five dimensions. In short, the definition of responsibility developed here should be just as useful to those who wish to understand variation between roles as it is in understanding individual variations in the acceptance of responsibility.

Individuals may, furthermore, occupy more than one role, which places competing demands on them to behave responsibly. Those who both work and have families most likely understand just what such competing pressures feel like. People, then, are often responsible for many different things and responsible to many different constituencies simultaneously. Balancing competing demands is a key feature of responsibility, as the families we interviewed know all too well (and as we discuss in more detail below). It follows, then, that a person may be responsible to one constituency while being irresponsible to another. Responsibility, as we define it here, is not a character trait that people either possess or lack. Responsibility must always be understood in a particular context. We have chosen (for reasons detailed in chapter 1) to focus on one empirical setting: parenting former NICU patients. While parenting is a particularly fundamental social obligation, there are, of course, many other settings that would be appropriate for an inquiry of this type. Our point here is simply to emphasize that our focus on parenting should not confuse our readers. This is certainly not the only responsibility that is encompassed by our theoretical discussion, nor is it the only responsibility worthy of scholarly attention. In fact, we hope our exposition below will stimulate other researchers to use these tools to examine other types of responsibilities.

Five Dimensions

People who take more responsibility can be differentiated from those taking less along five dimensions: (1) More responsible people tend to take account of others' interests as well as their own, balancing those interests against pleasures and interests of their own. Either the utility function being maximized is that of another person, or some institution, rather than the person's own, or at the very least it includes arguments describing others' interests as well.[2] (2) More responsible people think about long-term outcomes and maximize the utility function over a longer time horizon. (3) More responsible people tend to define their roles more diffusely. That is, such a person will maximize a utility function, trading off between many values, all of which he or she is responsible for, rather than a single value. (4) More responsible people use more discretion. The person chooses how to maximize the utility function rather than follows a rule or prescribed procedure. And (5) more responsible people cope with whatever contingencies arise. The person accepts the obligation to maximize the utility function under conditions of uncertainty about what exactly is entailed and what costs and benefits will accrue to him or her.

Below we discuss these dimensions in more detail, highlighting factors that support or undermine the acceptance of responsibility. Of course one or another of these attributes may characterize a person who accepts little or no responsibility; responsible people are distinctive in simultaneously taking account of others' interests, accepting a diffuse definition of a job, thinking about the long term, using discretion, and accepting resulting variations in their own welfare.

Taking Others' Interests Seriously

While to be "rational" is to choose trade-offs among values according to one's own preferences and tastes, to be "responsible" is to be rational on someone else's behalf, or at least not only on one's own behalf.[3] Behaving rationally and behaving responsibly may conflict; people are probably more likely to behave responsibly when rationality and responsibility co-

2. By a "utility function," economists mean a system of trade-offs among different values, or among the interests of different people. To "maximize a utility function" then one must decide how much of one value (e.g., the present happiness of a child for whom a trust fund has been set up) to trade to get more of another value (e.g., reserving resources for adulthood).

3. Here, we are arguing that responsibility is fundamentally social. Though we speak of people acting irresponsibly when they are shortsighted about their own future interests, or demand that people (perhaps especially their own children) learn to take responsibility for themselves, we would argue that this does not change the fundamentally social character of responsibility. In accusing people of irresponsibility, we may be charging such people with rationality on behalf of current selves at the expense of responsibility for future selves. The bitter tone of such comments suggests that shortsightedness about the future seems particularly irresponsible when people are squandering opportunities responsibly created by others or are setting up situations in which others will later have to take responsibility for them.

incide.[4] Being responsible (being rational on someone else's behalf) means thinking about the costs and benefits to the other party as well as to oneself and agreeing to bear some costs to improve the other person's welfare or to achieve the other's purposes. Being responsible may not entail complete self-sacrifice, but it often requires some compromise between others' interests and one's own. If responsibility involves taking others' interests into account, then correspondingly it is irresponsible to define too narrowly the group on whose behalf one is supposed to make choices and select trade-offs.

When a child is born, and to some degree before the child's birth, a new set of interests has to be incorporated into the family utility function. No longer is it sufficient to think about what the parents as individuals want or even what their other children need or want. The birth of a premature or congenitally malformed infant disrupts the delicate balance among the interests of various family members. Not surprisingly, parents may disagree about how to weigh the interests of the needy new child compared with the interests and needs of other family members. Strained marital relations may occur if the mother believes that she has changed her life to meet the child's needs but the father has not. In one family, the wife bitterly commented on how she was effectively confined to the house on weekends caring for the couple's disabled child while her husband continued to accumulate athletic trophies (1017). Another couple (whose case we discuss more fully later in the chapter) agreed on the priority they accorded their youngest child's acute medical needs, though they noted that the other children showed signs of neglect (2016). In this case, social service workers and teachers might have disagreed with the parents about how to allocate their resources: After one of their older children was taken to the police station for minor offenses, the parents worried that they had perhaps devoted too high a proportion of parental attention to the child with acute medical problems and hoped they could nip their older child's problems in the bud before he became a full-fledged juvenile delinquent. But the problem is more complicated than this. Not only is it difficult to balance

4. Mansbridge similarly argues that self-interested and altruistic motives can reinforce each other and that we err in suggesting that any hint of self-interest contaminates altruism: "Conceptually we distinguish among motivations by opposing them to one another. . . . Empirically, we demonstrate that people are acting for unselfish reasons by devising situations in which they are demonstrably acting against their self-interest. Yet in practice we often try hard to arrange our lives so that duty (or love) and interest coincide" (1990:133).

the interests of those who must be taken into account, but it is also often difficult to define the bounds of the group whose interests must be included.

Disagreements about how to take account of the critically ill infant or NICU graduate's interests without neglecting the needs of other family members may revolve around different assessments of what a baby really needs. A superficial understanding of developmental processes may lead a parent to underestimate how much cuddling, stimulation, or amateur physical therapy is called for. To take an extreme case, during our fieldwork a nurse at City Hospital reported to us that one mother was willing to go along with her suggestion that she should talk to her baby but seemed baffled. "But what should I say to him?" the mother asked.

La Rossa and La Rossa (1981) point to different notions about infant needs as a core explanation for why child care is more work for women than it is for men. Women, believing that an infant is a person and so requires and deserves the same consideration others are accorded, devote themselves to tracking and interpreting their infants' reactions. Fathers, in contrast, are more likely to see their infants as objects rather than people and are therefore much more comfortable leaving a baby in a crib while they do other things. Fathers may therefore have a different view than mothers about how much time one needs to spend visiting a hospitalized newborn or how much care an NICU graduate requires after his or her basic physical needs for food, clean diapers, and warmth have been met. When people's assessments of needs and interests differ so dramatically, it is hard to assess whether different patterns of behavior arise from selfish and irresponsible failures to value babies' needs equally with their own or whether they arise from radically different understandings of what babies really need.

In describing variations in parents' inclinations to value their child's needs equally with their own, we should be careful not to give short shrift to the social supports that undergird attention to others' interests. We can perhaps see this point more clearly by first looking beyond familial relations. In some instances, a legal requirement reinforces the fiduciary obligation to make sacrifices in one's own welfare for the sake of others to whom one has a responsibility. Laws against insider trading, for instance, make it clear that a board of directors is to defend stockholder interests and that board members cannot use inside connections and information in ways that would harm stockholder interests (Zey 1993). Similarly, professional privileges are partly justified by claims that professionals are altruistically oriented to their clients' needs and interests.[5] Parental obligations to take account of their children's needs are similarly buttressed by state laws about neglect and abuse of children (as we discuss more fully in chapter 4) but even more by a rich cultural tradition that stresses the appropriateness of feeling that one's own interests cannot really be regarded as fully separable from one's child's. If professionalism is part and parcel about valuing clients' interests above those of the professional, parenthood is even more deeply defined by parents' identification with their children and concern with meeting their needs, and others are not shy about pointing out lapses in parental (particularly maternal) devotion to meeting children's needs.

But social pressure and formal rules are not the only supports for taking account of others' interests. Mechanisms that increase information about others' interests or make them more salient also increase the chance that a person will take responsibility for others' welfare. Such mechanisms may create a community of fate in which the interests of the two parties are partially fused (Heimer 1985:201–6), and it is again useful to begin by briefly examining other settings where relations between the interests of various parties are laid out in contracts, and incentives to take account of others' interests are formally provided. Insurers worry that once insurance coverage is in place policyholders lose interest in avoiding accidents and reducing the costliness of accidents. How can insurers force policyholders to act in the insurers' interest? Insurers commonly stipulate that a policyholder cannot be compensated for a loss if he or she caused the loss or did nothing to prevent it. Because the policyholder's outcome depends on taking account of the insurer's interests, the policyholder will be more likely to take both sets of interests into account in deciding how much to invest in loss prevention (Heimer 1985). It is just such mechanisms that bring self-interest and responsibility into alignment.[6]

5. While some (e.g., Parsons 1968) believe professionals' claims, others (e.g., Freidson 1970, 1988; Starr 1982) are skeptical. Though professionals may generally believe that they and their colleagues protect client interests, professionals may nevertheless disagree about limits on the obligation to sacrifice their own interests. Bosk and Frader (1990), for instance, find that some medical students deny any obligation to care for AIDS patients if providing such care jeopardizes their own health. When altruism can legitimately give way to self-interest is apparently as much in dispute in other realms as it is in family life.

6. More generally, contracts make some outcomes of one person or organization dependent on the outcomes of the other, though as Stinchcombe (1990:194–239) argues, such interdependence is produced more easily in hierarchies and in contracts that incorporate hierarchical features. Similarly, pressure groups try both to inform policymakers of their

In families, it is usually not necessary to introduce artificial mechanisms to make parents take account of their children's needs. Daily contact makes parents sensitive to the needs and interests of their children. But when contact is reduced, as often occurs when parents separate or divorce, one or both parents may take less account of the children's needs, partly because of reduced information (Arendell 1986, 1995). Fathers (or mothers) may cease to feel that their child's happiness is their own and may even feel that looking out for the child is tantamount to providing for the happiness of a bitter enemy (the estranged partner). Similarly, when contact between parent and child is reduced because of a child's extended hospitalization at birth, parents may never learn to value their child's welfare in the first place—or so NICU staff members believe. One's child's pleasures and pains seem to have more motivational effect when observed firsthand than when experienced at a greater remove. An NICU nurse's phone report that a baby is longing to see its parents may then be just the hook needed to pull reluctant or frightened parents into the nursery and to get them to think of the baby as someone with needs, interests, and feelings that have to be taken seriously.

Thinking about the Long Term

In one of the very few social science investigations of responsibility, Elliott Jaques (1972) specifically linked responsibility to planning for the future. Pointing to the intimate connection between long-term performance and hierarchical differences in responsibility in industry, Jaques argued that higher-ranked employees are reviewed at longer intervals because short-run measures of performance distract executives from using long-term objectives to set priorities. Thus the more responsible the role, the more the performance measures embedded in the incentive and authority systems of industrial hierarchies will focus on distant outcomes. Responsibility necessarily entails thinking about the future as well as the present and making trade-offs between today and tomorrow, always with the full knowledge that no one can know what exactly tomorrow will bring.

Parenthood is perhaps the most future oriented of all social roles. Under most circumstances a parent who demonstrated an interest only in his or her present relationship with the child and showed no concern with the child's future would be regarded as an inadequate parent. When an NICU

members' interests and to remind them that their welfare depends to some degree on the goodwill of the pressure group.

nurse complained to us about how some young parents were interested only in dressing their babies in cute clothes, her moral outrage drew its force from her fear that such parents cared more about showing off an attractive infant than learning what they could do to enhance the child's prospects for the future.

Almost all parents are fully aware that parenthood is a long-term obligation requiring them to think about the child's future as well as its present. Despite this commonality, parents differ quite a lot in the degree to which they think it is their job to ensure that their child has a particular kind of future and in the extent to which they conceive of present events and actions as having future consequences. Without specifying intermediate steps, some parents predicted that by the time their severely damaged child was an adult he or she would be essentially normal. Completely missing the point of early milestones as indicators of developmental problems, one father of a very delayed one-year-old (who weighed only ten pounds at one year) told us that many premies ended up being "above average intelligence-wise" (1036M, p. 84). Referring to his son, he added, "His developmental stage is now—aside from [not] sitting up and [not] holding himself up—other than that he's just like a normal one-year old kid" (1036M, p. 84). His wife was similarly optimistic: "[At] five years old he'll catch up to everybody else; ten years old he'll be very smart, very intelligent, smarter than the rest. By the time he's fifteen he'll be passing everybody up as far as how big" (1036F, p. 50). Other parents were deeply concerned about the physical limitations their child would face and also engaged in agonized discussions about what it would mean if a daughter were unable to bear children or a son unable to participate in sports. Still other parents expected that psychological scars from the early hospitalization might well shape the child's future even if there were no obvious biological effects. Some parents, for instance, reported that their toddlers hated to have their feet touched, attributing this sensitivity to repeated heel-stick blood tests in the NICU.

Not all parents have a clear understanding of connections between present conditions and future outcomes. Better-educated and more middle-class parents were more likely to have basic information about developmental sequences. But regardless of class or educational background, parents who spent more time in the NICU were more likely to pick up information about developmental processes, about how to assess their child's progress, and about how they could intervene to help their child overcome deficiencies. Aware that early interventions might help a child compensate for medical insults or congenital abnormalities, parents with a strong orientation to the future worked hard to arrange for physical therapy or to place their child in a comprehensive zero-to-three program.

Parents concerned about their child's future were sometimes frustrated if they believed that the hospital staff seemed exclusively concerned with the present. Parents acknowledged that the staff had a better grasp than they of the causal relationship between present and future but noted that it was the parents who had to take the baby home. Thus, according to some parents, the inequality in knowledge was more than balanced by an inequality in motivation, this time favoring parents. As the party ultimately responsible for the baby's welfare, then, parents had to make sure that staff members kept their eye on the future as well as the present so that interventions now didn't damage the baby's future.

Among physicians, pediatricians are notable for their concern about the future of their patients.[7] But neonatologists are nevertheless sometimes faulted for worrying too much about saving infants and too little about the futures the infants are being saved for. Lending credence to this charge, one neonatologist asserted that every infant gets "the best," even when evidence suggests that the child is not neurologically intact (Guillemin and Holmstrom 1986:234). Anspach (1993) points to a central difficulty neonatologists face in taking responsibility: when connections between present indicators and future outcomes are poorly understood, reasonable people will disagree about the responsible course of action even when all agree that the future cannot be ignored. Intensive-care staff agree on the principle that life-sustaining treatment should be withheld from infants who would not survive or would survive only with serious neurological deficits, but this consensus disintegrates in practice because of disagreements about the prognosis of individual babies (Anspach 1993:58).

When the future is very uncertain, people are reluctant to take responsibility for long-term outcomes. This may be especially true in situations in which the social arrangements connecting one person to another (e.g., as a teacher, physician, therapist, or financial adviser) have rather short lives. Nevertheless, attention to the future is a core part of responsibility, and

7. Such concern has been manifested in political pressure, for instance in support of immunization programs and opposition to nuclear testing after strontium 90 was discovered in milk, and by the expansion of the jurisdiction of pediatricians beyond the early childhood years and into psychosocial areas. Pediatricians' definition of mission is anomalous. As Halpern notes, while most medical fields establish legitimacy by making narrow claims to expertise, early pediatricians "argued that pediatrics was legitimate precisely because it failed to designate a highly restricted arena of professional practice" (1988:54).

failure to plan for the future is regarded as irresponsible. Further, whether the sequence be the life cycle of a person or of a firm, others will be especially concerned that those who control the early parts of a sequence—as neonatologists do for hospitalized infants—feel responsible for the future consequences of present actions. Thus expectations about attention to future consequences are higher in occupations and roles concerned with providing services to children than those focused on the elderly, for instance. Pediatricians are expected to take a longer-term perspective than gerontologists, and teachers are expected to be concerned about preparing students for subsequent stages in the educational process and, ultimately, for adult life, not just about the quality of the classroom experience.[8]

Where there are relatively few rewards for taking a long-term perspective, a variety of mechanisms can strengthen the connection between present and future, reinforcing any naturally occurring incentives to plan. Annual reviews of a person's work make the tie between present performance and career prospects more real and predictable in the present. Planning committees provide some rewards in the present for thinking about the future and coordinate planning so that the schemes of one group do not undermine those of another.[9] Other incentive mechanisms, such as tenure, force people to internalize the long-term consequences of their decisions by forcing them to live with those consequences for the rest of their careers. Rules requiring insurance companies to maintain reserves to cover the losses of their policyholders and regulations about the management of pension funds both place a premium on being able to manage obligations for the future as well as the present.

Many of these mechanisms have counterparts in the NICU. Regular review of mortality and morbidity statistics, collection of information in follow-up clinics, expressions of concern from the hospital legal department about the possibility of malpractice suits, discussion of treatment practices in the light of newly published studies of long-term outcomes, daily review

8. Japanese schools are widely believed to take more responsibility than their American counterparts for launching students into adulthood; nearly half of work-bound graduates find jobs through semiformal contracts between employers and the schools from which they regularly recruit (Rosenbaum and Kariya 1989:1343).

9. Rewards can be arranged so that planners have a personal stake in the adequacy of their planning. When executives are compensated in stock rather than cash, their personal outcomes will vary with how well they have planned for the company's future. No doubt stock options are sometimes simply devices to provide higher incomes for top managers than stockholders would ordinarily approve. The complexity of schemes to encourage "responsibility" may make them especially vulnerable to corruption.

of individual cases in rounds, and evaluation of the performance of house staff, all serve to make staff members aware that they ignore the futures of their patients at their own peril. Parents may nevertheless remain nervous about the commitment of staff members to protecting their infant's futures. True, a variety of reviews and protections exist, but they may not require the medical staff to look very far into the future, and none of them are fully under the control of those who have the largest stake in the infant's future. And that, perhaps, is the central dilemma of planning for the future: all attempts to plan can be foiled not only by the inherent uncertainty of the future but also by the planner's inability to secure the cooperation of others whose contributions are indispensable to success.

Defining Obligations Diffusely

Taking responsibility typically means accepting a broad definition of one's obligations. Whether or not a person has behaved responsibly in performing a particular task depends on what function that task has in achieving some larger goal. The same act may then be praiseworthy or reprehensible depending both on the details of the situation and on whether the occupant of the role has been assigned specific tasks or is to be judged by more diffuse standards (Parsons and Shils 1951). But a steadfast orientation to diffuse standards is hard to motivate and sustain. A central difficulty with getting people to accept diffusely defined obligations is that if rewards are attached to more narrowly defined achievements, attention and effort are easily deflected from ultimate goals. Perhaps because the skills of parenting are well within the reach of most people, and because parenthood is decoupled from the work of other people and only loosely regulated, we ordinarily think of parenthood as immune to most of the perverse effects of incentive systems. But because the parenting of critically ill infants and NICU graduates may require both a substantial expansion of the repertoire of parents and a close coordination of parental activity with the work of medical staff, the question of how narrowly or broadly parents define their role has new significance.

There are strong cultural supports for a diffuse definition of parental roles—"You do what you've got to for your kids." How much care parents supply does seem to vary with how much children need, as we show later, so that the proportion of children's needs met by their parents may be almost the same for mildly and severely affected infants. Nevertheless, we find some variation in how far these assumptions extend. Even when roles are diffusely defined, their boundaries do not extend indefinitely. Often limits are defined by where the obligations of another role begin. As parents follow their responsibility for their children across organizational boundaries, for instance into the NICU, their roles as caretakers of their children overlap significantly with the roles of NICU staff members. The obligations of parents are, then, limited to some extent by where the NICU staff members' roles begin. Parents are not expected, for instance, to provide expert medical care. Likewise, the obligations of motherhood are limited by the assignment of some obligations to fathers, just as in the NICU obligations are divided between adjacent roles, such as doctors and nurses.

A role is composed of core tasks strongly associated with it and a penumbra of tasks more loosely tied to the position.[10] Both the core and the penumbra can shift through negotiation, but role incumbents' sense of their obligations may be resistant to change. For instance, in describing the division of work between themselves and their bosses, personal secretaries talk about "my work, your work, and our work" (Charlton 1983). While some tasks characterize all secretarial positions, others vary with the occupations of employers. While a boss may hope to convince a secretary that a lot of work is "our work," more negotiation will be required about that sphere than about tasks clearly defined as the secretary's. Secretaries who define "our work" and "my work" more liberally will likely be thought more "responsible" by their bosses. Resistance to diffuse definitions of a job will then vary with whether proposed changes lie in the core or the penumbra and will increase the more it seems that an employer (in this example) is attempting to redefine the core by making strategic assignments.[11] A nanny may be quite happy to take on new child-care tasks, such as arranging for a toddler to participate in play groups, which clearly fall

10. The penumbra is analogous to Barnard's (1938) zone of indifference. But while Barnard argues that workers are willing to do anything that falls within the zone of indifference, we argue that there are variations in consent even within that zone. Consent will be more precarious the further a task lies from the core of the job.

11. How workers respond to attempts to redefine their jobs will vary a good deal with the exact circumstance. Some attempts to assign tasks or to set performance standards may be undermined or modified by worker resistance (Burawoy 1979), which in turn may vary with how fairly management plays the incentive game. In other cases, the penumbra will be substantially defined by informal training, and conceptions of responsibilities will then vary with whether or not subgroups (e.g., women or minorities) are systematically excluded from some parts of professional socialization (White 1970). Worker resistance to more diffuse job definitions may then indicate fear of exploitation or variations in conceptions of the job rather than objections to diffusely defined jobs per se. In still other cases, workers may welcome redefinitions of their jobs, seeing such redefinitions as job enlargement or as opportunities for social mobility.

in the core, while resisting assignments that suggest that an employer is trying to turn her into a housekeeper.

NICU parents experience similar conflicts over the redefinition and expansion of parental roles. Were both parental roles going to be expanded, or was the change going to occur in one role only? Did acceptance of new assignments during the hospitalization imply acquiescence to more permanent shifts in the definition of roles? One source of tension within couples, for instance, was over questions about how far fathers' obligations extended beyond providing financial support. Fathers sometimes regarded themselves as having done their share if they provided adequate financial support and thus gave mothers the opportunity to spend more time with a hospitalized infant without worrying about also returning to paid employment. Though mothers were grateful for the flexibility, they sometimes felt that fathers had too quickly concluded that holding down a job was the entirety of the fathers' share. In such extreme circumstances as the hospitalization or illness of an infant, mothers suggested, a father might have to work and help care for the other children, and call medical equipment suppliers, and stay up all night during the weekend to watch the baby when no home nursing was provided. Parents simply cannot divide the work between themselves and assume that this initial division of tasks is carved in stone, mothers suggested. If one parent completes the work initially assigned to him or her and the other is still working (as is usual in these circumstances), there is an obligation to pitch in. Ultimately all of the work belongs to both parents. If motherhood is to be defined diffusely, then fatherhood must be to some degree as well, they insisted. And if the definition of motherhood changes permanently with the birth of a critically ill child, then perhaps fatherhood must undergo a similar transformation.

Mothers and fathers are peers. Together they encounter the unknown terrain of their child's hospitalization and discover how that reshapes their jobs as parents, and together they decide how much of the accommodation will occur in the role of mother and how much in that of father. But the division of tasks is also a division between the household and outsiders. The expansion of parental roles in other directions is somewhat different both because it entails negotiating with experienced role partners and because those role partners often treat parents as members of a category (perhaps with subcategories of mother and father) with whom standardized divisions of labor already exist. Parents differ among themselves, of course, in whether they regard chores assigned to physicians, physical therapists, or nurses as still "their business." Some parents reported that they trusted physicians and nurses and felt little obligation to check on their work. Other parents strongly disagreed, believing that because it was their child whose health was at stake, they had a duty to watch for signs of incompetence or inattentiveness among medical staff members and to confront these professionals if necessary. In addition, though, parents may encounter some resistance from staff members if they attempt to renegotiate the division of tasks between parents, on the one hand, and nurses, physicians, and physical therapists, on the other, or if they define their own role as overseeing the work of seasoned professionals. Following a problem across organizational boundaries is a key component of taking responsibility, but some features of organizations make it more difficult to do this. We discuss the struggles over the boundary between parenting and nursing or doctoring more fully in chapter 6.

Of particular concern to parents is the possibility that staff members will become fixated on the wrong indicators, inappropriately substituting intermediate for ultimate goals and shaping their behavior to produce the intermediate indicators whether or not these are still connected to the final goal. Clear demonstrations of this have been provided in other settings. Drawing on Merton's (1968:253–54) discussion of the displacement of goals, Blau (1963:44–47) showed how instrumental values became terminal values when employment placement workers used official indicators to claim they met organizational goals they had not actually met.[12] Bardach and Kagan (1982) provide innumerable instances of the perverse effects of narrowly focused regulations. In some cases otherwise admirable regulations were enforced in contexts where they were unnecessary or even harmful.[13] In other cases regulatory intervention ultimately led to lower standards than would have been achieved without intervention.[14]

When job descriptions are associated with multiple measures of perfor-

12. Employment placement workers would complete easier interviews in order to meet their monthly quotas, in the process undermining the official priority system for cases. They would also occasionally inflate measures of referrals by including cases in which an employee was merely returning to an earlier placement after an illness.

13. For instance, at a large aluminum plant with a good burn-prevention program, OSHA (Occupational Safety and Health Administration) required workers to wear protective clothing even though such garb increased the risks of heat exhaustion (Bardach and Kagan 1982:87).

14. In response to worker complaints, one large manufacturing firm had decided to install a new ventilation system. But after repeated OSHA inspections (to resolve a subordinate question) showing no violation of standards, the firm decided not to put in the new ventilation system after all (Bardach and Kagan 1982:107–8).

mance, people adjust their behavior to produce activities and outputs that are easily measured. A babysitter whose only obligation is to care for a child will be evaluated by the health, happiness, and development of the child; a babysitter whose duties include housework will be judged at least partly on the cleanliness of the house. Because it is easier to tell whether a house is clean than whether a child is well cared for, the babysitter may concentrate her efforts where her performance can most easily be evaluated. Because observability and importance are not likely to be perfectly correlated, accountability and responsibility may diverge. We must then worry, as Bardach and Kagan suggest, that "everyone will be accountable for everything, but no one will be responsible for anything" (1982:323).

But it is possible to enact flexible rule systems (focusing on terminal values) that do encourage responsibility.[15] Responsibility then arises because there is no fixed standard to hide behind—there are only such ill-defined goals as safety or overall improvements in health, and no authoritative checklist of tasks or standards. When only terminal values are articulated and few rewards are given for the achievement of instrumental goals, goal displacement is less likely to occur. Being responsible means being honest about accomplishment and about the function of any task in the overall system and continually adjusting measures of accomplishment and definitions of tasks to focus attention on core objectives. It means being true to the spirit rather than the letter of the law (or in this case, of the indicator). Assuming a responsibility means only rarely saying "not my job." When parental and NICU staff roles are defined sufficiently diffusely, then, a nurse cannot hide behind "doctor's orders" if she gives the wrong medication, physicians cannot claim success if a baby gains weight but is neurologically impaired, and parents may have to supervise home nurses and feed the baby through a nasogastric tube, as well as cuddling and bathing the baby, if that just happens to be what their child needs.[16]

However parents had conceived their role before the birth of a critically ill infant, they were quite likely to report that they had ended up doing

15. The standard of seaworthiness in marine insurance (Heimer 1985) is one such system. A ship must be seaworthy for a marine insurance contract to hold, but what constitutes seaworthiness varies with the season, the route, and the trade. In addition, insured vessels must be classed and inspected by classification societies, and these professional bodies modify their rules with the accumulation of information from research about safety, with the development of technology, and the like.

16. A nasogastric tube allows an infant to be fed breast milk or formula when the infant, for whatever reason, cannot be fed by mouth. The tube is inserted into the nasal passage, down the esophagus, and into the stomach.

things they had never imagined they would or could do. As parents soon learned, a diffusely defined role may stretch in unpredictable directions. Short of abandoning the baby or defining the tasks as belonging to the other parent or to some professional, a parent had little choice but to perform difficult, unpleasant, or frightening chores.

Using Discretion to Meet Contingency

Responsible adaptation to contingencies requires, first, adapting action and spending the right resources to deal appropriately with the flow of events and, second, deciding who should provide the resources for meeting the contingency. Though they have different causes and effects, the acceptance of responsibility requires that both problems of discretion be solved. These two aspects of adaptation to contingency may shape the experience of responsibility in different ways. For example, women who like the discretion of the housewife role will not necessarily welcome having to care for a sick child in the middle of the night.

Maximizing a utility function or choosing trade-offs between values and interests means doing different things under different circumstances. Taking responsibility thus entails monitoring the relation between output and input more or less continuously, adjusting one's own inputs (time, activity, effort, or attention) and using one's authority over a collectivity's resources to produce whatever result is required. Discretion then involves the right and the capacity to use appropriate means to respond to situational variations.

But others can grant or deny a right to use discretion, and lack of resources can curtail a person's capacity to respond. Access to resources affects the range of responsibilities that can be accepted and influences a person's tendency to think of responsibilities as costs or investments. The experience of taking responsibility is fundamentally shaped by whether a person owns or has authority over substantial resources or can call on others for assistance. Plentiful resources make it possible to be rational in one's own interest and responsible to others' interests or to institutional values.

Parents of critically ill babies are assigned rather limited roles while their infants are in the NICU. Their discretion about a range of matters is expressly limited by hospital staff members. Many of the decisions are simply outside the range of parental competence. Parents may participate in discussions about medical matters, but for the most part it is others who make the decisions. Matters that are ordinarily within the jurisdiction of parents often are not under their control in the NICU. For instance, NICU parents usually are not permitted to make decisions about how, when, or what to feed their babies, though in some instances mothers may be able to decide whether or not their babies will receive their own breast milk.

Medical staff members, in contrast, are given broad discretion. The technology of infant intensive care is relatively new, with the result that the balance between routine and nonroutine treatments is somewhat different than in other areas of medicine. In "frontier medicine," each case is in some sense an "experiment," particularly if the infant is especially premature, has a rare condition, or might be treatable with some new medication or machine. Such "experimentation" requires careful monitoring to calibrate doses appropriately, adjust for unexpected side effects, and determine whether the therapy is effective.

When an infant leaves the hospital, a great deal of discretion must be transferred from hospital staff members to parents or other care providers. Parents must learn how to tell whether the baby "looks sick" and when that means that it needs to be rushed to the emergency room. As much of the routine care is transferred to parents, the flow of children's problems often is a reminder to parents that now they have to use their discretion. They have to decide whether the baby should be awakened for a feeding, whether they should go ahead with a physical therapy session even when the baby has a cold, and so forth. But they also have to make assessments about what works and how to adjust when something isn't working. If the baby refuses to eat, as is common with infants who have had aversive stimulation to the mouth with endotracheal tubes, the parents have to develop strategies for getting enough calories into the baby.[17] The discharge planner at Suburban explained that parents need to master more than medical skills in order to care for their children after discharge. Parents need to learn how to suction their infant's tracheostomy tube, she noted, but they also need to learn when that skill is required (2010DP, p. 13). An attending physician at City Hospital similarly explained that caring for an infant requires more than simply following a care plan: "I think we like to give them [parents] a long-term picture and a global perspective, i.e., it's a whole baby, not just a schedule of medicines" (1001MD, p. 15). Parents must learn, then, how to use discretion. And they are more likely to make adaptations when they do not feel obliged to follow doctors', nurses', and therapists' orders too closely.

The smaller a person's resources or authority, the more the responsibil-

17. An endotracheal tube is inserted through the mouth and into the airway and is used for mechanical ventilation.

ity can be measured by the variability in the person's own inputs. As resources and authority increase, variations in responsibility are reflected in variability in attention, monitoring, and the allocation of other resources under a person's control. If accomplishing some result requires more time, more attention, or some particular performance, then that is the input that must be supplied. But the time commitment, attention, and activity of some subordinate may vary more than the inputs of the superior who holds ultimate responsibility.

Because NICUs are embedded in large, resource-rich organizations, we expect those holding positions of responsibility to adjust to contingencies more by varying the input of others than by varying their own contributions. Thus an attending physician will order physical or respiratory therapy, ask for a consultation from a gastroenterologist, and the charge nurse will vary the amount of nursing time devoted to patients (by adjusting the nurse-patient ratio) depending on how sick they are. In contrast, parents do not stand at the head of a child-care team. Adjustments for emergencies come out of their hides—only very rarely can someone else be called in to stay up all night with a sick baby once the child is home.

Formal responsibility in organizations is generally associated with both a high mean and a high variance in hours of work. But another measure of discretion is whether a worker is considered skilled; skill increases discretion by increasing both a worker's capacity to determine what needs to be done and his or her capacity to do it (Stinchcombe 1990). In contrast, people whose jobs are closely scripted have little discretion to adjust their activity to variations in the situation. As Leidner (1993) shows, the constraint of a script is imposed on McDonald's workers, whose responses to variability are not trusted; the purpose of the script is to curb responsiveness when it might lead to bad results. In NICUs, less skilled workers (e.g., phlebotomists, respiratory therapists) enact fewer routines and also are expected to follow their routines more closely than are more skilled workers (e.g., nurses and physicians). From a medical point of view, parents are the consummate novices. For this reason parents are provided with carefully worked-out routines (e.g., for administering medications or therapies) to follow when they take the baby home and are told to follow them exactly.

But while parents may be unskilled medical workers, they nevertheless must exercise a lot of discretion. They thus face what seem to them conflicting requirements both to use discretion and to limit their use of discretion. Such conflicting demands are not unprecedented and occur for (at least) three reasons. First, even relatively skilled workers may be precluded from taking much responsibility. Bosk (1979) shows how attending surgeons curb the discretion of residents, insisting that they rigidly follow the idiosyncratic preferences (the rough equivalent of medical scripts) of the attending they are working with. Such rules facilitate coordination, of course, but they also reinforce the notion that with ultimate responsibility goes the right to make decisions about how subordinates will perform their duties. Parents face similar requirements to knuckle under and accept limits on their discretion when they must coordinate their work with others and show respect for professional expertise. Although many parents are happy to defer to the greater experience and knowledge of medical staff, others are inclined to question and even resist medical authority.

Second, while organizational rules or scripts that reduce discretion may have the desired effects of increasing uniformity of outcomes and preventing the most flagrant failures to take responsibility, they may also lead to a ritualistic focus on means rather than ends (Merton 1968) and so undermine responsible adjustment to contingency. In hospital settings, ritualistic adjustment to insurance rules may have this sort of effect. Organizations often counter this tendency by arranging an overall assessment of how far the organization has achieved its goals (ignoring for the moment whether it has followed its rules). External examiners, accreditation reviews, site visits, and boards of directors all serve these functions. Parsons (1956) and Stone (1975) both comment on the importance of having a committee with some substantial outside representation to fulfill the function of refocusing attention on ultimate goals. In general, although accountability is increased by having a single individual (e.g., an attending physician) on whom to pin the blame, ultimate responsibility for tradeoffs between values is often lodged in committees composed of representatives of those values (e.g., the Joint Commission on Accreditation of Health Care Organizations, or a medical society). A single individual is too easily seduced into focusing on following rules rather than on achieving vague general goals that take account of the interests of several parties. These two separate types of mechanisms thus institutionalize pressures to use and to limit discretion.

Third, and finally, responsible and effective adjustment cannot be achieved if discretion is lodged in the wrong place. Chandler (1962) shows how the change from a functional to a divisional form at DuPont improved managers' capacity to adapt responsibly to individual product markets. In effect, managers had been adjusting to the wrong things because they did not tie engineering, production, and marketing together in a way that facilitated adjustment to individual product markets. Lodging discretion in the wrong place undermines responsible adjustment by focusing attention and rewards on the wrong things. Similar problems have occurred in NICUs when information about the effects of oxygen therapy were not properly collected and assessed (Silverman 1980) and when the effects of the constant light and noise (necessary to do the work) on the health of infants were not properly evaluated. Workers attend to immediate effects and to getting their work done, but no one has the overall responsibility of finding out what the net effect of such adjustments is and no one has the corresponding authority to undo all of the individual fixes if the net result is destructive. Responsible adjustment requires that discretion be lodged in a variety of places. Neither central control nor radical decentralization alone will result in responsibility.

Fundamentally, all parents must use some discretion when raising children. Parenthood is neither a highly regimented nor a highly regulated role. Interactions with children simply cannot be scripted to the same extent as other interactions, in part because children themselves are unpredictable interaction partners. Discretion, then, is a necessary, but not sufficient, condition of taking responsibility. After all, discretion may be used to maximize one's own interests rather than to take another's interests into account as well. In the sociology of professions literature, for instance, much is made about the danger of discretion (see, e.g., Freidson 1970). When the interests of client and professional clash, what mechanisms ensure that the professional's discretion will not be used in a way that compromises the interests of the client? When interests align, the use of discretion is less problematic. When interests do not align, however, the responsible course of action requires that discretion be used in such a way that the needs and interests of those involved are balanced.

Accepting the Consequences of Contingency and Discretion

While having discretion is important, being willing to accept the consequences is also crucial. In an organization, discretion thus entails having the right to gamble on the company's behalf. A responsible person will "go out on a limb" or "stick his (or her) neck out" rather than "pass the buck" and accepts that his or her own outcome (and even the outcomes of subordinates or family members) depends on the success or failure of the enterprise for which he or she is responsible. The rewards or penalties contingent on success or failure may be small or large—anything from temporary inconvenience, to the fortunes of a business empire, to the lives of people entrusted to one's care. Often the stake is an ill-defined reputation for competence, probity, or reliability; people with a reputation for responsibility are those whom others would want beside them in a crisis.

Although most parents are willing to go out on a limb for their child, parents typically do not regard the acceptance of parental responsibility as an investment in future opportunities.[18] Instead, parents accept responsibility for the child and bear the attendant costs because they have a strong sense that their fates are tied to the welfare of their infants, for better or worse. While they worry about costs to themselves and to other family members, what is really terrifying is the possibility of not providing the right care at the right time in a medical emergency. By the time they left the NICU, most parents were reasonably comfortable giving medications, inserting catheters, doing percussion therapy (pounding on the chest to

18. A partial exception to this rule that parents don't regard taking responsibility as an investment occurs when NICU staff members have doubts about a parent's capacity or commitment to care for a baby. In order to earn the right to take their child home, such parents must abide by contracts (specifying amounts of time to be spent on the unit and tasks to master) between themselves and the staff. Taking limited responsibility, as specified in the contract, during the hospitalization is then an investment that leads to the opportunity to take more responsibility later. (See chapter 5, and Heimer and Staffen 1995.)

In other situations, investment in future opportunities seems to play a crucial role in motivating the acceptance of responsibility. Because rights to assume important, interesting responsibilities are contingent on having met previous obligations, current responsibilities are investments in future responsibilities and authority. In some cases, required investments are very heavy. Coser's (1974) "greedy institutions," for instance, require heavy early investments if a person is to reap the reward of interesting opportunities later. Project work is also greedy, though projects have more limited lives. Kidder (1981), for instance, shows how devoted project members worked around the clock (often with little thought of how their schedules affected their families) to develop a new computer. Though they thrived on the excitement of the work, they also fantasized about the reputational effects of being associated with a fundamental breakthrough. Faulkner (1983) similarly argues that the career prospects of musicians producing musical scores for movie projects depend both on the quality of their music and on the success or failure of the film as a whole and that musicians are keenly aware that everyone listed in the credits gets a reputational payoff if the film is a success. The investments made by musicians producing the score for a film, by young computer scientists developing a new machine, or by entrepreneurs starting a business at least as often lead to failure as success. Sometimes investments nevertheless pay off in skills and experience, though such rewards may not compensate for the association with a box-office flop, a machine design that never went to production, or the loss of personal fortune in a bankrupt business. But because opportunities to accept subsequent responsibilities hinge on willingness to devote oneself to projects at earlier career stages, aspiring musicians and computer scientists must make substantial investments and accept heavy responsibilities even though the odds are usually against them. Parents of NICU babies are similarly constrained to make investments—even when the odds are against them—but for very different reasons.

help dislodge secretions in the lungs and ease breathing), or whatever their child required. They had rehearsed all this. But there was a crucial difference—at home *they* were responsible and would have to cope with any emergencies by themselves. Willingness to confront and accept this gut-wrenching fear was a core part of taking responsibility, and parents accepted the burden because they believed their child would be better off at home.[19]

In interviews, parents repeatedly told us how their lives had changed with the birth of the child, though noting that some of those changes would have occurred with the birth of any child. For some parents, especially those with adequate financial resources, sharing a resource pool with an NICU graduate was not terribly painful. But for others, the consequences were grave—all commitments and interests outside the home, including work, had to be abandoned, career plans had to be deferred, and friendships were sacrificed. Some of these changes led to substantial shifts in identity—one man had to give up bodybuilding (2024), another couple had done martial arts together but could no longer afford the time away from the children (2015). Other changes were positive, and parents glowed as they told about their new career plans, their heightened sense of competence given the evidence that they could care for a child with medical and developmental problems, and their pride that they had gotten through the rough period in a responsible and humane way.

Though most parents would initially have described the price they paid as a "cost," after the fact many said that they had reaped unexpected benefits. The benefits were not enough to make them glad that they had had to go through a child's hospitalization, to be sure, but they were often substantial enough for parents to feel that they had come out the other side better, more mature, and more competent people. In these circumstances,

19. To some degree, this terror about whether one would be able to cope in a medical emergency is simply an intensified version of what all parents face. And, of course, some NICU parents conclude that they are not up to it, either abandoning the child to the care of the other parent, relinquishing custody of the child, or retaining custody but placing the child in a long-term-care facility.

Anxiety about the consequential nature of responsibility is not limited to parents, of course. One recently promoted secretary one of us interviewed, for instance, found her new responsibilities as personnel manager too burdensome because others' fates hinged on her activities; she had carried out the same activities with equanimity when her supervisor bore ultimate responsibility. Others are apparently pleased at the consequential nature of their acts and report that their jobs are satisfying because of the responsibility they have. Reports of promotion are often described as "the usual increases in *responsibility* and pay" (emphasis added) (Heimer 1984).

when costs ultimately led to benefits, parents commented on their experiences with less bitterness, and though no parent we interviewed wished the child had never been born (and selective refusals of interviews by less committed parents, especially fathers of out-of-wedlock babies, are surely important to the sample result here), many felt enriched rather than impoverished by having tied their fate to their critically ill infant. It is hard to know how to think about this—outside observers might argue that parents have simply constructed rationalizations for their behavior and might not agree that it was so clearly "all worth it."

The five dimensions that differentiate more responsible from less responsible behavior are also the dimensions around which accusations of irresponsibility and rewards for taking responsibility are organized. We have suggested how each of these dimensions renders responsible behavior problematic and what incentives and institutional arrangements increase the likelihood that people will take responsibility. This cursory look at how we might distinguish responsible from irresponsible parenting now needs to be fleshed out with an account of how actual people meet the challenges of parenthood, particularly when parenting has turned out to be especially challenging.

Who Takes Responsibility? Portraits of Seven NICU Graduates and Their Families

The parents we interviewed faced burdens that covered a wide range. At one extreme were parents whose dreams had become reality: Their children were essentially healthy and normal, and they had weathered the initial crisis. And at the other extreme were parents whose worst fears had been realized: Their children continued to suffer from disability and disease, and their lives were forever changed. Such parents also had a variety of reactions to the burdens they faced. Some parents embraced their responsibility, no matter what the magnitude, but others simply rejected it. Here, we provide portraits of seven former NICU patients and their parents, illustrating the range of variation we find in our interviews along these two dimensions: how onerous the responsibility is and how much responsibility the parents assume.

We begin with Isaiah and Gregory, who represent our first category: those children who are relatively healthy and whose parents embrace their responsibility. Isaiah was quite healthy at the time of our interview, and his mother Sarah in many ways represents the model of responsible parent. Gregory was also doing quite well at the time of our interview and had quite responsible parents, but his illness had created a great deal of tension between his parents, as sometimes occurred between other parents. Not every child is as well as these two, however, and not every parent is as committed or as competent. Robert and Lily, whom we describe next, provide a contrast to Isaiah and Gregory on both fronts and represent our second category: those children who are still very ill and whose parents limit or reject their responsibility. But not every parent of a sick child is quite as resigned to their child's condition as Robert's and Lily's parents are, however. Our third category includes those parents who have quite sick children but are also quite responsible. Jason's parents, Cindy and John, and Tammy's parents, Grace and Roger, illustrate that sometimes even very large burdens are shouldered admirably. We conclude by describing Stephanie and her son, Jayjay, who illustrate our fourth category: those children who are relatively healthy but whose parents nonetheless assume very little responsibility. Table 3.1 provides quick portraits of our seven families and may be used as a guide for the rest of the chapter.

Isaiah (1002) was a normal, healthy toddler when we interviewed his mother, Sarah. Interviewing her in the cafeteria of a downtown college campus, however, made watching Isaiah a chore. Sarah had suggested we meet there because she wanted to visit her thirteen-year-old daughter, who was attending a week-long summer academic program for gifted children. What is interesting about Isaiah's case is that although Isaiah was "normal," his mother was extraordinary.

When Isaiah went home from the hospital, it was to join a large, working-class African-American household. In the seven years between her fifth child and Isaiah's birth, Sarah had finished her bachelor's degree and been employed as a clerical worker. Isaiah's father (who declined to be interviewed) worked full-time in construction, and his mother had been home full-time managing the household since his birth. Sarah described her anxiety when she took Isaiah for a routine visit to the pediatrician a week after his birth only to learn that he was severely dehydrated and needed to be rehospitalized. Sarah noted that she had not had much of an appetite following the baby's birth and speculated that her supply of breast milk had probably been adversely affected. Isaiah ended up at City Hospital, where his medical course was rather uneventful. With some IVs and supplementary feedings, he recovered quickly, and tests uncovered no deeper problem.

But a child's hospitalization is never uneventful for the family, particularly not when there are five other school-aged children and the hospital is

Table 3.1 Seven NICU graduates and their families (grouped according to the magnitude of the burden and how much responsibility the parents assume)

	Smaller Burden: Initial Crisis/ Child with Few to Some Ongoing Problems	Larger Burden: Initial Crisis/ Child with Many Ongoing Problems
Less responsible	1024: Stephanie/JayJay—single mother, African-American/abdominal surgery, healthy	1018: Gloria/Mike/Robert—parents not married, Caucasian/spina bifida, hydrocephalus, quite delayed
		2001: Vicky/Steve/Lily—parents not married, Caucasian/premature, respiratory problems, somewhat delayed
More responsible	1002: Sarah/Isaiah—parents married, African-American/dehydration, healthy	1001: Cindy/John/Jason—parents not married, Caucasian/genitourinary surgery, surgery still needed
	2012: Laura/Greg/Gregory—parents married, Caucasian/premature, respiratory problems, some delay	2016: Grace/Roger/Tammy—parents married, Caucasian/spina bifida, multiple congenital anomalies, surgery still needed

several hours away by public transportation. Sarah spent most of Isaiah's ten-day hospitalization at his bedside, staying in the parent room and going home only rarely to make sure that the rest of the family was managing without her. By the time of Isaiah's birth, Sarah's older children had learned to supervise and assist the younger ones, and they pitched in during the crisis. Sarah described how she managed to juggle the demands of all of her children, for instance when five children all had parent-teacher conferences at the same time or when there were too many school plays and athletic events for her to see them all. Sarah was not simply the mother of all these children, but she was also the very effective manager of the household, contributing her own efforts when necessary but substituting the children's own labor when appropriate.

Isaiah, because he was the child who needed it, got a lot of maternal attention during his hospitalization. Sarah believed it was important for her to visit the NICU, both because she felt she should check on the care her son was receiving and because she believed Isaiah needed her there. She had read that babies recover more quickly when their parents are close to them, and she believed there were indications he responded to her presence. In support of this view, she noted how Isaiah had "refused" to go to sleep when she planned to go home for a bit when he went down for a nap. Because he had been home for awhile before his hospitalization at City, Sarah felt that Isaiah was already firmly attached to her and would miss her if she were absent.

Such attentiveness to the children's responses and needs characterized Sarah's relations with all of her children. Sarah described differences among the children in loving detail, illustrating her unusual blend of protectiveness and advocacy, on the one hand, and respect for autonomy, on the other. It was Sarah who had located the class her academically gifted daughter was attending, for instance, and who had persuaded the child's reluctant father that it really was okay for her to spend several weeks at a downtown college campus. But Sarah was now there to reassure herself that the stimulating program did not come at the cost of her daughter's safety.

Though Isaiah showed no signs of his early illness, it seemed clear that Sarah would have risen to the occasion had he been more seriously ill. Nevertheless, Isaiah's case is extremely important in illustrating that a lushly developed set of parental routines and a fully articulated set of principles about parenting can emerge without the stimulus of a sick or disabled child. Some parents may become responsible when faced with a challenge, but others are responsible whether faced with an unusual challenge or not.

Many of our families fit the model just described: mothers who provide most of the day-to-day care for their children and fathers who "pitch in" with child care, but are primarily breadwinners. Though much has changed over the last few decades, much has also stayed the same. Fathers may be doing more than their own fathers, but many mothers are also doing more than their own mothers—combining paid employment outside the home with child care and household responsibilities.

While most of the couples we interviewed were sanguine about the division of labor in their households, others were considerably less so. Several described marital strain following the birth of a sick infant. Some separated for brief periods, at least one couple divorced, and another planned to. Though Laura and Greg (2012) managed to keep their family intact, it was not without great effort. A white, married, two-income couple who were buying a home, Laura and Greg wanted very much to have children. Gregory was born by emergency C-section at just twenty-eight weeks gestation after Laura was stricken with preeclampsia (a condition in pregnancy that causes dangerously elevated blood pressure and edema, or swelling). He was hospitalized for three months and was sent home with oxygen and an apnea monitor (a device that displays the infant's heart rate and respirations and sounds an alarm if either one becomes too high or too low). Laura had returned to work while Gregory was still in the hospital so she would be able to stay home with him after discharge. Trusting only herself to care for her sick son, Laura extended her leave from her job at a local hospital for three months while he grew and was eventually weaned from the supplemental oxygen. Greg was working as an apprentice learning a trade and was unable to take time off during Gregory's hospitalization and continued recovery at home.

Though Gregory was doing well at the time of our interview, Laura still had some concerns about his physical development and was seeking a consultation with a physical therapist. Gregory's right-sided weakness, she noted bitterly, would never have been noticed by her husband. She described Greg as being afraid of the baby when he was first sent home and seemed so small and fragile. This initial reluctance soon developed into a pattern: "He got used to not doing anything" (2012F, p. 21). And by the time of our interview, Laura was filled with resentment that their son was her responsibility. Though she had returned to work, it was she who coordinated Gregory's medical care, took time off from work to take him to the doctor, sought physical therapy consultations, and the like. Greg would help, if asked, but Laura wished he would take more responsibility. When asked about the division of responsibility for Gregory, Greg admitted he could probably do more, but he showed no awareness of the anger his wife revealed.

Though there was more harmony in Isaiah's home (at least according to Sarah's account), both Gregory and Isaiah were paired with committed and competent mothers, and they were both quite healthy at the time of our interview. Robert (1018), in contrast, was not doing what a normal eighteen-month-old should at the time we interviewed his mother. Born with spina bifida (a spinal cord defect) and hydrocephalus (an accumulation of fluid in the brain), he was paralyzed below the waist. Not only was he unable to walk, but he was also unable to turn over or even to sit up. Although his mother, Gloria, described Robert as being very strong, our observation was that he was too weak to hold a bottle by himself. He did manage to feed himself, as was demonstrated to us, but only when his bottle was propped up against a pillow. Though seriously developmentally delayed, Robert was described by his "aunt" and part-time caretaker (his mother's brother's live-in girlfriend) as an "easy" baby because he didn't move around much and so caused little trouble. Robert's cognitive development also was not what it should have been for his age, though this serious delay might have been partly due to an infection (following the malfunction of the shunt that drained fluid from his brain) that occurred shortly before our interview. Before the malfunction he had been babbling, his parents reported, but he had become largely silent since then.

Robert lived with his twenty-year-old white mother and two half-siblings, a four-year-old brother and three-year-old sister. In addition, his mother's seventeen-year-old stepbrother and his sixteen-year old girlfriend shared the apartment. Robert's parents had been living together at the time he was born, but Robert's father, Mike, was now reunited with his ex-wife and their three children. Gloria had never been employed and had dropped out of high school when her first child was born. She had been happy to have a child, she said, because she then had a family—her parents had not been at home much, and she had felt lonely as an adolescent. Gloria supported her children with public aid and Robert's disability payments, and occasional gifts and loans from her stepfather. Mike was employed, but contributed little to Robert's support, a pattern strongly disapproved by both Gloria and Mike's ex-wife.

Our information about Robert's situation comes from interviews with both parents, from our observations during the interview with Gloria, and from Robert's medical record. Not all of the information is fully consistent. Each of Robert's parents gave more glowing assessments of his or her own parenting and harsher assessments of the other parent's contribution. Gloria, for instance, described herself as spending nearly all of her time caring for her children, though Mike reported that she frequently went out, leaving Robert and his siblings in the care of the sixteen-year-old "aunt." Not that this was so bad, Mike hastened to add, given that the aunt was probably at least as competent and loving as Gloria. Further, he complained, Gloria had done little to get the help that Robert needs. His own employer suggested that they take Robert to the local Shriners' hospital, which they have since done, and so the child's condition may improve.

But Mike was rather clearly not deeply invested in his son's progress. He seemed to think that it was entirely possible that Robert would be fine in the long run. When asked what he thought Robert would be like at age fifteen or twenty, Mike answered vaguely: "Really I couldn't say, cause I don't know. I haven't seen him for awhile now, so I couldn't tell. From the last time I talked to Gloria she said that all the doctor's going to do is put braces on his legs and they're going to straighten him out. He might just turn out to be normal. I don't know" (1018M, p. 7). At another point he commented: "To me he [Robert] seems normal, I mean all but his legs and the shunt that's in his head. Other than that he seems normal to me" (1018M, p. 38). He didn't know even approximately the schedule of visits to Robert's various doctors, didn't know whether Robert got physical therapy, believed that the final outcome would depend entirely on what the doctors could do and not at all on what he did, and though he claimed he would "never abandon Robert," he also believed he would lose contact with him if Gloria were to move farther away.

Ironically, Mike's ex-wife was pressing him to take his paternal obligations to Robert more seriously. She urged that they care for Robert regularly and believed that Mike should have his name put on the birth certificate so that his access to his son would depend less on Gloria's goodwill. Mike seemed not to have understood that her proposal would do a lot to solve the problem of his losing contact with Robert if Gloria relocated. Mike's brief against Gloria also included suggestions that she misused "Robert's" money, spending it on rent and other things that benefited her and the other children rather than Robert exclusively. He also complained that she asked him to buy diapers when there were still diapers "sitting right there" (1018M, p. 35). Citing his mother as an authoritative source, Mike suggested (repeatedly) that Robert's spina bifida was perhaps caused by Gloria's behavior—allegedly the "tight clothes" Gloria wore during her pregnancy made it hard for the baby to move and explained why he was "all hunched up" at birth (1018M, pp.12, 17, 30–31). During our interview, Mike had little to say about Robert himself or about his relationship with his son.

Gloria was more resigned than accusing in her discussion of Mike's neglect of Robert (and her).[20] She presented herself as a woman who wanted

20. Interestingly, Gloria gave Mike some of the blame for Robert's health problems. Shortly after his first discharge from City Hospital, Robert had to be rehospitalized for pneumonia. But, Gloria noted, this was not surprising given that "all of his [Mike's] kids ended up with pneumonia when they got home from the hospital" (1018F, p. 7).

children—perhaps even another one eventually—and would like to work in a preschool someday. She clearly saw the children, all of whom have different fathers, as her responsibility rather than their fathers'. Yes, it would be nice if a father contributed in some way, but one shouldn't count on that. "Women don't need men," she asserted. "That's all there is to it! We don't need 'em. I mean, I'm doing a lot better off by myself now without Robert's father than I was doing *with* him" (1018F, p. 33). By her report, Mike "cannot handle his son's problem. He cannot handle it. He doesn't, he just, you know, blocks it out completely" (1018F, p. 16). Gloria saw it as her job to keep the children fed and clothed, to keep a roof over their heads, and to take them to the doctor when necessary. And she clearly had preferences about where to get medical care. Though she had to use part of her rent money to pay the $47 cab fare, Gloria took Robert to City Hospital when his shunt malfunctioned rather than have him treated at a nearby hospital where she believed the care would be inferior. Since Gloria barely made ends meet between her social security and welfare payments and had no money set aside for emergencies, she flatly admitted that had Robert gotten sick after the rent had been paid, she would have had no choice but to take him to the local hospital.

Despite some indications that Gloria put the children's needs first, the children seemed more like they were Gloria's roommates than her charges. Though she did what she could for them, Gloria didn't arrange her life so that she could do more. She didn't try to expand the household economic resources, find ways to ensure that the children would always be able to get the medical care they needed, or learn about what she or anyone else could do to increase the likelihood that Robert would lead a normal life. Her understanding of child development was quite superficial. Though she had learned how to assess the functioning of the shunt (which she claimed to do faithfully three times a day) and how to tell if her child was ill, she seemed not to have understood how spina bifida might affect Robert's development. This poor understanding also showed up in her comments about the other children. She noted that one of them had speech problems but didn't seem to think that she should be doing anything about it. Although Robert was behind on his shots and was not enrolled in a program to stimulate his development, this could not be attributed entirely to his mother's ignorance. Gloria admitted that Robert's doctors at Shriners' had lectured her on these subjects, but she was waiting for the zero-to-three program to get back in touch with her rather than pursuing this option more aggressively (p. 16). She explained that she loved her kids and talked movingly about worrying about how Robert would interpret his father's abandonment of him: "When Robert gets older, what's Robert gonna think? 'Daddy leave me 'cause,' you know, 'I can't walk' or 'I'm crippled' or 'I'm a freak.' You know, I think for Robert right now I just shouldn't think that way. Because, you know, [I should] just tell Robert, 'Your father was no good.' [laughs] It's not easy to sit there and tell your kid why [his] father is not around" (p. 26). But Gloria also sometimes had trouble taking care of their needs "outside the home, such as doctors—things like that I'm not very good at" (p. 52). Gloria's life was far from easy—each month she faced the problem of stretching her meager income to cover the family expenses. But because she defined Robert's problems either as temporary and self-rectifying, as problems to be solved by doctors rather than by her, or as conditions that could not be corrected or even ameliorated, the job of parenting Robert was far less burdensome than it might otherwise have been.

Though Lily (2001) was considerably less developmentally delayed than Robert, her future was still far from certain. Like Gloria, Lily's mother Vicky was young, white, unmarried, and struggling to make ends meet. Estranged from the father of her two young children and recently divorced from another man, Vicky had moved in with Steve several months before our interview. Though Steve didn't mind that Vicky had children of her own, he told us he was still getting used to the idea of having an instant family. They shared expenses, but the children, she explained, were largely her responsibility.

Vicky's pregnancy with Lily was plagued with complications right from the beginning. This was an unplanned pregnancy she was ambivalent about carrying. Vicky began to bleed early in the pregnancy and was eventually hospitalized until the delivery. Six weeks after being admitted, Vicky delivered Lily at just twenty-nine weeks' gestation, eleven weeks premature. Lily required mechanical ventilation and suffered a bleed in her brain while on the ventilator but after two months was discharged from the hospital with a monitor, medications for a heart problem, and instructions to have her followed closely by the physicians at Suburban Hospital. Since her discharge, her mother reported she had been rehospitalized several times with bouts of pneumonia. Though her heart problems had resolved by the time of our interview, she was still moderately developmentally delayed—beginning to talk and walk quite late—and required nebulizer treatments for asthma.

Though Vicky expressed concern about Lily's health problems and developmental delays in our interview, she often failed to follow through to ensure that Lily was receiving appropriate medical care. She didn't pursue a referral to a physical therapist, though she admitted to being worried about her daughter being "slow," so Lily never received the extra stimulation that might have improved her motor skills. Though Vicky said she worried quite a bit, she also seemed to believe there was nothing she could do that would improve Lily's outcome. When Lily was discharged home, Vicky was scared and overwhelmed. She admitted having trouble learning how to use the apnea monitor. She frequently mispositioned the sensors and got several false alarms, but rather than ask for more instruction, she simply stopped using it. Though Lily was rehospitalized a number of times because her prematurity made her prone to pneumonia, Vicky didn't have either a regular pediatrician or medical insurance. Vicky had gotten off public aid and begun to work part-time. Her earnings, combined with Steve's, rendered them ineligible for medical benefits. For the seven months before our interview, all of Lily's medical care had been received at the local emergency room.

Both Gloria and Vicky provide adequate homes for their children: they provide shelter and food and somehow manage to stretch the meager household resources to make ends meet. However, they also seem quite resigned to their children's medical difficulties. They furthermore seem not to have much of an orientation to the future or an idea of how their actions may help shape that future. Even when faced with quite heavy burdens, however, not all of our parents view their roles this way. Jason's parents, John and Cindy (1001), are also white, young, and unmarried. However, their similarities with Gloria and Vicky end there.

Jason was born with severe bladder and urinary tract problems, necessitating numerous surgeries. Early repairs led to further problems, including blockages of the urethra by scar tissue. The blockage was misdiagnosed as a simple urinary tract infection. Had Cindy not been alert and suspicious, more serious complications, such as kidney damage, could have ensued. Repairs to excretory systems are particularly problematic because of the delicacy of the muscular and nervous system control over the bowels and bladder. In addition, for males repairs to the urinary system raise questions about future sexual functioning and about aesthetic matters such as the appearance of the genitalia and the disruption of the growth of pubic hair. By the time we interviewed John and Cindy, Jason was a toddler, developing normally in most respects, but facing unusual uncertainty over potty training, since it was still unclear whether repairs to his ureter would work as intended. The uncertainty was particularly difficult for his parents, who were repeatedly told by physicians that an entire course of surgeries could not be mapped out since each subsequent stage depended on how successful the previous surgery had been.

The period just after Jason's birth was especially difficult. The shock of discovering that he was "not normal" coincided with transfers from one hospital to another as several physicians declared themselves incapable of repairing the damage. Cindy described how unprepared they were for the birth of a sick child: "We were ready for this child in every sense, but we just weren't ready to deal with any more than having a child. You know, there is having a child, and having a child with *problems*" (p. 35). But they quickly adjusted. Cindy got herself discharged almost immediately and then began following her baby from one hospital nursery to the next. John's employer did not give him much time off work, so Cindy faced this ordeal mostly alone. When Jason was admitted to City Hospital, several hundred miles from home, Cindy arranged to stay nearby. With the help of a national charitable organization that gave her a room while her son was ill, she was able to see Jason every day. Cindy's older sister, Diana, took care of Timmy, Jason's older brother, though Timmy made it dramatically clear that he felt abandoned and unloved when his mother more or less disappeared from his life. To compound the difficulties, Cindy was herself ill during this early period, experiencing debilitating headaches. Though she was given a variety of drugs to reduce the headache pain, she ultimately concluded that she couldn't take the drugs because they made her too drowsy to care for the kids. The headaches eventually went away, perhaps because the stress and sleeplessness of the early days after Jason's birth gave way to a more routine existence. Jason came home from City Hospital, doctor visits became less frequent, trips to the specialty hospital were also less frequent, and Jason began to sleep more than forty-five minutes at a time.

To say that Jason consumed more than his share of the family resources is an understatement. John and Cindy were poor and struggling but doing their very best for their children. Jason was Cindy's second child. She had been a troubled adolescent, responding to a move and her own mother's illness and death (from multiple sclerosis) by dropping out of school, abusing alcohol, and becoming pregnant at sixteen. A friend, not the baby's father, convinced her to marry him to "give the baby a name," but the marriage never worked and the couple divorced after a few years. Cindy later began seeing John, but they had a stormy relationship and she had moved to another state to live with an aunt while she sorted her life out. In the meantime, Cindy's sister, Diana, a crucial stabilizing influence in her life, was keeping Cindy's son, Timmy. Timmy was to join Cindy only after she provided strong evidence, in the form of savings, that she had gotten herself on track. Cindy was working two jobs in order to accumulate savings more quickly. It was during this time that she discovered she was pregnant.

The pregnancy was a turning point both in Cindy's life and in her relationship with John. John, who had been visiting Timmy regularly and telephoning him nightly in Cindy's absence, was thrilled about the pregnancy and immediately began stocking up on baby supplies. Cindy reported a variety of changes in them as individuals, in their relationship, and in her child-rearing and household management. Cindy and John had not married—John especially saw no advantage to a legal tie—but regarded themselves as committed to each other and to the children. Cindy continued to receive some public assistance and was especially concerned that they eventually have health insurance. John had a steady working-class job and was taking classes that would enable him to get a better one. Cindy was unwilling to leave the children in someone else's care at the time of our interviews but had been equipping their house so that she could expand her babysitting jobs. Family assistance had been very important to Cindy and John. They lived in a house rented from a relative. When they accumulated sufficient savings, they would be able to purchase the house. Cindy's sister and her husband were considerably more financially secure than John and Cindy, and they gave the children generous gifts as well as contributing to savings accounts in their names.

Diana's assistance had been important in other ways as well. She and her husband both worked in medicine and had guided Cindy's search for information and medical expertise. Where most high-school dropouts would not venture to the medical library, Cindy had sought medical journals for information about her son's condition and state-of-the-art therapies. While Diana's encouragement had been important here, Cindy's spunk and John's steadiness were crucial as well. Cindy learned the skills of advocating for her child, confronting the medical team when necessary, and making judgments about when local hospitals could provide treatment and when she needed to draw on the resources of City Hospital, several hundred miles away. Here, we see that despite many difficulties, Cindy was able to learn how to become an effective participant in a foreign organization.

John and Cindy's concern about Jason's medical problems needs to be examined in the context of their parenting style. Cindy talked movingly about what kind of a parent she used to be and how she has been transformed, rather abruptly coming to grips with the seriousness of her responsibility for her children: "I grew up when I had Timmy. It helped me grow up a little bit. But I *really* grew up when I had Jason" (p. 23).[21] She talked not only about what they need now but was intensely concerned about their futures. During John's interview, Cindy and John talked about which of them could better understand the difficulties Jason might face in a locker room as an adolescent. John insisted that no woman could understand this; Cindy insisted that a mother could empathize with essentially any trouble her child must face. Cognizant of the differences among family members, Cindy tried to find resources to provide what each needed. For a while she stocked up on the foods Jason could eat, reasoning that the rest of them could get by on whatever was around, but that he had to have special foods. Timmy had some speech problems and was often difficult for others to understand, but Medicaid would not cover a speech therapist for him. Cindy tried to scrimp to cover that herself. Recognizing how dropping out of school limited their own employment opportunities, John and Cindy had begun saving for their children's college educations and insisted that their boys would go to college.

While she regarded herself as an adequate parent before, Cindy was now an unusually attentive and thoughtful one, and proud of it. One important indicator of their pride: John and Cindy had half hoped that we would use their actual names in our writing. Though they were sensitive to the dilemma of exposing Jason to the gaze of the world, they also felt that they had done a superb job.

While John and Cindy still face some uncertainty about Jason's long-term prognosis, Tammy's parents, Grace and Roger (2016), faced the kind of ongoing uncertainty that makes planning for the future—for instance, thinking about college—seem like a fantasy. After two years of nearly constant medical intervention and repeated surgeries, their daughter Tammy's health was still quite precarious at the time of our interviews with them, requiring great sacrifices from her family to provide the care she needed.

21. In her book on the meaning of motherhood in women's lives, McMahon (1995) finds that motherhood transforms all women's lives, but it transforms them in different ways. Working-class women like Cindy are more likely to report that having children made them feel more grown-up, whereas middle-class women are more likely to report that having children made them feel more fulfilled.

Tammy's case was quite complicated. She was born with a long list of congenital anomalies, some of which could be repaired with surgeries, others she would have to try to live with. Her parents first learned that their daughter was not developing normally when a routine ultrasound revealed at least three abnormalities affecting her heart, her bladder, and her abdomen. Her parents were nevertheless relieved when further tests indicated no signs of Down's syndrome or spina bifida. Grace and Roger briefly considered terminating the pregnancy. They had three older children at home to consider. But they decided against it. Since then, Grace especially has often wondered whether she should have spared Tammy the pain of repeated surgeries and hospitalizations. Hindsight did not lead them to conclude that they had made a mistake. They both still believed they wouldn't have made any other choice given the information they had at the time.

Tammy's situation was worse than her parents had feared. When she was examined after birth, three congenital anomalies turned out to be fourteen. She required immediate surgery and had undergone countless surgical interventions since. Only after several weeks in the hospital and months of follow-up care did Tammy's parents learn that she had spina bifida, after all. In the mass of medical details these parents were trying to comprehend, the term "myelomeningocele" was lost on them. Grace understood that Tammy had a lesion on her back, but did not understand that this was commonly known as spina bifida. To medical specialists, the difference between a myelocele (spina bifida in which the neural tissue of the spinal cord is exposed) and myelomeningocele (spina bifida in which the neural tissue and the membranes that envelop the spinal cord protrude from the spinal column forming a sac under the skin) is an important distinction. To the parents, however, what mattered was that their child had spina bifida. Spina bifida was something these parents could understand. And it was also something they thought they had escaped.

Tammy's condition tested the skills of even the best physicians. Taken singly, her health problems were manageable, and even correctable. However, in combination they presented a challenge that her physicians regarded as unprecedented. But Tammy's parents were undaunted. Rather than throw their arms in the air and surrender when faced with physicians who said they had done all they could, these parents searched for other solutions. They became experts in their daughter's health. Though Grace was "scared to death" (2016F, p. 24) at taking Tammy home from the hospital the first time, both she and Roger learned to care for her ileostomy and to change the dressings on her surgical wounds.[22] They rose to the challenge of complicated home-care routines (later including frequent bladder catheterizations), became proficient at detecting the earliest signs of infection and illness, and became advocates for their daughter when she was hospitalized (as we describe in more detail in chapter 6). Roger and Grace firmly believed they could not leave others to worry about Tammy's medical problems; instead they felt they had to fight for her. Grace was fired from her job as a nurse's assistant when she left work for six weeks during one of Tammy's hospitalizations, showing how difficult it is to balance multiple responsibilities. If Tammy needed her, she was there. Though the family has suffered financially, and even moved into a smaller house to save money, they always insisted on the best care for Tammy. When a physician at Suburban Hospital suggested he didn't have the skill to correct one of Tammy's more complicated problems, Grace and Tammy flew several hundred miles to see one of the nation's top pediatric specialists, and she underwent the surgery there.

Just as Cindy and John were transformed by their child's illness, so too were Grace and Roger. Before Tammy's birth, Grace claimed, she didn't think of herself as an advocate for her children and didn't believe their outcomes were especially contingent on what she did for them. After Tammy's birth, however, she learned to use tremendous discretion and developed into a fierce advocate. But the family had been transformed in other ways, as well. The older children in this family were feeling the neglect that follows when parental resources are simply stretched too thin. Because Tammy demanded so much of the family's resources—including time, money, and attention—there was little left for the other children. Roger especially talked at length about how their eight-year-old son had suffered and how they worried about his delinquent activities. Although they had gotten medical help for him and enrolled him in a program at the police station, they remained very concerned. What would become of a boy who is breaking the law at his young age? his father wondered: "All the kids suffer, but he needs medical help that we can't give him. Maybe one day, if we can keep him out of trouble long enough, he'll either outgrow it or

22. An ileostomy is the surgical formation of an artificial anus by connecting the ileum to an opening in the abdominal wall. Because the ileum is one of the lower parts of the small intestine, an ileostomy is located higher on the torso than a colostomy, which forms an artificial anus by connecting the colon to an opening in the abdominal wall. In both cases, feces collect in a specially designed plastic bag which is changed as necessary.

we can deal with it" (2016M, p. 33). Tammy was getting a disproportionate share of the family's resources because she needed them. For her, it was literally a matter of life and death. But when resources are stretched thin, as in this case, being responsible to Tammy's needs meant being less responsive to other family members'.

While some parents seem acutely aware of what their children need and make great sacrifices to provide it, others seem much less oriented to thinking about their children's welfare. Surely not every parent would have risen to the challenge faced by Grace and Roger. Many would have been unable or unwilling to master the medical details, travel great distances and spend days on end living in the hospital at their child's bedside, or learn to care for their child at home. Extraordinary burdens are just that—extraordinary. However, even when not faced with extraordinary burdens, some parents demonstrate little capacity to take their children's welfare seriously, to think about and plan for their children's futures, to conceive of their role as parents broadly, and to set goals and use their discretion to meet them.

Stephanie (1024), like Gloria, Vicky, and Cindy, started having children when she was just a teenager. The first of her four boys was born when she was just sixteen, and she dropped out of high school shortly after becoming pregnant. When we interviewed her, Stephanie lived in a multigenerational African-American household with her maternal grandmother, her mother, her mother's sister, and several of their children (some of whom, like Stephanie, had children of their own). Stephanie and her family lived in the midst of urban poverty, crime, and blight in a dark, crowded home that seemed to have been neglected for many years. Employment opportunities were few for a young woman like Stephanie, and she had only been employed once since leaving high school in the tenth grade, and then only briefly. She worked as a cashier at a small grocery but was fired after a short time for reasons that were unclear. She attempted to get her GED (General Equivalency Diploma), but was unsuccessful and has never searched for other employment.

In this large, extended, welfare-dependent household, Stephanie's grandmother provided much of the stability. She cleaned the house and looked after the scores of small children, leaving the other adults more or less free to come and go as they pleased. Stephanie was openly ambivalent about her children. Even though her grandmother provided much of their care, she flatly admitted to times when she wished she hadn't had them. When asked what she would like to do, she answered simply, travel. She fantasized, like many parents, about being able to just pick up and go. Her feelings of confinement were especially acute following the birth of her first child, when she resented not being able to be "on the street" with her friends: "I couldn't do this and I couldn't do that because I had a baby. I was gettin' depressed" (1024F, p. 16). Her depression eventually led her to some involvement with drugs and a suicide attempt, after which her grandmother assumed much of the responsibility for her children.

Just before she became pregnant with Jayjay, Stephanie had an abortion. She didn't want to have any more children, she said, but her boyfriend at the time told her having an abortion was pointless because she was sure to get pregnant again. She did become pregnant again, just as he predicted, but their relationship deteriorated by the time Jayjay was born. Jayjay's father didn't attend the birth or visit Jayjay in the hospital and provided only intermittent financial help in the form of occasional small gifts. He visited Jayjay episodically but did not play a prominent role in the child's life, and Stephanie had contact with him only rarely. Though Jayjay's paternal grandmother expressed some interest in seeing Jayjay and having a part in his life, Stephanie resisted. Without much elaboration, she declared that she simply didn't want any of his family to have contact with her baby.

At the time of our interview, Jayjay was a seemingly happy, healthy toddler. He had round cheeks and smiled at us frequently during the interview. In spite of his mother's repeated attempts to shoo him away, he stuck nearby throughout our visit. He lifted his shirt and showed us the scar on his abdomen, the only visible sign that he had been ill. Stephanie recalled her devastation when she learned the results of a routine ultrasound at seven months' gestation. The ultrasound indicated that the baby's intestines were protruding through a hole in the abdominal wall and that he would need surgery immediately after birth. She considered giving the baby up for adoption, saying that she just "couldn't deal with it if he were handicapped" (p. 9). However, she gives credit to her grandmother for convincing her to keep the baby. As it turned out, his stay at City Hospital was relatively brief, and he recovered well from his surgery.

By her own account, Stephanie was overwhelmed by the responsibilities of parenthood and unprepared for them. When describing Jayjay's illness, she mainly talked in terms of how her life would be affected if he were sick rather than what it would mean to him. Rather than describe his pain, she described hers. She gave very little thought to planning for the future. For her, the future was something that just happened (like getting pregnant even when a child was unwanted), not something one planned. In her own words, "You never know what the future's gonna be like. You might not live to see tomorrow, so you gotta live by day-to-day" (1024F, p. 25). She had a fairly narrow conception of her role as parent, letting others, especially her grandmother, provide much of the day-to-day care and nurturing. Rather than see her role as doing whatever was necessary, she admitted, "I didn't wanna have nothin' to do with no handicapped baby" (p. 3). In many ways, Stephanie was still a child herself. Though she did manage to take Jayjay to the doctor and to keep appointments with the follow-up clinic, Jayjay was getting adequate, even if not exemplary, care largely because of the efforts of others.

Though Stephanie is low on our scale of responsibility, it is important to note that she has managed to ensure that Jayjay is cared for, even if she is not the one providing most of the care. Other parents, like Jayjay's father, take no responsibility even for finding suitable alternative care providers. Unfortunately, as we have already noted, we had great difficulty contacting such absentee parents and getting them to consent to be interviewed. Robert's father, Mike, is rare in this regard. Of the nine biological fathers who did not reside with the mothers of their children, only two consented to be interviewed.[23] Stephanie, Vicky, and Gloria, while far from models of responsibility, are all doing far more than the biological fathers of their children.

We have discussed responsibility as a general category here, but it is important to remember that paternal and maternal responsibility are really quite different. As we emphasized in chapter 1, gender is a strategic resource. Maternal obligations are less often shed than paternal ones. Capturing the sentiments of many women, one mother explained that while she had "never once" felt that she had a choice about whether to take on the burden of caring for her son, she believed that her husband had: "He had a choice. . . . If he couldn't handle it, then he'd walk" (1036F, p. 74).

23. The levels of involvement of these nine fathers varied a good bit. Three fathers (1024, 2001, and 2021) had little or no contact with the child. In three other cases (1018, 1019, and 1031), the child had some contact with the father, but the mother had no expectation of support or assistance beyond an occasional gift. Finally, three of the mothers (1014, 1032, 2023) could expect some financial help from the baby's father as well as some help with child care, and the child sometimes spent the night in the father's home. Of these nine mothers, one was living with another man, and one anticipated that she would eventually be reunited with her child's father after his release from prison.

We stress that these are only rough indicators of levels of paternal contribution, and that it is important to remember that there are equally important variations, both in parental contributions and in the stability of the parents' relationship, among the forty families in which the parents were living together at the time of the interview.

But maternal and paternal obligations differ in other important respects as well. Even when paternal obligations are not shed, they often differ in content from maternal obligations. In many of our intact families, fathers defined their role in the family as breadwinner, even if both parents worked outside the home, and restricted their participation in other parenting activities.[24] Together, parents may constitute a very responsible pair, but each contributes something different. In the next section, we explain how we categorized each parent we interviewed on our scale of responsibility, we will explore the differences between parents who faced "normal" burdens and those who faced far more onerous responsibilities, and we will present further evidence on the differences between mothers and fathers.

Who Takes Responsibility? Rating the Parents We Interviewed

The seven portraits above give a good indication of the wealth of information we uncovered in our interviews. Though the parents we interviewed all thought of themselves as good parents, what it meant to be a "good parent" varied quite a lot. In parenthood, the minimum standard is set and enforced largely by the state, and that standard is quite low. Here, we see that parents sometimes exceed the minimum standard by a great deal, but at other times just barely manage to meet it, and occasionally even fail to meet it. Our first task, then, is to describe in some detail what indicators we used to categorize parents on the five dimensions we discussed above. After providing an explicit definition of what it means to be responsible, we then present several tables that summarize our findings by grouping the parents we interviewed according to how much responsibility they accept and how needy their children are.[25]

We began with the five dimensions discussed above. Responsible parenting requires, first, taking account of the child's interests as well as one's own; second, thinking about and planning for the child's future; third, defining one's obligations with respect to the child broadly; fourth, using

24. While Coltrane (1996) argues that fathers in intact families have become more involved in the domestic sphere over the past three decades, and even suggests that this trend is likely to continue, Hochschild's "second shift" (1989) still belongs primarily to women. Walzer (1996) argues that women do a disproportionate share of the "mental labor" in the home, including worrying, processing information, and managing the division of labor, as well.

25. We interviewed eighty-six parents in eighty-three interviews. Eighty parents were interviewed separately; six parents were interviewed jointly. Of the parents we interviewed separately, forty-six were women and thirty-four were men. Two of these interviews (one mother, one father) did not contain enough information to code the parents on all five dimensions of responsibility.

discretion to adjust to the child's needs; and finally, being willing to accept that one's own welfare is contingent, varying with what proportion of the family resources has been consumed by the more pressing needs of others. Each parent interview was read in its entirety, and then we scored the parents as either low, medium, or high (0, 1, or 2, respectively) on each of these dimensions, taking into account the full context of the interview and the information we had collected from the medical record. We also averaged the parents' scores on the five dimensions to create a summary variable (also ranging from 0 to 2) capturing the parents' overall orientations to their obligations. The mean on this summary variable is 1.25, indicating that most of the parents accept an intermediate level of responsibility. Women score somewhat higher than men, although the average for both remains within an intermediate range (mean score of 1.36 for forty-five women; mean score of 1.14 for thirty-three men). This summary measure is strongly correlated with our more impressionistic global assessments from reading the interview as a unit. As we reread our interviews, we coded parents as "not very responsible," "somewhat responsible," and "extremely responsible." The Pearson correlation of this global assessment with the average of the five items described above is .849. Finally, we categorized parents according to how the responsibility of caring for their child compared with caring for a normal, healthy infant or toddler. For some the burden was about the same, for others a bit heavier than usual, and for still others the burden was very heavy. The mean scores on these variables are presented in Table 3.2. Below we describe more fully how we coded the interviews.

Taking Account of the Child's Interests

Our first measure is an assessment of the extent to which the parent shows concern for the child's welfare. Analytically, there are two separate parts to this. We ask whether the parent thinks of the child as a full human being. We also consider whether, once the parent realizes that the child has needs and wants, can experience pain and pleasure and the like, he or she is willing to try to meet those needs. In practice, of course, these two components are often conflated. Parents were rated "low" if they showed little or no empathy with the child's experience and had difficulty even identifying, let alone meeting, the child's needs. Mike (1018) is an example of a parent who rated low in this category. In the interview he spent very little time discussing Robert but instead focused on how his own life had been altered. In contrast, parents were rated "high" if they identified so strongly with their child's interests that those interests became essentially their own.

TABLE 3.2 Percentage of parents who accept low, medium, and high degrees of responsibility and whose children have few, minor, and serious sequelae following discharge from the NICU

Parental acceptance of responsibility[a]	Percentage of Parents Who Score			
	Low	Medium	High	Mean Score (0–2)
Dimension (defined by high end)				
Concerned with child's welfare	5	23	71	1.68
Has long-term orientation	22	46	30	1.09
Defines parental obligations diffusely	20	42	35	1.17
Uses discretion to adjust means to ends	30	36	31	1.04
Accepts contingency and interdependence	19	31	47	1.29
Summary measure of responsibility (mean of individual items)	11	42	45	1.25 (SD = .57)
Magnitude of burden to be assumed[b]	Percentage of Parents Whose Child Has			
	Few or No Sequelae	Minor Sequelae	Serious Sequelae	Mean Score (0–2)
Current level of impairment of child	54	19	26	.75 (SD = .85)

Note: Based on data from 83 interviews with 86 parents (49 mothers, 37 fathers). Three interviews were joint (one interview for two parents). Eighty interviews were individual (46 mothers, 34 fathers). Note that 34 *children* are counted twice because we have two interviews for the child (one with the mother, one with the father) and have coded each parent for this table. Percentages do not sum to 100 in some rows because of missing data. Two interviews (one mother, one father) did not contain enough information to code the parents on all of the dimensions.

[a] Verbal codes were assigned numerical equivalents on a scale from 0 to 2. A very occasional parent was given an intermediate value (.5 or 1.5). These intermediate values were retained for purposes of computing means, but not for forming the main categories of this table. Thus, $0 \leq \text{low} \leq .5$, $.5 < \text{medium} \leq 1.5$, and $1.5 < \text{high} \leq 2$. "Low," "medium," and "high," correspond to "limited," "intermediate," and "very responsible," respectively, in Table 3.3.

[b] The categories for magnitude of burden correspond exactly to the three categories used in Tables 3.3 and 3.4, although the labels there are "initial crisis/well baby," "initial crisis/some consequences," and "initial crisis/continuing problems."

Parents, like Cindy (1001), who modified their behavior because they identified so strongly with their child's suffering and pain are included here. In the intermediate category, then, are parents who provided some commentary on their child's experience and needs but were not so empathetic that they experienced the child's needs or pain as their own. Parents who note that the child has needs, but don't seem to feel that obliges them to do anything in particular, would fall into this category.

Of the parents we interviewed, about 5% showed relatively little concern with the child's welfare and were coded "low" on this variable. Another 23% expressed a moderate degree of concern for the child's welfare, and 71% were coded "high" because they expressed a great deal of concern with the child's well-being. The mean score on this variable is 1.68 (on a scale that runs from 0 to 2), somewhat higher than the mean on the other items. Mothers scored slightly higher than fathers on this dimension. For the forty-five mothers for whom we have data on this, the mean score was 1.74; the mean score for the thirty-four fathers was 1.59. Most parents, then, are quite concerned with their child's well-being whether or not they manage to act on this concern.

Planning for the Future

We are also interested in whether a parent seems to be oriented to the future. Of course, thinking only about the future can be just as irresponsible as focusing only on today. But connecting present actions to future outcomes, and adjusting those actions as necessary, is one hallmark of responsibility. Parents were rated "low" if they gave very little thought to the future or if their plans for the future seemed unrealistic, with little understanding of the intervening steps required to make them reality. Stephanie (1024) fell into the low category on this variable. She explained that she wasn't oriented to the future, because in her experience the future was quite uncertain, not something to plan for but rather something to watch unfold. Sarah (1002), on the other hand, was quite oriented to the future. She talked at length about how to ensure that her children had educational opportunities and about how, after Isaiah was in school, she herself planned to return to school to get a master's degree to increase her own job opportunities. Parents like Sarah who seemed to be thinking fairly concretely about what their child's current situation implies for what the family will be able to do in the future were rated "high" in this category. The intermediate category included those parents who either had only some plans for the future or whose plans seemed somewhat detached from their current situation.

As Table 3.2 shows, about 22% of parents were concerned mostly with the present and devoted little attention to planning for the child's future. About half of the parents (46%) were coded "medium" on this variable because, though quite grounded in the present, they nevertheless were making some plans for the future. The last 30% of parents were actively engaged in planning for their child's future, thinking carefully about the long-term consequences of whatever decisions they were now making. The mean score on this variable is 1.09, indicating that while most parents do spend some time thinking about the future, we could not say that they are carefully planning or that they weigh future consequences very heavily when making decisions. Again, the forty-five mothers for whom we have data scored slightly higher (1.17) than the thirty-three fathers (1.06) on this dimension.

Defining Obligations Broadly

With this variable, we attempt to capture whether parents have a narrow or a diffuse sense of their obligations to their children. Parents may think of their obligations as being fundamentally about providing shelter, warmth, and food and then protecting their children from disasters as they grow up. Or they may think of parenthood as providing what an individual child needs to help it flourish—whatever that may be. Parents, like Gloria (1018), rated "low" on this variable by defining their obligations narrowly. Rather than try to master the "outside stuff," as Gloria called it, she left those details to others or simply left tasks undone. These parents provide basic, more or less standardized care that is not much tailored to the child's individual needs and takes little account of variations between children.[26] Parents with a broad conception of parenting, in contrast, are willing to master the medical details even if they find them difficult. Even though

26. Alternative school movements, including especially the individualist branch of the home-school movement richly described by Stevens (1996), argue that because there is no such thing as an "average" child, it is inappropriate to construct educational systems that cater to the average child. For some, the answer is to take children out of formal educational systems and school them at home, where appropriate adjustments for individual variations can be made more easily. From that perspective, it is ironic to find that some parents raise their children with little regard for individual differences. Standardized educational and parenting practices may be more common in institutionalized settings, but they are clearly not restricted only to those sites. Pressures for standardization occur elsewhere as well.

Grace (2016) was at first repelled by her daughter's ileostomy and was scared to take her home from the hospital, she learned to change Tammy's bag and eventually mastered far more complex medical details to ensure that her daughter was receiving the best possible care. Parents rated "high" when their repertoire of activities and skills expanded with their children's needs. In the intermediate category are parents who demonstrate some flexibility in their definition of parenthood, expanding their role to include some tasks but not others or only taking on the tasks that are assigned to them.

Roughly 20% of the parents we interviewed defined their obligations to their child quite narrowly as providing financial support, food and shelter, and some help growing up; 42% showed some limited flexibility in how they defined their roles; and 35% had very broad conceptions of parenthood as providing whatever care their child needed. The average parent has a score of 1.17 (on a scale from 0 to 2) on this variable, indicating some willingness to adjust notions of parenthood in the light of a child's special needs. Mothers defined their roles somewhat more broadly than fathers (mean score for forty-five mothers, 1.29; mean score for thirty-three fathers, 1.02). As we will see below, it is on this dimension that parents whose children are really ill are most different from those whose children were essentially normal by the time of our interviews. Having a critically ill infant, especially one whose illness strongly shapes the child's future, requires a parent to do a lot of rethinking about what parenthood entails.

Using Discretion to Adjust Means to Ends

Parents vary in how actively they monitor their child's progress and intervene to reach desired outcomes. The variation we are trying to capture has two parts, because those who have not at least implicitly formulated goals have no standard by which to assess their child's progress or the appropriateness of their own intervention. We are interested, first, in whether parents have goals for their children. If parents do have goals for their children, then, second, we are interested in whether they evaluate their children's progress toward those goals and make needed adjustments along the way to increase the chance of reaching the goal. In some senses, this dimension and the previous one are nested. A parent who doesn't feel that he or she has to adjust inputs for variations between children is not likely to believe that he or she has to watch carefully to see whether the inputs are producing the desired result. But this is a matter of degree. Even parents who have a narrower conception of parenthood still have some sense that inputs have to vary—not all children eat the same amount, nap for similar lengths of time, or have the same temperament. Parenting requires at least some use of discretion. What we are interested in capturing, then, is the difference between people who rather rigidly follow routines (especially when those routines are developed by others, like doctors or therapists) and those who try to understand what the routine is supposed to accomplish, look for evidence of whether it seems to be working, and modify the routine when the evidence suggests it isn't.

Parents rated "low" in this category because, like Mike (1018), they seemed to have no goals for their child or because, like Gloria (1018) and Stephanie (1024), they seemed to make very little connection between their own actions and what happened to the child. Parents rated "high," in contrast, if they had very clear goals for their child, demonstrated a good understanding of developmental milestones and the role of intervention in assisting a child's progress, and had a sense that they should monitor the child to see whether current therapies and other interventions were effective. Grace and Roger (2016) used a tremendous amount of discretion in managing their daughter's chronic illnesses. Not convinced that their daughter would receive the best possible care if they always deferred to the medical authorities, they became astute observers of her condition and intervened when they thought an adjustment in her treatment was necessary. Other parents fell in the intermediate category: they only occasionally adapted routines to produce better results, they did relatively little adjusting but seemed to have some sense that intervention might be appropriate, or they continued to monitor the effectiveness of interventions even if they felt powerless to modify routines established by "experts."

Among the parents we interviewed, roughly a third (30%) fell into the "low" group because they either had no particular goals for their child or adapted their activities very little in order to achieve those goals they had. Another 31% were categorized as "high" on this variable because they had well-articulated ideas about what their child should be able to accomplish, monitored the child's progress, and either intervened with health-care providers or made modifications of their own routines to increase the chances of the outcome they thought appropriate. Finally, 36% of parents fell into an intermediate category either because they had less fully articulated views on what should be happening or because they were unable for a variety of reasons to intervene effectively or to modify their own routines in appropriate ways. The mean score on use of discretion is 1.04, squarely at the midpoint, suggesting, we believe, the difficulty of adapting means to ends in these complicated situations. Gender differences were quite large here, with the forty-five mothers scoring 1.20, and the thirty-three fathers .88.

Accepting the Contingency of One's Own Welfare

The core of what we are interested in here is the extent to which parents feel that the welfare of each family member is interdependent. That is, do parents feel that the total family's welfare (including their own) must be balanced according to what each family member needs? Initially, we conceived this as a measure of the parents' willingness to defer their own plans or gratification while they dealt with the crisis of a sick baby. For many of our parents, however, the crisis was relatively brief and plans didn't have to be put on hold for long. And for other parents, there wasn't a big conflict between meeting the baby's needs and carrying on with the rest of their lives, because the parents were neither deeply invested in their careers nor passionately consumed with hobbies, clubs, or volunteer work that took them outside the home. There is still some variation among parents on this dimension, but it is subtler than we had expected.

We rated parents "low" in this category if they either displayed no sense that adjusting their own lives or delaying their own plans might be appropriate or if they gave no indication that the welfare of one family member depended on what the other family members needed. Though Stephanie (1024) had no career to defer, she did have an active social life, and she described her difficulty accepting that her life had to change when she became a mother. Gloria (1018) also rated "low" here. She did not describe how to balance her children's needs with her own but instead glossed over the differences between them, presenting her life as having changed relatively little, because she treated Robert just as she would any other child. In contrast, both Cindy (1001) and Roger (2016) described in moving detail how difficult it was to try to balance the needs of each of their children. Both families had made sacrifices and adjusted their lives with the addition of a sick child (though the sacrifices were greater for Grace and Roger). Parents like these rated "high" when they demonstrated a clear recognition that every family member's welfare was contingent and that sacrifices were sometimes necessary. In the intermediate category were parents who believed that some adjustments and deferrals were necessary but that sacrifices would be made by others before they would make them themselves. Here we included parents who, for instance, believed the spouse's career, friendships, and interests could be sacrificed while their own should be protected, or who said that their willingness to make sacrifices for their children had limits.

About 19% of the parents we interviewed felt little need to adjust their own plans and dreams to take account of a child, apparently believing that little accommodation was needed for a child who had a very rocky start. Most parents, however, felt that some adjustment was necessary. For 31% of parents, these accommodations were rather limited, perhaps because sacrifices were made by others (other children or the other parent) first. Finally, we categorized 47% of parents as falling into the high category, because they very clearly expressed their sense of the interdependence of family members and showed their willingness to defer cherished plans and to accept sacrifices so that they could meet their critically ill child's needs. The average score on this variable was 1.29, indicating that most parents saw some need to make substantial sacrifices and adjustments. Mothers were more likely than fathers to believe that they had to make changes in their lives to adapt to their child's needs (mean score for forty-five mothers, 1.41; for thirty-three fathers, 1.12). In many cases, though, parents had few plans to defer and few outside interests to drop or hoped that someone else (e.g., a spouse) would do a disproportionate share of the adjusting.

Measuring the Burden

Finally, we noted how heavy the responsibility of caring for a particular child was compared with caring for a normal, healthy newborn. Taking into account the parents' descriptions of what their children required, the information gathered from the infants' medical records, and our observations during the interviews, we categorized the parents in three groups. In the "low" category are parents of children like Isaiah (1002) and Jayjay (1024). These children were very ill during the initial crisis but went home requiring essentially normal newborn care. In the "intermediate" category are parents of children like Gregory (2012) and Lily (2001). The initial crisis was not resolved by the time they were discharged home, and their health has been somewhat precarious since their discharge. Gregory was discharged home requiring oxygen, and though he was weaned from the oxygen successfully, he still required some physical therapy and was prone to lung problems at the time of our interview. Lily had been briefly rehospitalized several times for pneumonia and was slightly developmentally delayed. In the "high" category are parents of children like Robert (1018),

Jason (1001), and Tammy (2016), who experienced both an initial trauma and many serious sequelae, some of which were life-threatening.[27] Included here are children with spina bifida or hydrocephalus (like Robert), children with serious gastrointestinal or genitourinary defects (like Tammy or Jason), children with serious mobility problems, ventilator-dependent children, and any others who were seriously ill.

About half of the parents (54%) we interviewed had children with only minor continuing problems. This is not to say that the hospitalization wasn't a traumatic experience, only that the baby was essentially a "well baby" by the time of discharge or at least by the time of our interview a year or more later. For these parents, the responsibility of caring for their NICU graduate was not substantially greater than the responsibility a parent ordinarily accepted in having a child. For another 19% of the parents, the responsibility was intermediate, because although their child had some continuing problems, they were neither life-threatening nor of the sort that required repeated medical interventions. For 26% of the parents, though, medical and developmental problems continued more or less unabated after the child's discharge from the NICU. In these cases, the magnitude of the burden parents faced was well above that faced by ordinary parents. Among the children of the parents we interviewed, the average level of impairment was .70 on a scale ranging from 0 (essentially normal, or small burden) to 2 (continuing serious problems, or heavy burden), indicating that most parents in this group faced some (though usually not substantial) burdens beyond those faced by typical parents.[28]

On average, the mothers we interviewed had healthier children than did the fathers we interviewed (mean scores of .75 for forty-six mothers and .82 for thirty-four fathers).[29] We hasten to add that this gender difference does not arise from differences in how the parents talked about their children but instead from somewhat different routes into our interview group. When parents are not married or co-residing, the medical record (our source of information about how to locate parents) only very rarely con-

27. We use the word *sequelae* here because it includes both consequences of medical treatments and events or conditions that are merely further developments or manifestations that flow from the baby's premature birth, illness, or congenital condition. Thus sequelae would include both the vision problems that are sometimes a result of oxygen therapy and developmental delays or cerebral palsy, for example, that are further developments not directly "caused" by anything done in the NICU.

28. Each child was counted only once for this calculation (N = 49).

29. Recall that we interviewed all of the mothers of these children but were only able to interview a subset of their fathers.

tains information sufficient to locate fathers. We therefore had to ask mothers for help in soliciting the participation of fathers in our study. Because mothers with very needy children had more reason to maintain ties with their babies' fathers, they were typically more able and willing to help us contact fathers as well.

Is Level of Parental Responsibility Explained Simply by the Magnitude of the Burden?

In some senses our measure of the magnitude of the burden to be assumed is an indicator of how hard it is to take up the responsibility of raising and responding to the special needs of a particular child. Thus, one could argue that the cost of being concerned with a child's welfare is lower when the child is a healthy baby who needs mainly to be cuddled and loved than when the child is repeatedly subjected to painful surgeries. One can easily imagine that a parent might become detached in one way or another from a child whose health continued to be precarious. The parent might either deny that the child was experiencing pain (or asserting, as pediatricians and neonatologists long did, that the child would not remember the pain in any case) or decrease contact with the child so as not to be confronted with the graphic evidence of the child's suffering. Similarly, it is less costly to plan a future that can be expected to follow a normal path than to worry about the very uncertain consequences of newly developed medical treatments.

It is costlier for a parent to define obligations expansively when that means regularly taking the midnight shift with a ventilator-dependent child than when it means staying up an occasional night with a sick, but usually healthy, child. It is more difficult to adjust means to ends when the parent has to master the rudiments of physical therapy or modify techniques for the insertion of a catheter than to find out what tricks work for potty training a healthy two-year-old. And of course it is quite a different matter to defer career plans to stay home for a couple of years with a young child than to defer dreams indefinitely to care for a seriously compromised infant facing a very uncertain future.

To put it somewhat differently, the standard economic assumption is that parents would be reluctant to "pay" more for the "same good." Under this assumption, we would expect that as a given level of responsibility became harder to achieve—or "cost" more to achieve—fewer parents would attain that level. Parents of "normal" children should then look more responsible than those of children who continued to need a lot of

TABLE 3.3 Percentage of parents accepting responsibility for children by variations in the magnitude of the burden (N in parentheses)

	How Large is the Burden?[a]							
How Much Responsibility Do Parents Accept[b]	Initial Crisis/ Well Baby		Initial Crisis/ Some Consequences		Initial Crisis/ Continuing Problems		Total	
Limited acceptance of responsibility	7	(3)	19	(3)	14	(3)	11	(9)
Intermediate	58	(26)	38	(6)	14	(3)	42	(35)
Very responsible	33	(15)	38	(6)	73	(16)	45	(37)
Missing	2	(1)	6	(1)	0		2	(2)
Total	100	(45)	101	(16)	101	(22)	100	(83)
Column percentages	54		19		26			

Note: Based on data from 83 interviews with 86 parents (49 mothers, 37 fathers). Three interviews were joint (one interview with two parents). Eighty interviews were individual (46 mothers, 34 fathers). Note that 34 *children* are counted twice because we have two interviews for the child (one with the mother, one with the father) and have coded each parent for this table. Percentages do not sum to 100 in some rows because of missing data. Two interviews (one mother, one father) did not contain enough information to code the parents on all of the dimensions.

[a] The categories for magnitude of burden correspond exactly to the three categories used in Table 3.2, although the labels there are "few or no sequelae," "minor sequelae," and "serious sequelae."

[b] Acceptance of responsibility is a mean of assessments on five dimensions. "Limited," "intermediate," and "very responsible" correspond to "low," "medium," and "high," respectively, in Table 3.2.

assistance and sacrifice from their parents. But our evidence suggests that parents don't think of their children as they do other goods.

In Tables 3.3 and 3.4, we provide evidence about how the level of responsibility assumed by parents is related to the burden parents face. Once again it is important to remember that the parents we interviewed were on the whole quite a responsible lot—presumably those who were less inclined to accept responsibility for their unusually needy children refused to be interviewed. We believe that such self-selection has little bearing on the differences between the parents that we report in these tables, though. Self-selection should raise all of the mean scores on the responsibility items but should not disproportionately affect one or another category of parents. Table 3.3 shows what percentage of parents with essentially well babies, babies with some continuing medical problems, or babies with serious continuing difficulties take on only limited responsibility, accept intermediate levels of responsibility, or act very responsibly. Rather clearly, there is no simple relationship between the magnitude of the burden the parents face and how responsible they are. That is, one is not necessarily "more

Table 3.4 Mean responsibility scores for parents of children with different degrees of impairment

	How Large Is the Burden[a]		
	Initial Crisis/ Well Baby (N = 44)	Initial Crisis/ Some Consequences (N = 15)	Initial Crisis/ Continuing Problems (N = 22)
Dimension (defined by high end)			
Welfare	1.65	1.56	1.82
Long-term	1.08	1.00	1.18
Diffuse	1.02	1.07	1.52
Discretion	.92	1.03	1.27
Contingency	1.20	1.20	1.59
Summary measure of responsibility mean of individual items	1.17	1.18	1.46

Note: Based on data from 83 interviews with 86 parents (49 mothers, 37 fathers). Three interviews were joint (one interview with two parents). Eighty interviews were individual (46 mothers, 34 fathers). Note that 34 *children* are counted twice because we have two interviews for the child (one with the mother, one with the father) and have coded each parent for this table. Percentages do not sum to 100 in some rows because of missing data. Two interviews (one mother, one father) did not contain enough information to code the parents on all of the dimensions.

[a]The categories for magnitude of burden correspond exactly to the three catgories used in Tables 3.2, although the labels there are "few or no sequelae," "minor sequelae," and "serious sequelae."

responsible" when facing a lighter burden or, conversely, "less responsible" when facing a more onerous one. If anything, parents facing a larger burden are somewhat more likely to act very responsibly. While 33% of parents facing a relatively light burden (because their child had become essentially a well baby) act very responsibly and 38% of those facing an intermediate burden (because their child continued to experience some medical or developmental problems), fully 73% of those facing a heavy burden (because their child had continuing difficulties of a serious nature) act very responsibly.

Table 3.4 again categorizes parents by the magnitude of the burden they face, but this time shows the mean responsibility levels (by individual dimensions and for the average of the five items) for each of the three groups of parents. This table suggests that there may be some modest tendency for parents faced with heavier burdens to take their responsibilities more seriously. On the average, the parents of "well babies" take less responsibility (with a mean summary score of 1.17) than those whose children continue to have serious problems (whose mean summary score is 1.46). We find some evidence, then, that parents, rather than assume a constant responsibility, not only adjust their contributions to the demands but in fact do more the greater the burden is.

Interestingly, these differences between parents whose children are relatively healthy and those whose children remain quite ill are only a bit larger than the differences between mothers and fathers. Fathers' mean scores are all very close to the mean scores for parents of healthier children (although fathers that we interviewed on the average had slightly sicker children, as we noted above), whereas mothers' mean scores are closer to the scores of parents with the sickest children (although mothers on average had healthier children, as we noted above).

We hesitate to make too much of any of these quantitative results both because of the relatively small size of our sample and because we suspect that we are better at seeing evidence of a responsible orientation when it has had a chance to blossom than when it exists only in nascent form. Thus, for instance, parents facing a heavy burden are more often required to use discretion than those who have essentially normal children. Despite our attempts to ask questions in a way that would elicit statements about the use of discretion even when less discretion was needed, we may not have compensated fully for differences in people's situations. An alternative explanation, though, is that parents' understandings of what is involved in parenting changed when the shock of having a critically ill infant was followed by the realization that their child would continue to have serious problems. According to this interpretation, the higher mean scores of parents faced with heavy burdens are a reflection of their changing (and more responsible) orientations to parenthood.

Conclusion

We argue in this book that parents are not all equal and that some parents shirk their obligations to their children while others throw themselves heart and soul into meeting their needs. The mission of this book is to account for these variations by showing how they arise and how such variations in orientations and levels of contribution are rewarded or punished, supported or undermined. As a first step in such an undertaking, it is crucial to demonstrate both that the alleged variations exist and that they can be measured with some reliability.

Our dependent variable, taking responsibility, is morally charged, and that makes the task of this chapter particularly difficult. We have no wish to join forces with those who believe that children should always be cared for by their biological parents because blood ties are inviolable, nor with those who believe that any parent, whether biological or adoptive, is always better than a shelter or foster home, nor with those who believe that poor, young, or badly educated parents are always suspect. Instead, we are arguing for a careful investigation of what is entailed in accepting responsibility for a child, a nuanced view of variations in the extent to which people take responsibility and a fuller examination of the role of such larger entities as families, formal organizations, and government bodies in fostering and sustaining individual responsibility.

We began the chapter by elaborating our definition of responsibility. We identified five dimensions of responsibility: taking account of others' interests, planning for the future, defining obligations diffusely, using discretion, and coping with whatever contingencies arise. And we argued that these five dimensions can be used to understand two different types of variation. The first type is between roles. That is, some roles require more responsibility than others. The second type is between occupants of roles. That is, occupants of the same role may assume more or less of the responsibility associated with their role. In seeking to understand variations in parental responsibility, we are focusing on this second type of variation in responsibility between occupants of the same role. Though our focus is on the NICU, we believe our definition of responsibility to be a general one that should apply equally well to other empirical settings. Though many roles may require one or more of these dimensions of responsibility, more responsible roles are identified by simultaneously requiring all five dimensions. Similarly, more responsible individuals are those who simultaneously take others' interests seriously, take a long-range view, define their obligations broadly, use discretion to adjust means to ends, and accept the contingent nature of their obligations.

Having developed the theoretical apparatus for understanding responsibility, we then moved on to a systematic analysis of variations in the acceptance of responsibility among the parents we interviewed whose children had been hospitalized in the NICU. We rated the parents we interviewed along the five dimensions of responsibility, noting that they varied both in the magnitude of the burden they faced and in how responsible they were. We have four main findings we wish to highlight. First, we found that there is significant variation in the amount of responsibility parents assume and that this variation can be measured systematically. Second, women were on average more responsible than men. And, third, the larger the magnitude of the burden parents faced, the more responsible they were likely to be. These last two findings together suggest that while part of taking responsibility is undoubtedly linked to persistent cultural notions about gender, another part of taking responsibility is emergent, demonstrating that many parents use their agency to meet unexpected contingencies as they arise. And finally, we found that some parts of taking responsibility are more difficult than others. As our empirical analysis shows, while most parents took their child's needs seriously, far fewer of them demonstrated that they used their discretion to adjust means to ends. Attachment to their child is not the stumbling block for assuming responsibility for most parents. The stumbling block is translating that attachment into meaningful action on the child's behalf.

Now that we have fleshed out our definition of responsibility, we turn our attention, first in chapter 4, to the tools that parents and hospital staff have at their disposal both to take responsibility and to induce others to do their part. And we follow this with a detailed analysis in chapters 5 and 6 of what it means to take responsibility in the organizational context of the NICU. What parents and medical staff regard as the responsible course of action will not always coincide. Attempts at social control are made by each party to induce the other to behave in what each regards as appropriate. But parents vary both in how much scrutiny they receive from NICU staff and in how closely they in turn scrutinize the care their infants receive in the NICU. As we will argue, parents' experiences in the NICU are shaped in part by how long their infants are hospitalized. Parents whose babies are quite sick are more likely both to become objects of social control in the NICU and to engage in social control efforts of their own.

Furthermore, when we examine social control in the NICU in chapter 5, we find that some parents who are "responsible" may still find themselves or their behavior labeled "inappropriate" by the NICU staff.[30] Most of the parents we rated as "responsible" would be similarly regarded by the NICU staff (though the staff don't explicitly use the five criteria outlined above in making their evaluations). However, otherwise responsible parents may be labeled "inappropriate" because the NICU staff is concerned not just with the parents' competence to care for their infants after discharge but also with how well the parents fit into the organizational rou-

30. The infants whose parents we interviewed were in the NICU before our observations in the two units began. We, therefore, don't have both interviews and field observations for the same parents and infants. We do, however, find a great deal of congruence between our observations and parents' accounts in interviews. For more on this and other issues related to our research methods, readers may wish to consult the Appendix on Methods.

tines of the NICU. For instance, by defining their obligations broadly, parents may overstep the rather limited role defined for them by the NICU staff. Of course, parents who don't visit or ask questions or take an interest in learning about their infants' illnesses and what care will be required at discharge will be more likely than other parents to become objects of social control in the NICU. But our point remains the same: social control decisions by the staff in the NICU depend on their organizationally driven definition of responsibility. So both parents who would be rated as very responsible along our five dimensions and those who would be rated as quite irresponsible are likely to be the objects of social control in the NICU, though for different reasons. The former parents may become objects of social control for violating norms about how parents should fit into the organization of the NICU and the latter for violating norms of adequate parenting. Parents, then, receive instruction about what it means to take responsibility for their infants in the NICU, but this instruction is geared to the requirements of life in the NICU, and what is required after leaving this organization may be something quite different indeed.

Parents also vary in how likely they are to be agents of social control in the NICU, monitoring, evaluating, and intervening in the activities of the staff. Here we find that those parents who define their obligations broadly, for instance, are more likely to believe that their role as parent in the NICU includes overseeing the care their infants receive. In short, responsible parents are very likely to become agents of social control in the NICU—visiting often, asking questions, educating themselves about their infants' illnesses, monitoring the care their infants receive, and intervening when they feel it's necessary. And parents who have a narrow definition of their role, who believe that everything will be taken care of by somebody else more expert than they, will be far less likely to become agents of social control in the NICU. Part of the variation we observe in whether parents view themselves as social control agents is due to the individual characteristics of the parents. Those parents who are unable to visit, are poorly educated, and have little experience with large bureaucracies will find it more difficult to navigate in this strange world of high-tech medicine. However, part of the variation we observe is due to the characteristics of the organization. Organizations vary in how easy or difficult they are for outsiders to penetrate. As we will show in chapter 6, the NICU presents parents with many obstacles, but with grit and determination, many parents find a way to take responsibility nonetheless.

Once parents take their infants home, we find that a key component of taking responsibility continues to be the ability to secure necessary goods and services from others. Parenting is in some senses a unique responsibility. Not only are the health and welfare of a child at stake, but the responsibility is of a long duration and broad scope. So while taking others' interests into account is, for instance, an essential component of taking responsibility, the mechanisms that work in one organizational setting to encourage actors to do so may not be present or effective in another. In chapter 7, we revisit our five dimensions of responsibility, this time detailing how such responsible orientations are encouraged or undermined in parents. Here, we find that there are multiple routes to responsible parenting but that responsible parents share a belief that their contributions are crucial.

Our task in the rest of the book is to understand variations in the acceptance of responsibility for critically ill children. Although we focus intensely on one empirical setting, our definition of responsibility remains a general one. As a foundation for the rest of the book, this chapter has examined what it means to take responsibility, how responsibility can be investigated empirically, and, briefly, how variations in responsibility appear in the lives of parents whose infants spent their first days in an NICU.

FOUR

Responsibility as a Joint Enterprise: The Role of the State in the NICU and the Home

PARENTS VARY in how much responsibility they assume for critically ill children. But responsibility in the NICU is, in fact, a joint enterprise—shared by the families into which the babies are born and to which they are eventually discharged (if all goes well), the staff members who care for them during hospitalization, and the state, which often pays for the care and sets and enforces standards for both medical care and parenting. Each of these parties has a stake in ensuring that the infants who are the focus of this study are well cared for. Although the family, the hospital, and the state share this responsibility, the jurisdictions and perspectives of each are unique.

The division of responsibility among these three parties affects the capacity of each to do its job. The general problem here is that no one can meet extensive obligations adequately without drawing on essential goods and services provided by others. A first task for someone who has a heavy responsibility, then, is to construct a network that includes those who can supply crucial goods and services and to fashion those ties to facilitate some orchestration and supervision of others' activities by this central person (who is ultimately responsible). No actor can behave responsibly unless he or she can intervene authoritatively to encourage or induce others to do their part in a timely and competent fashion.

In the case of critically ill infants, the network consists of three main groups of actors—family members, hospital staff members, and such representatives of the state as judges and child-welfare workers. But whereas hospital staff members are repeat players incorporating a new family and a new child into well-established routines, the family often is in the process of being constructed and only very rarely consists of people who are repeat players experienced in managing the care of critically ill infants. Child-welfare workers and judges are more likely than families to be experienced repeat players but are not as familiar with NICUs and their patients as hospital staff members. This asymmetry of experience, we argue, gives hos-

TABLE 4.1 The family, the hospital, and the state: The infant's relationship to three key participants, and the nature of their obligations to the infant

Participants	Infant's Relationship	Nature of Obligation
Family	Child	Particularistic Direct Long-term Broad scope
Hospital/NICU	Patient	Universalistic Direct Short-term Limited scope
State	Young citizen	Universalistic Indirect Long-term Limited scope

pital staff members a decided edge in constructing and deploying a network that fits their needs.

The roles of the three main categories of participants vary along a number of crucial dimensions, as summarized in Table 4.1. Each of these participants has a distinct relationship to the infants who are the focus of this study. These infants are children to the families into which they are born, patients to the hospitals and their staffs, and young citizens to the state. And the nature of the obligations of each of the main participants varies accordingly. Both the family and the hospital staff have direct responsibilities for the infants, but the state has a responsibility only to see that other parties meet their obligations. It usually has no direct responsibility itself, only a regulatory one. And while the hospital staff and state have a universalistic obligation to the patient and the citizen, respectively, the family has a much more particularistic obligation to its child. Finally, the commitment of the hospital staff and the legal system is considerably narrower in scope than is the family's commitment to the infant, and the hospital's obligation is of a considerably shorter duration than either the family's or the state's.

From a Kantian or Rawlsian perspective on responsibility, we have no business putting our own child's welfare before that of any other child. And indeed, the state and the NICU are supposed to treat each child equally. Theirs is, as we have noted, primarily a universalistic obligation.

However, the universalism of the philosopher's formulation of responsibility seems absurd when we examine responsibility from the perspective of the family. It is precisely the parents' tie to a particular child that is the foundation on which their responsibility rests. From a sociological point of view, then, particularism is not less morally sound than universalism but is simply another way of assigning responsibilities.

We have already introduced two of the core participants in the drama of getting a critically ill infant home: the families into which the infants are born and the NICUs where they are treated. In this chapter, we focus most of our attention on the role of the third core participant, the state. We argue that anyone who accepts a large responsibility must also ensure that other key participants do their part. In our case, the work of getting a critically ill infant home cannot be accomplished by either the family or the hospital alone. Each must rely on the contributions of the other. But how does each ensure that the other does its part? In order to answer this question, we must understand the role of the state, which both helps set and enforce minimum standards of parenting and doctoring and grants each party some limited authority to intervene in the activities of the other.

We begin with a brief theoretical discussion of how responsibilities come to be assigned to different parties and how rights to intervene are allocated and enforced. Our goal in this chapter is to develop the rudiments of a theory of how legal regulation shapes responsibility. We analyze in particular the crucial role of rights to intervene and the problem of consent or submission to intervention. But the legal foundation for intervention is of only limited importance, of course, because rights to intervene are quite circumscribed and because the use of legal tools is shaped by factors other than rights. In the NICU, physicians' rights to intervene also depend on the patient's condition, and in practice parents' rights to intervene vary with parental competence (especially in using legal tools) and resources. How rights are exercised and by whom further depend on whether interested third parties are able to generate more "distant" rights to intervene, as, for instance, are embodied in the Baby Doe Regulations or the Child Abuse Amendments to the Child Abuse Prevention and Treatment Act. In addition to laws and regulations that specifically govern relations between parents and children and between parents and health-care providers, the state also supports responsible parenting by facilitating access to resources through its regulation of contracts between insurers and policyholders, its provision of welfare assistance to poor parents and children, and its sponsorship of health and educational programs. The state thus supports responsible parenting less by intervening directly than by allocating rights to intervene and providing usable routines that shore up commitment, facilitate access to resources, and guarantee contracts.

Responsibility for a critically ill child is assigned jointly to the hospital staff and the infant's family. When responsibilities overlap significantly, the chance of conflict rises, and the role of the state as referee grows accordingly. After outlining the jurisdictions and perspectives of the NICU staffs and the families, we describe the complex role of the state—as protector of young citizens' rights to life, health, and happiness; as mediator in disputes between families and hospitals; as promulgator of the laws that govern activity in the NICU; and as the financer of last resort that covers the medical bills of the uninsured (or inadequately insured) and foots the bill for many child-welfare programs. We distinguish between four types of law—civil, criminal, regulatory, and fiscal—that are relevant to activities in the NICU and discuss how each type of law variously affects parents and hospital staff. We can also distinguish between four corresponding conceptions of the state as well: the state as guarantor of relations among strangers through civil law, the state as protector of public order through criminal law, the state as defender of the weak through regulatory law, and the state as agent of public policy decisions through disbursement of money for authorized purposes.

"The state," as we're using it here, then, should be understood not as a unitary entity with a single purpose but as an aggregation that includes legislative bodies, welfare bureaucracies and their agents, and the judiciary. Each piece has a different role to play in regulating parents and hospital staff, and they sometimes pull in different directions. It should also be noted that the laws that govern medicine and family life are primarily state, not federal, laws. However, there is a great deal of agreement between states on many of the key issues discussed in this chapter, so we emphasize the points of agreement rather than discuss state-by-state variation in any detail. Our use of "the state," then, while often really the states, is a shorthand way of capturing the many legislative and judicial authorities that variously regulate medicine and family life, all in the name of protecting the child as young citizen.

The state has not just one role in the NICU, then, but many. First, the state, in its various guises, defines the floor, or minimum standard, of acceptable role fulfillment for the two other core participants. But taking responsibility, as we argue throughout this book, entails exceeding minimum standards, and the state does little to compel performances that rise above the floor. What is the state's role, then, in encouraging responsibility? In addition to defining the floor, the state also provides tools that can be used by participants to intervene authoritatively in the activities of others. In other words, the state provides both parents and NICUs with some of the tools needed to take responsibility. But participants vary both in their competence at using tools such as the law and in their motivation to use them. Because state agents are not routinely in NICUs, where decisions are being made, or in parents' homes, where neglect or abuse may take place, the law must be used by someone who has both the motivation and the competence to do so. What role the law plays thus depends largely on what role others give it. If people employ legal tools frequently and cleverly, the law will play a much more substantial role than if they either ignore legal tools or thwart others' attempts to use legal tools.

As infants are discharged home, the perspectives and jurisdictions of the three core participants necessarily shift. What was once an overlapping responsibility for the infant patients, shared by parents and hospital staff, is now a singular responsibility, shouldered primarily by the parents. Although the hospital's job includes training parents for the discharge home, once this training is complete, the parents are largely on their own. The state retains its interest in protecting the health and welfare of its young citizens, but state intervention in enforcing the floor for parenting is now quite unlikely for most parents. In general, the state is much more likely to intervene in the NICU than to invade the sanctity of the home. Although our rights to privacy demand such respect, this also means that the law is less effective as a tool for parents once they have gotten their infants home.

In the NICU, the law gives parents and NICU staff members a way to manage their interdependence. Each depends on the other for a contribution that it cannot provide itself but also cannot do without. Parents cannot provide high-tech medical care and hospitals cannot provide homes. In general, when accomplishing something depends on contributions from others, one's capacity to take responsibility for the outcome is dependent on having some enforceable right to intervene. This enforceable right is provided by the law in the NICU. However, when infants are discharged home, parents must construct alternative ways to secure contributions from others. The law is, for instance, silent about whether fathers as well as mothers must perform unpleasant medical tasks at home and so helps little in managing parents' overlapping responsibilities. Even if one is highly motivated to use a tool and is skilled in using it, a tool may not prove equally useful in all settings. Instead, parents must fashion other tools and employ other mechanisms to construct a network that will meet their needs. State intervention, therefore, is a necessary, but not sufficient, condition for promoting responsibility after discharge home.

Conceptual Foundations: How Are Responsibilities Assigned and Who Has Rights to Intervene?

Organizations assign obligations, rights, resources, and incentives to encourage actors (whether they be individuals, departments, or other organizations) to take responsibility for getting things done.[1] But such assignments are problematic. Not everyone who is assigned a task takes the obligation equally seriously. Rights to intervene may be contested by others. Resources, especially time, are often in short supply. Incentives designed for a system with slack (unused capacity and somewhat more than adequate resources) may not work well in a system with more pressure. When obligations, rights, resources, and incentives do not coincide, actors are less likely to take responsibility.

Further, not all responsibilities lie inside the borders of formal organizations. When responsibilities span organizational borders or fall in the domain of less formally organized groups, assignments of responsibility may be even more problematic. Often responsibilities will not be formally assigned; instead people may assume that responsibilities have been assigned by custom or even by nature. When responsibilities fall "naturally" to a person or have been customarily assigned to a person in a particular category, it may be harder for others to intervene when things go wrong. Adjustments of resources to fit responsibilities may also be more difficult when responsibilities are not formally assigned and are not subject to negotiation.

We might therefore wish to distinguish between three kinds of obligations: *Contractual* responsibilities are explicitly assigned to actors in working out a division of labor. Within organizations, contractual responsibilities might be spelled out, for instance, in a formal contract, department or organizational handbook, job description, or meeting. In relations between organizations, formal contracts often are used to specify the rights and duties of each party, although as Macaulay (1963) has noted, details of formal contracts are not always heeded. In less formally organized groups, a division of labor may be worked out in a meeting or even in a

1. The arguments of this section are developed more fully in Heimer (1986).

casual discussion. Because of their positions in a hierarchy or legal system or because of their professional status or relationship with some other person, actors sometimes have an *ultimate* responsibility to see that particular jobs get done properly even though they are not supposed to do them themselves. A boss may bear formal responsibility for the activities of subordinates, an organization may have to answer to public authorities for the activities of suppliers or subcontractors, or a professional may have an obligation to report on any irregularities in others' performances. Finally, actors who depend on others' inputs to do their own jobs may have *contingent* responsibilities if they must take over responsibilities that are the (unmet) contractual obligations of others. People may then feel responsible for tasks that are formally assigned to others. It is thus entirely possible that more than one actor will have an obligation to see that some responsibility is met. Although these three kinds of responsibilities are logically separable, they are not always empirically distinct, since a responsibility is often shared by several actors and which category it falls into depends on whose perspective one adopts.

In our case, the parents are, of course, ultimately responsible for their children, but physicians and the state also each have an ultimate responsibility for infants who are treated in the NICU. During the infant's hospitalization, the physicians have ultimate responsibility for providing expert medical care. Unlike parents, however, their responsibility is contractually based. The attending physicians, in particular, are responsible for overseeing the care administered to patients by subordinates, like residents and nurses, even if they do not administer that care themselves. And the state bears an ultimate responsibility for protecting the health and welfare of its citizens. Because of the division of labor in the NICU, staff members must rely on the contributions of others to provide adequate medical care. Staff members, therefore, have contingent responsibilities. Even though it is not the nurse's job to make treatment decisions or write orders in a chart, for instance, during our fieldwork we often observed nurses taking responsibility for getting orders from residents when they felt a medication was needed, a treatment plan required adjustment, and the like. Because nurses must rely on the contributions of residents to give adequate medical care to the patients, they often assumed responsibility for tasks that were not formally assigned to them.

The distinction between ultimate, contractual, and contingent obligations is important partly because obligations incurred in various ways are likely to be differentially associated with the rights, incentives, and resources necessary to meet the obligations. Actors with contractual responsibilities may or may not have adequate resources and incentives, but they typically have some right to take responsibilities. Actors who have ultimate responsibility may or may not have resources, but they typically have incentives and some rights to take responsibility even when this interferes with the discretion of subordinates or contractors. Actors who have contingent responsibilities will often have an incentive to take a responsibility but may lack the resources (e.g., because the organization will have assigned the resources corresponding to the responsibility to someone else) and will quite often lack the right to intervene.

When an actor has a contractual or an ultimate responsibility, he or she typically has some right to take that responsibility or to see that whoever has subordinate obligations is doing an adequate job. Rights to intervene are clearest when written into contracts or organizational hierarchies but can be secured in less formal ways. Dotted lines appear on organization charts; informal relations supplement hierarchies. We might thus distinguish between rights according to where they fell along a continuum between *formal* rights—clearly laid out in laws, contracts, organization plans, and job descriptions (with those earlier in the list being more formal than those later in the list)—and *consensual* rights that arise during informal negotiations about who will do what, governed by precedents and customs about who has what obligations, or through the development of working relationships or friendships.[2]

This distinction between formal and consensual rights to take responsibility is important for two reasons. First, more consensual rights tend to be more precarious and can more easily be contested. Second, as one moves along the dimension from formal to consensual rights, one finds actors asserting their rights to take responsibility in ever more delicate form. Orders are replaced by requests, memos by discussions in meetings, formal schedules and timelines by suggestions about when it might be convenient to receive a response or by a promise to call about the matter on a particular day. These diplomatic assertions of a right to be interested in an outcome tend to be more time consuming than their more authoritative

2. Lempert (1972) argues that contract law can be used as a model to understand more informal agreements. Although there are important differences between contractual agreements and more informal agreements, the principles of contract law can help us determine whether an agreement will be binding and whether social sanctions will be brought to bear if an agreement is violated. The idea is that the law formalizes fundamental social values, and through the law we can learn the conditions under which even informal social agreements will be considered more or less binding.

counterparts and to require more sensitive interpersonal negotiation, and are more likely to be done face-to-face. They rely on embarrassment and shame (about not having the job done) as much as on the logic of the schedule or legal rights to intervene and tend to underplay authority relations between the various parties interested in getting a particular job done.[3] Because rights to intervene are easier to establish when an actor has contractual, rather than contingent, obligations and still easier when the actor has ultimate, rather than contractual, obligations (largely because of the backing of the state), we would expect some tendency for actors to turn important and problematic contingent obligations into contractual ones and an increased emphasis on the connection between contingent or contractual obligations and ultimate obligations when rights to intervene are important and otherwise precarious.

Contractually based responsibilities arise when people or organizations form relationships with one another. When contracts are formalized in one way or another, enforcement mechanisms such as the law become available as tools to sort out disagreements and to press others to meet their obligations. Although both marital relationships and relationships between patients and health-care providers are contractual, in both cases there is empirical variation in the extent to which people choose to establish the relationship in the first place and in how formal they make it. By choosing to seek care from physicians, patients and their families enter a legally regulated relationship in which both parties implicitly accept the intrusion of the state, avail themselves of legal tools, and accept the use of legal tools by the other party. The relationship between the parents of hospitalized infants and the neonatologists responsible for their care is somewhat anomalous in that, with few exceptions, parents have not chosen to seek treatment for their child. Parents are thus thrust into a legally regulated relationship with their child's health-care providers which they might not have otherwise chosen.

The legal regulation of family life varies to some degree with whether the conjugal pair has chosen to marry. Couples who do not marry invite less legal scrutiny and have fewer legal tools at their disposal. Similarly, the legal enforcement of parental (and particularly paternal) responsibilities is facilitated by the marriage of the parents. Parents who have formalized

3. In his book *Street Corner Society,* William Foote Whyte (1993) uses the phrase "initiates action" for the informal capacity to intervene in the course of action of a group of young street corner men. This mechanism is an example of the informal right to intervene to assume responsibility that we are discussing here.

their union are more likely to meet obligations to their hospitalized infants in any case (e.g., see Tables 2.3 and 2.4 for evidence about the visitation patterns of married vs. unmarried parents). It is far from clear that the formalization of ties is what causes the acceptance of responsibilities, of course. Instead it seems more likely that people who intend to take up obligations to a spouse and children are willing to formalize the tie, while those who are more ambivalent are reluctant to marry. The existence of a formal contract is thus mostly an indicator of the existence of a strong tie, but it may nevertheless reinforce an already robust tie.[4]

As we will show below, although families have an ultimate responsibility of long duration and broad scope, hospital physicians also have an ultimate responsibility for the health of their young patients—at least during the time that the children are patients. Because both parents and medical staff have legal responsibilities for the infant, when they disagree about treatment decisions, each party has legal tools at its disposal. Each of these parties also has contingent responsibilities should others fail to meet their obligations. But because many more of the hospital staff's responsibilities are grounded in formal contracts, hospital staff are more likely to have well-established rights to intervene to get work done competently, whereas parents will often have to negotiate delicately or resort to threats if negotiation fails.

NICU Views on the Division of Responsibility

Among the main categories of participants, those associated with the NICU have the most clearly articulated sense of who has what responsibilities for the infant patient. The state and the family step on to medical turf in claiming some right to make decisions about the baby. State representatives, for whom the child-welfare issues of critically ill babies are but a small portion of their work, and families, armed with little more than their biological tie to the child and their sense of the rights that are theirs by custom, confront hospital staff members, who are armed with vast clinical experience, medical textbooks, and administrative and medical protocols and who are backed by the authority of professional associations, medical and allied professional training programs, certifications by the Joint Commission on Accreditation of Health Care Organizations (JCAHO), and,

4. We can see the same pattern in business contracts. Civil law facilitates the formation of contracts. And while trade can occur between two parties who have not formed a long-term contract with each other, the volume of trade tends to increase when such contracts are formed.

ultimately, by a state license to practice medicine (or some ancillary profession).

Fundamentally, the NICU interest in the baby is as a patient that to one degree or another requires the intervention of the experts who work there. The NICU's main job is to treat the baby for its primary medical problems and to discharge the infant as soon as possible. The motto in the NICU, we were told during our fieldwork, is that discharge planning begins on the day of admission. The NICU's tie to the infant, then, is of a relatively short duration. But while the infant is in the NICU's custody, it is the NICU staff members, and not the parents, who make the decisions. The NICU's job includes both medical care and the nonmedical special care that flows from the child's medical needs (e.g., special feeding protocols). Some of this care can be done by nonspecialists such as parents, but NICU personnel are the ones who decide who will participate and how in caring for their patient. They are, quite simply, in charge of the division of labor. Parents need not ask staff members to feed, change, and bathe the baby for them in their absence. Such routines will be carried out more or less automatically (with the occasional glitches of any large, complex organization). Instead, parents must request permission (at least initially) to take over some tasks from staff members. The default care providers are staff members, and parents are the most ancillary of ancillary care providers.

Even though innovations take place quite rapidly in neonatal intensive care medicine, many decisions about the patient's course of treatment still flow almost mechanically from standards of care that mandate particular treatments for particular problems, with important modifications and adjustments to take account of the patient's reactions to interventions, treatments, and medications, and with fine-tuning to take account of the particular combination of presenting symptoms. Fundamentally, though, the patient may be thought of as the "raw material" upon which the NICU production system operates, and each of the workers in the NICU has his or her assigned role in the productive process.

The NICU production system does have subroutines to take account of variations in its clinical raw materials, however. As much as they might like to treat only the medical problems of their patients, they inevitably must also confront the social problems presented by their patients' parents (Heimer and Stevens 1997). The variations in subroutines are responses to two contingencies—first, the families are also consumers and, second, the NICU cannot finish its work without the participation of families. The NICU staff, then, has an ultimate responsibility for the medical care of their patients—and they attend to this responsibility first. But this ultimate responsibility ends abruptly at discharge. The NICU's *patients* must also be somebody's *children* if their work is to be finished.

The NICU thus requires something different from each of the other two groups of participants. For its responsibility to be discharged smoothly, the NICU requires the parents' cooperation. It needs parents who do not interfere with the staff's ability to provide the necessary medical care, families who are sufficiently supportive of NICU activities that they neither appeal too often or too vigorously for state intervention nor object so strongly to its treatment of the patient that they file suit or have the patient moved to another facility. And it needs parents who commit themselves to taking the child home (if that is feasible) and participate sufficiently to learn to care for the baby before discharge. From the state, the NICU needs legal backing for its insistence that parents be fully prepared to take the child at the end of the process and for its right to decide what medical care is appropriate whether or not the parents approve of those decisions. It also needs some further protection from interference by others who might wish to shape medical decisions (e.g., to prohibit the withdrawal of life support or to mandate some kinds of care). And the NICU needs the state to foot a substantial portion of the bill for neonatal care, given that many infants are not covered, or not fully covered, by insurers.[5]

Families' Views on the Division of Responsibility

A key difference between the NICU and the family is that while the NICU has a direct responsibility of short duration, the family has a direct responsibility of long duration. The NICU, furthermore, has a regular production system designed specifically to manage the medical and developmental problems of critically ill neonates, but only a very exceptional family has organized itself in advance around these tasks. The family finds itself essentially without any system to deal with an unanticipated disaster—nearly always a one-time event for which no rational family would have planned. While the infants are patients to the NICU staff, they are children to their parents. Parents are unusually vulnerable when they face the NICU. They

5. As Table 2.1 in chapter 2 shows, 40.9% of infants from City Hospital and 17.7% from Suburban Hospital were either on public aid or uninsured. These figures understate the financial contributions of the state. Some families who have insurance nevertheless end up receiving some financial assistance from the state when their insurance runs out or when their disabled child qualifies for special federal programs such as social security or the Katie Beckett program, or state-level programs for early childhood education (zero-to-three programs) or for children with particular kinds of disabilities.

have just experienced a disaster, and fairly often it is a disaster that affects the health and sometimes threatens the life of the mother as well as of the child. Often they are inexperienced, first-time parents, sometimes even a new couple (if they are in fact a couple at all). As they learn what medical problems their child has, parents must learn the medical language and the facts (insofar as the facts are known) about phenomena whose existence they had not even imagined. And at the same time they must be unceremoniously initiated into a whole new social system.

In other situations, parental claims to a significant role can be legitimated by either the parents' preexisting relationship with the child or their knowledge about the child. A long-standing relationship makes the parents' claims to have the child's best interest at heart more credible than they are in an NICU, where staff members have physical custody of the child and may question the commitment of parents to a sick or handicapped newborn. Usually the parents' knowledge about the child can make them experts in interpreting symptoms, in supplying a context for a new crisis, in predicting the child's physical and emotional reactions, and in managing the child (e.g., feeding or comforting and calming the child). But in the NICU, parents cannot claim any special knowledge of the infants themselves and must offer evidence of their commitment. The best they can do is to supply relevant family medical history or details about the pregnancy. The claim of parents to their infants is, thus, in some respects precarious during the child's hospitalization in the NICU. One mother describes the frustration that can result: "He was my son, yet I had no parental responsibilities. I had no control over him at all. I mean, I could not even change a diaper. . . . They did everything for him. It became a battle of wills where she [the doctor] had all the control and we were working against each other" (1026F, p. 21). Comparing the situation to a custody battle, this mother had a strong sense of her parental obligations, but felt she had few parental rights while her son was in the NICU's custody.

Although parents have ultimate responsibility for their children, they have little capacity to intervene while the infant is hospitalized. Because they do not occupy positions in the organizational hierarchy of the NICU, parents have neither the contractual nor contingent responsibilities associated with such positions. With few formal rights to intervene, parents must cultivate their consensual rights, but these rarely have time to develop. Both the parents and the hospital have an ultimate responsibility for the infant, but their responsibilities are different. Whereas the hospital is responsible only for the patient, the parents are responsible for the child.

That is, the hospital's responsibility is limited to the medical care of the infant, and only while it is hospitalized, but the parents have broad responsibility for the child's welfare, both during the hospitalization and beyond. These responsibilities overlap during the hospitalization, often creating considerable tension and conflict. Parents feel that they, too, have an obligation to protect the interests of their children, as one father's thoughtful response indicates: "I think it was our obligation as parents to have some input and decide the fate of our child. I realize we're not doctors, but I think we're looking out for the best for our child" (1026M, p. 21). Parents may have felt similar obligations in the past, but they did not always exert their rights. At one time, in what Eliot Freidson (1988) has described as the "golden age" of American medicine, the responsibilities of parents were largely surrendered when their children became patients. Now, however, parents (and, under other circumstances, patients themselves) are claiming more rights to be involved in medical decision making. Whereas physicians once were entrusted with decisions and parental rights were more or less suspended, now parental rights are being asserted, sometimes quite vigorously.

As we will discuss in more detail in the next section, the parents' position in the NICU has been significantly bolstered by the state, which defines their legal rights to participate in NICU decision making. Such regulations as the laws of informed consent mandate the patient's (or parents', in our case) right to participate in treatment decisions. Over the last few decades, patients and families have increasingly asserted that right, arguing that physicians are not always the best representatives of patients' interests. Disagreements about who represents the patient's best interests are no longer negotiated between patients, families, and physicians only on the medical ward or in the doctor's office but are occasionally matters to be settled in courts of law. Although the courts have stopped considerably short of granting patients full autonomy, they have ruled that in some cases patients and their families have the right to refuse treatment (Anspach 1993; Cook County State's Attorney's Task Force 1990; Newman 1989; Zussman 1992).

Parents, therefore, require something different from each of the two other core participants. From the hospital and the NICU, the parents require skill and expertise in treating the child's medical problems. But because the obligations of the parents and the staff overlap during the child's hospitalization, the parents also require a system of care that allows their participation. The state provides parents with legal rights to act as parents while their children are hospitalized—as long as doing so does not interfere with the child's health and well-being. Among its many roles, the state becomes the arbiter in disputes between the parents and the hospital, disputes which sometimes require swift intervention.

Adjudicating Parental Rights and Professional Responsibilities in an Organizational Context: The Role of the State

The state shares an ultimate responsibility with the parents and the NICU. However, the role of the state is qualitatively different from the roles of the other two. While both NICUs and parents have direct responsibilities for caring for their patients and their children, respectively, the state has primarily an indirect role. Only intermittently, and then usually only briefly, are any state agents directly involved in NICU cases. However, the law's presence is felt even when no state agents are present, because the law helps define the rights and responsibilities of both of the other primary participants in the NICU. What happens in the NICU, then, happens in the "shadow of the law" (Mnookin and Kornhauser 1979).

Parents stake their claims to participate in decisions in the NICU on their rights to family autonomy and privacy, their right to freedom of religion, and their ultimate responsibility for their child. They are the ones who will have to bear the burden of raising a disabled child, balancing its needs against the needs of other family members within the constraints imposed by family resources. And physicians' claims are based on their traditional rights to make treatment decisions, mastery of arcane medical knowledge, and clinical experience. Each claim has a long and distinguished legal history. But decisions in the NICU are not left simply to parents and physicians; the state reserves the right to intervene. The state, through legislatures, regulatory bodies, and courts, claims, as *parens patriae,* the power to make decisions as the disinterested protector of infant citizens, because its interest in the lives and health of its citizens takes precedence over the parents' interest in control over their own children. As the following account illustrates, the state may be called in, as the ultimate authority, to settle disputes that occur when what the parents think is best for their child conflicts with what the doctors think is best for their patient.

When a critically ill newborn was transferred to Suburban Hospital, a serious dispute erupted between her parents and the doctors charged with saving her life. The physicians argued that their patient required at least a transfusion and perhaps ECMO (a machine that does the work of the heart and lungs) to save her life, but her parents resisted on religious grounds.

As faithful Jehovah's Witnesses, they refused to consent to the proposed treatment. Stressing that he was pursuing the only course of action he felt was morally defensible, the father gravely pronounced to the head of neonatology, "God has given *me* responsibility for this child's immortal soul." For the young father, the rejection of blood products was a moral imperative, the only responsible course of action given his family's religious beliefs. However, on this fateful day, as his parents-in-law and several ministers from his church watched, the father's vision of the responsible course of action collided with the hospital's and eventually the state's. During the day-long crisis, we observed a series of tense, but respectful, meetings during which the family called in a variety of church members, some of them religious authorities, others with special expertise in medicine. Many members of the hospital staff attended as well—the attending physician, the resident, the social worker, and sometimes a nurse or two, the head of neonatology, and a member of the hospital's legal staff.

The hospital attorney explained the legal situation and the procedures that allow an attending physician to take temporary custody of a patient and administer medical treatments in spite of the parents' opposition.[6] The attending physician repeatedly explained the infant's condition, patiently discussing the proposed medical treatments, explaining why substitutes for blood products would not be medically acceptable here, and stressing that unless the infant's condition improved dramatically, she would shortly reach the point where a transfusion would be essential to save her life. With treatment, the infant's prognosis was excellent. But the father and mother (who was still hospitalized and participated in the meeting by telephone) repeatedly asked the physicians not to administer the blood products, and the physicians agreed to delay until they believed they could wait no longer without jeopardizing their patient's health. In the early evening, the attending neonatologist decided that further delay was impossible, and she took legal custody of the infant and ordered a blood transfusion. The patient's condition did not improve adequately with the blood transfusion alone, however, and she eventually required ECMO. Within a few days, her condition had improved dramatically, and she was soon discharged to her parents. Despite the tense negotiations, all those involved (including her parents) were quite pleased with the infant's outcome.

6. It is interesting to note that the hospital attorney takes the position of the "state" here (protecting the health and welfare of its young citizens), making state intervention possible even though no state representatives are present. However, it should also be noted that be-

Not all dramas about medical decisions in the NICU have such happy endings, however. Many babies either die or survive with impairments; families and staff members may be unable to resume cordial relations after the dispute; staff members and family members may not behave as honorably or sensibly during the crisis as members of both groups did in this instance. And the state may not always intervene so efficiently or effectively. In general, the state will not intervene in medical decisions, including the refusal of medical care, if the individual is both legally competent and the decision does not adversely affect the interests of a third party. Jehovah's Witnesses may forgo blood transfusions on religious grounds as long as they are legally competent and they act only for themselves. However, if a woman is pregnant or a minor child is involved, the state will routinely intervene to protect the life and health of the unborn or minor child.[7] In cases such as these, the state is unusually effective, because it has adapted to the timetable of medicine and aligned itself with high-ranking medical actors to protect the infants from being denied life-saving medical intervention. The cooperation of hospital staff members, who saw how appropriate legal tools could facilitate their work, is essential if laws are to be translated into workable hospital routines. However, state intervention does not always go so smoothly, nor does it always support the hospital or physician points of view about the responsible course of action.

The cases that led to the now-defunct Baby Doe regulations are perhaps the most notorious of neonatal legal disputes.[8] In one such case, the Indiana Supreme Court decided that the parents of an infant with Down's syndrome—a genetic disorder that is not in itself fatal—had the right to refuse surgery to correct the infant's throat obstruction, a condition that if

cause the attorney is an employee of the hospital, this is more likely to happen in situations where the interests of the hospital and the state align. See Heimer (1996a).

7. Frohock (1992) describes the role of the state in regulating alternative medicine and spiritual healing, asking when the state should override religious and other beliefs to preserve the life and health of its citizens. Jehovah's Witnesses reject only the administration of blood products, yet this rejection of mainstream medicine has led to some landmark court decisions that have helped define when the state's obligation to protect its young citizens from harm should take precedence over the right to religious freedom. For instance, in *Jehovah's Witnesses in the State of Washington v. King's County Hospital Unit 1* (1967), the U.S. Supreme Court held that the state "may justifiably intervene to protect the health and welfare of minors participating in religious practices because 'the right to practice religion does not include the liberty to expose the child to ill health or death'" (Frohock 1992:305, 266n).

8. The literature on the Baby Doe cases and the resulting regulations is voluminous. See n. 22 for a summary of the Baby Doe Regulations and relevant citations.

left untreated would result in the child's death. Here, the court intervened to support the parents in their battle with the hospital and its physicians, who favored treatment. The controversy that ensued helped focus the public's attention on the sometimes tragic outcomes in the NICU. In contrast to the case we observed, the parents' right to determine the fate of their child took precedence over the physicians' right to make decisions on their patient's behalf.

In general, though, the courts are ill suited to the task of resolving medical disputes, and they have been reluctant to shift the burden of decision making from families and physicians to the courtroom. This is partly a recognition that such decisions are often better left to the consciences of families and the medical expertise of physicians and partly the result of the incongruity between medical and legal timetables. Medical decisions can—and must—be made at any time of day or night. Dire consequences may result from the long delays that take place in courts of law. The courts have in some instances adapted their routines to accommodate medical timetables, but this adaptation is not distributed evenly to the hospital and its staff, on the one hand, and the parents, on the other. Instead, as repeat players, the hospital and its staff have had a stake in developing innovative legal routines that will help them do their jobs. Moreover, as an organization with a legal staff, the hospital is well equipped, and can afford, to use the law as a tool when necessary, which gives it the advantage over parents. Families have no corresponding organizational routines to facilitate their use of law.

The capacity of the state to intervene in the NICU extends beyond court settlement of disputes between parents and medical-care providers about treatment decisions. In state and federal legislation, the state promulgates some important ground rules for NICU activities. The state may pay many of the hospital bills (e.g., through Medicaid), the courts may decide whether parents are competent to care for their children, and when the child becomes a ward of the state, state agents (child-welfare workers) may make decisions about who will care for the child after discharge from the hospital.

The state, then, has many concerns. In its various guises, the state is concerned with whether children are deprived of appropriate medical treatment either because hospital staff members discriminate against disabled infants or because parents have religious objections to potentially life-saving treatment. The state is furthermore concerned with such issues as whether someone else needs to take over the parental role because the biological parent is incompetent or insufficiently committed, whether parental resources really need to be supplemented by the state, and whether the hospital has correctly charged the state for the services it has provided. The last would not be especially important to us here except that such fiscal concerns provide an important incentive for hospitals to ensure that parents are ready and able to take a child home at discharge. Because the state (and private insurers) may refuse to pay the bills beyond a certain point, a hospital will be reluctant to keep a patient hospitalized after discharge is medically appropriate just because parents are unprepared to take the child home.

We can group the laws that govern activities in the NICU into four different general categories: civil law (e.g., medical malpractice cases), criminal law (e.g., state laws against homicide or prohibiting the abuse and neglect of children and requiring that they be reported), regulatory law (e.g., state law governing professional practice or requiring informed consent), and fiscal law (e.g., federal law denying certain funds to states without programs to prevent medical neglect of handicapped infants; state and federal medical aid and welfare regulations). Though all four types of law govern the activities of hospitals and their staffs, parents are governed mainly by the limits set by criminal law (against homicide and child abuse or neglect) and fiscal law (regulations for welfare and medical aid). While the consequences of violating these laws may be quite serious, very few parents will in fact experience those consequences directly, although such laws have important indirect effects on the experience of parenting a critically ill child. As we will demonstrate in more detail below, the law is much more oriented to governing the activities of the hospital and its staff than of the parents.

Civil Law

The activities in the NICU are governed first by ordinary civil law. Under the law of torts, medical personnel and organizations are accountable for harms they cause to others. Medical malpractice suits are brought against physicians, other health-care providers, and hospitals, and insurers sell expensive policies to cover losses from malpractice suits. Lieberman (1981:69) notes that the sources of liability for a health professional parallel those of a manufacturer: actual performance of medical tasks (corresponding to defects in construction), the choice of a course of treatment (corresponding to errors in design), and the information given to the patient and his or her family to aid their decision making (corresponding to the warnings on product labels and associated leaflets). The standard to which a physician is held varies with the source of liability—for performance of medical tasks, the standard is negligence;[9] for the choice of the course of treatment, the standard is the "standard of care" in the medical community, though in a few cases courts have found that a physician was at fault even when the care provided was in line with the standard at the time;[10] and for informed consent, no clear standard seems to exist (Lieberman 1981:69, 71, and 81, respectively).

As in all medical malpractice suits, the fundamental question is whether the health professional could have prevented or limited harm, in this case to the baby.[11] In their chapter on perinatal brain injury and neurological impairment, Pegalis and Wachsman explain when a physician will be liable: "Failure to anticipate, prepare, monitor and/or apply appropriate skills or techniques in caring for the fetus and newborn may be judged a

9. The standards for negligence are knowledge sensitive, and decisions are based on assessments not of what a physician actually knows but of what a physician should reasonably be expected to know. Physicians, like other experts, are held to different standards than laypeople in determining negligence. See Scheppele (1991) for an insightful discussion of tort law.

10. In general, the question about the design of a course of treatment is whether or not the physician provided care that met current standards of the medical community. But two questions may be raised about medical standards. Courts may ask what the relevant medical community is and whether standards are local or national. Since the late 1960s, courts have recognized that the medical community is national, not local, and have relaxed previous requirements that local experts testify about the standard of care. In addition, courts can ask whether the medical standard is appropriate and in a few exceptional cases (e.g., *Helling v. Carey*, 83 Wash. 2d 514, 519 P.2d 981 [1974]) have overruled the medical standard.

A quite different issue arises, though, when medical standards are evolving, as often happens in cutting-edge fields such as neonatal intensive care. For instance, Gail Kalmowitz, who became blind from the oxygen therapy she received as a premature infant in 1952, sued the hospital for malpractice even though she had received standard care. Many premature infants were blinded from oxygen therapy during the 1940s and 1950s, but it was not until 1956 that physicians understood that it was the oxygen therapy that was the problem. (See Silverman [1980] for an argument that physicians could have arrived at the answer sooner had they been more careful scientists.) Kalmowitz had persuaded the jury, but accepted a settlement just before the jury returned its verdict (O'Connell 1979).

11. Two studies of malpractice claims (which are of course not a good sample of all neonatal cases) suggest that harm might have been preventable in many cases. Nocon and Coolman, reviewing twenty-five perinatal malpractice cases, concluded that in those cases, "fifty-six percent of professionals failed to recognize a high-risk pregnancy or fetal distress. Of those who did, 44% failed to treat properly" (1987:89). Cornblath and Clark, reviewing 250 claims involving neonatal brain damage, concluded that in 31% of the cases harm was preventable, in 42% it was not preventable, and in the remaining 27% it was impossible to attribute responsibility for the outcome (1984:298–302).

'departure' from the standard of care. If the 'departure' causes injury and/or deprives the child of a substantial opportunity to avoid injury, then liability will exist. Under such circumstances, the injury is deemed 'preventable'" (1992:499). In neonatal intensive care, causal relationships are difficult to establish, and there is ambiguity both about whether substandard medical care caused, or failed to limit, harm and about whether that substandard care was provided by NICU staff or by other health-care professionals (e.g., an obstetrician who provided prenatal care or delivered the baby).[12] But, as Pegalis and Wachsman note, "Absolute precision is not the legal test" (1992:501). They argue that, instead, cause must be established only on a "more likely than not" basis (1992:387, 501) and that liability would arise "if obstetrical or neonatal care were substandard in the context of some foreseeable harm to the fetus/newborn" (386).

The emphases on "foreseeable harm" and "standard of care" suggest where we should expect to find the biggest effects of tort law, and medical malpractice insurers, like other insurers, encourage medical practitioners and hospitals to engage in a variety of loss-prevention activities. Innumerable inspections, certifications, reviews, and rules flow from the purchase of insurance or the decision of a hospital to self-insure. Just as the simple decision to get a mortgage to purchase a home leads to entanglement in a net of rules about title insurance, fire insurance, escrow accounts, late payment penalties, and the like, so decisions about malpractice insurance are coupled with JCAHO (Joint Commission on Accreditation of Health Care Organizations) inspections, certification of professionals, continuing education programs, development of medication and procedure protocols (the core of a "standard of care"), rules about reporting particular "incidents,"

12. In addition to ordinary medical malpractice suits, suits have been brought for "wrongful conception," "wrongful pregnancy," "wrongful birth," and "wrongful life" (Lyon 1985:195–196; Pegalis and Wachsman 1993:69–84; Weir 1984:116–17). Generally, wrongful conception and pregnancy suits are brought by parents who conceived and bore healthy, but unwanted, infants because of physician negligence or error in prescribing contraceptives, performing sterilizations, or attempting abortions; wrongful birth suits are brought by parents (of impaired children) who would have avoided or terminated pregnancies had they been adequately informed about the likelihood of defects; and wrongful life cases are brought by or on behalf of impaired children who, but for physician negligence or error, would not have been born to bear the pain and suffering associated with their impairments. Because the alternative for the child is not to have been born at all, the courts have thus far not allowed any impaired children to recover general damages in wrongful life suits. Though an NICU might be implicated in a wrongful life suit (for prolonging an infant's life), the main effect of this group of suits is probably to emphasize to physicians the importance of prenatal testing and of providing parents with an opportunity for informed consent.

rules about "gowning" (even though gowning has been shown not to influence infection rates) and scrubbing, and the creation of positions for risk managers and legal counsel.

Civil law is designed to hold individual physicians, medical staff, and hospitals accountable for their actions. However, the effects of civil law extend far beyond those who are found liable. Though professional associations would undoubtedly press for some inspections, certifications, and protocols whether or not malpractice claims made them necessary, and many of the effects are consistent with what medical personnel would want in any case (e.g., good record keeping), the threat of medical malpractice lawsuits increases the pressure for hospitals and physicians to conform to the "standard of care." Hospitals and their staffs have a strong incentive, then, to develop a standard of care, to revise that standard when appropriate, and to ensure compliance.

Parents are much more likely to be plaintiffs in civil suits than defendants. It is the patients (and in our case, their parents) who bring civil suits against hospitals and physicians. Though, in theory, parents could also be found negligent in civil court, parents are hardly ever sued *as parents.* Civil suits require a party other than the state to bring the suit to the attention of the courts. This is the meaning of civil law, and the only way it is applied. And while children could, in theory, sue their parents in civil court, they hardly ever do and certainly not during infancy. Civil law, then, governs the behavior of hospitals and their staffs to a much greater extent than that of parents.

Criminal Law

In addition to civil law, criminal law also shapes what happens in the NICU. Parents, as ordinary citizens, may not legally cause the death of another person, and neither may physicians or other health-care providers. Laws prohibiting murder and manslaughter are invoked to prevent physicians from withdrawing life support from (let alone giving fatal injections to) infants. Though no physician has yet been tried for causing an infant's death by withholding or stopping treatment, nevertheless physicians and hospital lawyers are acutely aware that such legal actions are possible.[13]

13. Weir comments that "no physician has yet been prosecuted for having withheld ordinary medical treatment from an infant with a serious birth defect" (1984:101), and Fost states that "never in the history of this country, as far as I have been able to determine, has any doctor ever been found liable for deliberately withholding or withdrawing any life-sustaining treatment from any patient for any reason" (1989:330). But in at least one prominent case where the father went to extreme measures to withdraw life support from his child,

Parents also could be prosecuted for first- or second-degree murder or manslaughter for deciding to withhold medical treatment from their child, though prosecution for withholding or withdrawing treatment is extremely rare and preliminary hearings only a bit more common.[14]

State laws prohibiting child abuse and neglect are invoked more often, and they govern the behavior of both parents and hospital staff members, though cases are much more commonly brought against parents (and especially mothers) than against health-care providers or hospital social workers. The state where this research was conducted is typical in that there are several statutes that address the issues of child abuse and neglect. Though there are some differences between states, these statutes typically define what is meant by neglect and specify categories of people who are legally required to report abuse or neglect to the state agency charged with protecting children. Statutes also specify the penalties for failure to report and make some provision for hospital staff to assume temporary custody of a patient in an emergency medical situation if treatment is necessary to save the patient's life.

With respect to the practice of neonatal medicine in our state, neglect is defined broadly. First, the statutes classify as neglected any child from whom medical treatment is withheld, any child abandoned by parents or other persons responsible for the child, and any newborn whose blood or

---

the physicians were ignorant about the law (see Goldman, Stratton, and Brown [1989] and Gostin [1989] on the case of Baby Linares). Lieberman (1981:89) also comments on misinformation about the law and physician anxiety about prosecution. The few "close calls" (e.g., the initial conviction, overturned on appeal, of a Massachusetts obstetrician for failing to ventilate an aborted, but possibly viable, fetus and the preliminary hearing on the charge of conspiracy to commit murder in the case of the Danville conjoined twins) (Weir 1984:101; Lyon 1985) no doubt fuel physician fears. But physicians are not the only ones who have had "close calls"—several parents have also received court scrutiny (see n. 14).

14. See Weir (1984:91–115) for a careful discussion of relevant legal questions and cases. Weir stresses that there is "considerable uncertainty regarding the legal status of nontreatment decisions" and that nontreatment decisions are "legally risky" for both parents and physicians. Though most nontreatment decisions receive no legal scrutiny, some are brought before the court for review. Until recently, no parents had been prosecuted for withholding treatment from their newborn child, although in a few cases parents were threatened with prosecution. For instance, the parents (and the attending physician) of the conjoined twins born in Danville, Illinois, in 1981 were charged with conspiracy to commit murder; charges were later dismissed (Weir 1984:95–97). The case of Rudy Linares, who removed his infant from a respirator and held the staff at gunpoint until the baby died, was brought before a grand jury. The grand jury decided not to indict Linares for murder (Cook County State's Attorney's Task Force 1990:1). Finally, in early 1995 a Michigan father, whose child died after the father unplugged the respirator, was tried for manslaughter but quickly acquitted (Frey 1995; *New York Times* 1995).

urine contains illegal drugs. The statutes also specify that it is illegal to withhold care from impaired children but allow some leeway for religious opposition to particular medical treatments.[15] Second, the laws in this state specify categories of people, including social workers and a variety of health-care workers, who are required to report abuse or neglect to the state child-welfare agency and classify failure to report those as a misdemeanor for people other than physicians. Physicians who fail to report suspected abuse or neglect are to be referred for disciplinary action to the state medical disciplinary board.[16] Third, the laws in this state specifically recognize that abuse can occur in settings other than the home and thus acknowledge that health-care professionals might be among those who could neglect and abuse children. Finally, state laws specify the occasions when others may take custody of a child to prevent harm to the child. For instance, a statute specifically provides that "a physician treating a child may take or retain temporary protective custody of the child without the consent of the person responsible for the child's welfare" in order to provide emergency medical treatment (when that treatment is not itself high risk and is essential to prevent permanent harm or death) when there is insufficient time to apply for a court order.

In practice, NICU staff members make three uses of statutes on child abuse and neglect.[17] First, physicians take temporary custody of infants in order to give medical treatments opposed by their parents. Second, as required by law in the state where we conducted this research, physicians and other staff members report evidence of maternal drug use during pregnancy. In this state, the child-welfare department is informed when the results of a drug screening test conducted at birth suggest maternal drug use or when the child has clear withdrawal symptoms (even without a positive drug test). And third, staff members start the process of hearings

15. Specific statutes are not cited here because such citations would reveal the location of our research.

16. State statutes further specify that the body that regulates professions should take disciplinary action against physicians, nurses, and social workers for willful failures to file reports in instances of suspected abuse or neglect and lay out a range of possible sanctions.

17. See Haralambie (1987, 1:584–98, 2:293–298) for a good discussion of statute and case law on medical neglect. The problem of medical neglect is also discussed extensively in literature on informed consent, which is covered in more detail below. Interestingly, much less attention has been given to how child-abuse and -neglect statutes are used by staff members wishing to encourage parents to prepare for the discharge of their hospitalized children. See chapter 5 for a discussion of how the law undergirds the staff's attempts at social control in the NICU.

on custody when the parents of a child who is ready for discharge have not met the training requirements to take the child home.

Whereas civil law is much more likely to be applied to hospital staff members, criminal law is much more likely to be applied to parents. While the likelihood of having the criminal law applied to physicians and other health-care workers is rather remote (Nelson and Cranford 1989; Fost 1989), the charges, should they be made, are quite serious. For parents, in contrast, charges are considerably more likely, though the crimes charged are typically abuse or neglect, not manslaughter. Parents may have a child removed from their custody, and this can be because either the hospital or the state believes that they are truly unfit parents or physicians believe that parental religious beliefs should not prevent a child from getting necessary medical treatment.

The effect of criminal law, through its threat to parents, is thus probably greater than the effect of law that works through its threat to physicians and other health-care providers. In part, this is because an interested party, namely the physician or social worker, acts to bring parent misbehavior to the attention of the law, while parents do not ally themselves with the state against physicians.[18] Further, in at least some states (including the one where we conducted this research), some of the mechanisms needed to translate decisions about withdrawal of life support into legal actions against physicians and parents have not been put into place (Lantos, Miles, and Cassel 1989). And, as we discuss below, with the passage of statutes about surrogate decision makers, some protection is provided even to parents and physicians who decide that life support should be withdrawn.

Regulatory Law

The third category of law that affects the NICU is regulatory law. The relevant laws in this category include those about certification of health professionals and restrictions on who may practice medicine, regulation of the distribution of drugs, laws defining death (in some cases, recently revised to clarify questions about the timing of the harvest of organs, and then extended to apply to when life support may be withdrawn whether or not organs are being harvested), and laws requiring informed consent for med-

18. This is partly because physicians will almost always treat a hopelessly ill or medically compromised infant if that is what the parents wish. Parents therefore do not need the assistance of the law to get physicians to treat infants. See Anspach (1993) and Guillemin and Holmstrom (1986).

ical treatment. This category of law sets many of the ground rules for the practice of medicine and so has mainly to do with the regulation of medical practice rather than the standards of parenting. However, the laws of informed consent, while not granting parents full participation rights, at least guarantee them minimal rights to participate in medical decisions.

Until the mid-1970s, the rules about informed consent were developed almost entirely by the judiciary. Though the consent requirement had long been part of the common-law tradition, more recent cases, such as *Canterbury v. Spence* (1972), had shifted the focus from simple consent to informed consent. This shift, coupled with the medical malpractice "crisis"[19] of the mid-1970s, seems to have spurred medical professionals to press for statutory definition of the requirements of informed consent.[20] Meisel and Kabnick review the statutes of the twenty-four states that enacted informed-consent laws between 1974 and 1977, concluding that though, on balance, the laws did not change the rules much, "they will preclude the possibility of judicial liberalization of common-law rules in a manner that might favor patients" (1980:563); Faden and Beauchamp (1986:140) draw the same conclusion.

In the state where we conducted this research, for instance, a 1979 law establishes a patient's right "to receive information concerning his or her condition and proposed treatment, to refuse any treatment to the extent permitted by law." On many of the central issues of informed consent this statute is silent. No comment is made about who is required to give information about medical procedures and for which ones, whether the standard of disclosure should be a professional or lay one, what elements must be part of the disclosure (must the health-care provider discuss the nature of the procedure, the risks, appropriate alternatives, the benefits of the procedure?), or what exceptions there are to the duty to disclose information. Several other statutes elaborate related points. For instance, another act

19. Lieberman (1981) concludes that the medical malpractice crisis was more a product of insurer practices than of changes in the likelihood that dissatisfied patients would sue.

20. Meisel and Kabnick (1980) offer some evidence of pressure from medical organizations for legislation on informed consent and on other topics related to the malpractice crisis. In some cases informed-consent statutes were drafted by attorneys for medical groups. The American Medical Association drafted a model statute, which Meisel and Kabnick describe as "an example of the unfortunate tendency of organized medicine to view informed consent as nothing more than a legal hurdle to be surmounted by a consent form, rather than a recognition of the fundamental human rights of bodily integrity and self-determination" (1980:561). Other observers tend to agree that most, though not all, medical groups have taken a defensive stance on informed consent (Katz 1984; Schuck 1994).

primarily protects the rights of hospital personnel not to perform procedures that violate their moral or ethical views but is worded to protect the rights of patients to refuse treatment as well. Two other acts deal with questions about who can give or withhold consent. One specifies that for most purposes the consent of a parent is required when the patient is under eighteen years of age but that a patient who is younger than eighteen has "the same powers and obligations as a person of legal age" if he or she is married or if she is pregnant. Further, minor parents are empowered to consent to medical treatment for their own children. In cases of emergency, a physician need not get parental consent to treat a minor. Though it was enacted toward the end of our research, a state law now provides a statutory basis for the termination of life-sustaining treatments without judicial review, laying out who may make such decisions, what procedure should be followed and under what medical circumstances such decisions can be made, and protecting parents and physicians from charges of murder if they decide that withdrawal of life support is appropriate.[21]

Statutes vary somewhat from state to state, but the doctrine of informed consent strikes an uneasy balance between the competing rights of the patient and family to make medical decisions and of the physician to make treatment decisions. Although there is some disagreement about how to think about the relationship between normative statements (e.g., codes of ethics) and actions, most commentators seem to believe that there is a substantial gap between the ideal of informed consent and its practice and that the gap has likely increased with the routinization of informed-consent procedures (e.g., informed-consent forms presented to patients or their families upon admission to a hospital or before major procedures) and with the increasing social distance between physician and patient (Faden and Beauchamp 1986; Heimer 1992b; Katz 1984; Rothman 1991; Schuck 1994).

Anspach (1993) has argued that consent procedures in the NICU do not produce full, informed consent but instead simply fulfill the legalistic requirement of having a consent form signed. The accounts of our parents support this point. One mother described the consent process before her son was transported: "They brought forms in for me to sign, but I was half

21. Two separate state acts, concerning power of attorney and living wills, further protect people's rights to make their own medical decisions. Though these acts obviously do not apply to neonates, they do suggest legislative sympathy with the dilemmas of individuals and families who do not wish to use life-support systems to prolong dying.

unconscious at the time. They made me sign them . . . they told me what it was, but I was so leery . . . and they needed me to sign this right away" (2002F, p. 5). A father felt he was rushed through the procedure of consenting to surgery: "They didn't explain too much to us. They just told us, 'Here, sign these papers. We have to operate right now.' We signed them and they were gone" (1004M, p. 20). Many of the parents we interviewed felt they had very little information at the time their consent was required. Rothman (1991) points out that in previous generations patients received little information and were not routinely asked for their consent, but he argues that the pervasive silence of physicians on the exact nature of a person's illness and possible treatments occurred in the context of a lifelong patient-physician relationship and joint participation in a community. Without such a shared history, physician silence is considerably less acceptable. For one thing, Schuck (1994) argues, without open discussions between physician and patient (or the patient's parents in our case), the physician will not have sufficient information to know what the patient's interests are and so will be unable to fulfill his or her fiduciary obligation to the patient.

This symbiotic relationship between regulatory law and medicine is not new, of course. Indeed, the law contributed much to the institutionalization of medicine long before the laws of informed consent. In practice, regulatory laws often work in tandem with other kinds of laws. For instance, when parental consent is required for medical treatment, parental refusal of medical treatment may constitute abuse or neglect and the hospital can petition a court for custody of the child so that it can provide the disputed treatment. Though consent procedures are important in themselves, they are also significant as one link in the chain of actions by which hospitals use the law to wrest control from parents or by which parents use law against health-care providers and hospitals they believe have mistreated their children. Considerable institutional attention is thus focused on the consent process (see Heimer 1992b) and on documentation that parents have been fully consulted about orders to withdraw or withhold treatment. This does not, of course, mean that all relevant information has been disclosed, that parents have been made to feel comfortable asking "dumb" questions, or that anyone has addressed parents' concerns about how their child will function at age ten or how siblings will be affected by bringing a damaged child into the family. Rules about informed consent, like other regulatory laws, surely play an important role in the life of the NICU—but they do not always serve their manifest function.

Fiscal Law

Finally, what happens in NICUs is shaped by fiscal law—regulations about the expenditure of federal and state monies. Both parents and hospitals are subject to the constraints imposed by fiscal laws. Not every parent is dependent on state subsidies (in the form of welfare checks and medical aid), but every hospital is. The most notorious of the fiscal rules imposed on hospitals are the Baby Doe Regulations and the Child Abuse Amendments to the Child Abuse Prevention and Treatment Act. Based on the 1973 rules prohibiting discrimination against the handicapped by programs receiving federal funding, the Baby Doe Regulations were initially brought to the attention of NICU staff members in a May 1982 notice from the Department of Health and Human Services. However, the Baby Doe Regulations failed to pass court scrutiny, and the Child Abuse Amendments were subsequently passed in 1984 and reauthorized in 1989.[22]

22. The scholarship on the Baby Doe cases and the subsequent regulations is extensive and the history convoluted, involving actions by President Reagan, the Department of Health and Human Services, the Congress, and the state and federal courts. In May 1982, following instruction from President Reagan, the Department of Health and Human Services (HHS) published a notice to health-care providers ("Discriminating against Handicapped by Withholding Treatment or Nourishment") advising them that under Section 504 of the 1973 Rehabilitation Act, it was unlawful for hospitals receiving federal funds to withhold medical or surgical treatment or nutrition from a disabled infant if an otherwise similar infant without the disability would have received treatment or nutrition. In March 1983, HHS published its Interim Final Rule, "Nondiscrimination on the Basis of Handicap," requiring hospitals receiving federal monies to post notices describing federal protection of the handicapped against discrimination and providing a toll-free telephone number to report violations. This rule also provided for on-site investigations by HHS personnel. In April 1983, the Federal District Court for the District of Columbia invalidated the Interim Final Rule because HHS had violated procedural requirements about provisions for public comment. In January 1984, HHS published its Final Rule, "Nondiscrimination on the Basis of Handicap: Procedures and Guidelines Relating to Health Care for Handicapped Infants." This was subsequently invalidated by a lower federal court, and that decision was upheld by the Supreme Court. The court argued that a hospital's withholding treatment when no parental consent had been given for treatment did not violate the 1973 Rehabilitation Act, that the regulations were not based on any evidence of discrimination and were outside the authority of the secretary of HHS, and that the secretary could not dispense with the 1973 Act's focus on discrimination and use federal resources to save the lives of handicapped infants whether or not they had experienced any discrimination.

A second approach, ultimately successful, was to introduce legislation amending the Child Abuse Prevention and Treatment Act. The Child Abuse Amendments of 1984 were first introduced into the Congress in 1982, signed into law by President Reagan in October 1984, and reauthorized by President Bush in October 1989. The statute required that states set up programs for monitoring and reporting on medical neglect, making such programs a condition for receipt of federal funds supporting child protective services systems. In April 1985, the Department of Health and Human Services issued its Final Rule to implement the

All hospitals receive federal funds through Medicare and Medicaid as well as through other programs, and the Baby Doe Regulations used this funding as a lever, on the grounds that hospitals receiving any federal funds were prohibited from discriminating against the handicapped in any of their activities, whether these activities were themselves federally funded or not. A second route, employed after the Baby Doe Regulations were struck down by the courts, uses the lever of federal funding for state programs to prevent child abuse. But the enforcement mechanism is an indirect one—states receiving funds for child-abuse prevention programs are the direct target of the Child Abuse Amendments, and compliance with the federal requirements is a condition for continued funding. Hotlines, threats of investigation, pressure to set up Infant Care Review Committees, and the like all resulted from the application of fiscal law, though some of these mechanisms quickly passed from the scene.[23]

Though the initial effect of these fiscal laws seemed likely to be large, in practice their effect probably has been quite small, for a variety of reasons. Fiscal pressure is a relatively blunt instrument here. For the Baby Doe Regulations, the federal government would have to demonstrate a pattern of discrimination in the NICU before funds could be withheld. For the Child Abuse Amendments, the funds that might be withheld are relatively modest and in any case go to the state rather than to any one hospital. Further, the pressure is being applied to the wrong problem—the bulk of cases in NICUs are not "handicapped" infants but premature ones. And because the strong predisposition of physicians and parents is toward treatment rather than nontreatment in any case, there was no substantial "problem" to be corrected by the regulations and statutes in the first place. In the case

---

Child Abuse Amendments of 1984 ("Child Abuse and Neglect Prevention and Treatment Program"). Under this legislation, Infant Care Review Committees are encouraged but not mandated.

See Bopp and Nimz (1992); Gerry and Nimz (1987); Kopelman, Kopelman, and Irons (1992); Lyon (1985); Newman (1989); Shapiro and Barthel (1986); and Walman (1992) for discussions of these regulations and the very common misperceptions about their applicability to NICU care. The appendix of Caplan, Blank, and Merrick (1992) gives a chronology of the events in the legal history of the 1984 Child Abuse Amendments (though they have misdated the final event in the series). Lyon (1985) provides more detail than most about how key cases unfolded and what happened to families and infants subsequently. He and Harrison (1986) also discuss the case of Brian West, whose medical problems resembled those of Baby Doe, and whose court-ordered surgeries left him in agony for several years before he died.

23. See Fost (1992) for an assessment of the effectiveness of the Infant Care Review Committees.

of parents, fiscal pressure can only be applied to those parents who are dependent on the state for welfare or medical aid. And, in any case, the requirements for receiving funds are based primarily on need and are not used to shape parents' behavior.[24]

The Law as a Tool

Compared with the roles of parents and staff members, the role of the state (or states) in the NICU is hard to understand, partly because it plays numerous roles—as guarantor of relations among strangers through civil law, as protector of the public order through criminal law, as defender of the weak through regulatory law, and as agent of public policy decisions through disbursement of money for authorized purposes. In its various guises, the state defends the rights of children as individuals, mediates between families and medical teams, and regulates the activities of parents and various professions. But the role of the state is even more difficult to understand than this complexity would suggest, because the relevant law is ever-changing, as legislators and judges attempt to make the law speak to the dilemmas created by contemporary medicine. Keeping these difficulties in mind, we can nevertheless draw several conclusions about the role of the state in neonatal intensive care.

While the state regulates the activities of both the parents and the hospital and its personnel, it plays different roles with respect to each of these two main participants in the NICU. Though the state is more rigorous in its regulation of the hospital and it staff, it plays an important role in defining the floor for both acceptable parenting and acceptable medical care. The floor for medical care is somewhat higher than the floor for parenting, however. Civil and regulatory law combine to compel hospitals and their staffs to provide care that at least meets the "standard of care" of the medical community at large. This standard of care is a flexible one that is continually under review as new knowledge is accumulated and reviewed by a community of medical specialists, scientists, and scholars. Hospitals are,

24. Though not enacted during the course of our research, the 1996 welfare-reform measures try to use fiscal law to shape parents' behavior by, for instance, setting limits on the number of consecutive months that a woman and her children can be on the welfare rolls and requiring that recipients either continue their educations or work in order to continue to receive benefits. There has been much debate about the effectiveness of the proposed reforms and about the potentially deleterious effects of ending the state's guarantee of financial assistance to poor women and children. We have yet to see whether a blunt instrument is better than no instrument at all. See Levine (1996) on how poor women respond to pressure to seek employment.

furthermore, situated in institutional networks that include insurers, accreditation bodies, and professional organizations and work in tandem with the law to compel behavior that exceeds the state-specified minimum standard. No law requires JCAHO certification. But insurers require such certification, and hospitals and health practitioners carry malpractice insurance because of the possibility of lawsuits.

Parents, in contrast, not only have lower floors but also have no institutional network to set and enforce a flexible standard of care that exceeds the state-specified minimum standard. The state has few sticks and even fewer carrots to compel parents to do more than simply not neglect or abuse their children. Though the state does grant parents some participation rights in the NICU, it does little to encourage parents to use those rights and must rely on the hospital to inform state agents of suspected neglect or abuse. There is no license to revoke, no job to be taken away, and only sometimes is there any financial pressure to exert (though we have already seen what a blunt instrument such financial pressure can be). And there is no competition in the market for parental services—infants do not look elsewhere if they are dissatisfied with what their parents provide.

Despite this, most parents exceed the state-specified minimum standards. Our task in the remainder of the book is to explore how some parents manage to construct a network that includes those who can supply crucial goods and services that cannot be supplied by the parent alone. In order to secure such crucial goods and services, parents will often have to deal with actors in many different organizations, including pediatricians, insurers, medical equipment suppliers, follow-up clinics, visiting nurses associations, and the like. No actor can behave responsibly unless he or she can intervene in some authoritative way to encourage or coerce others to do their part in a timely and competent fashion. The state provides parents with some authority to coordinate and intervene in the activities of others, like medical professionals, but parents must first define their obligations broadly enough to include supervision of and intervention in those activities. On the necessity of defining responsibility broadly, the state is silent.

If having flexible standards and the capacity to intervene in the activities of others to meet those standards are keys to taking on large responsibilities, then the law figures prominently in both the parents' and the hospital staff's capacities to take responsibility. In the NICU, the law may be thought of as a tool that can be used by either parents or hospital personnel to intervene authoritatively in the activities of the other. Parents have some rights to participate in medical decision making, may refuse some medical treatment, sue hospitals and doctors in civil courts, and alert state agents if they suspect medical neglect or abuse (though this is rare, because insofar as there is a bias, it is toward overtreatment, as we have noted). And hospital staff can take temporary custody of infants to administer emergency medical treatment and have the obligation to alert state agents if there is evidence of neglect or abuse. Though both parents and hospital staff are motivated to use the law as a tool, hospital personnel have a distinct advantage. They are more experienced and competent at its use. Because hospital staffs are made up of experienced, repeat players (often with in-house counsel), they are much more likely to be skilled at using the law as a tool to settle disputes or coerce parents to behave appropriately. Indeed, as the example above of the Jehovah's Witnesses illustrates, the use of the law to take temporary custody of an infant has become a routine hospital procedure. For some parents, in fact, the NICU seems to have become an extension of the state—with unit social workers and state child-welfare workers setting up conditions that must be met before their child will be discharged home.

Parents, in contrast, have no routine procedures for taking legal action against the hospital or its staff. Though in our interviews parents often vaguely alluded to their rights to participate in decisions in the NICU, very few of them used the law as a tool to coerce staff members to do as they wished. Only four parents said that they had thought about suing their child's NICU doctors at one time or another (1026F, 2012M, 2024M, 2025F), but all had decided against doing so. At least three other parents threatened to sue various hospital personnel in order to underscore the seriousness of their wishes for their children's care (2025M, 2033F, 2033M). And one father still intended to sue "the doctors, the hospital, everybody" (1036M, p. 28, also p. 42) because the team at the referring hospital had "left [his son] for dead" (p. 24) rather than treat him or transport him to a facility equipped to manage his grave condition. "They were just waiting for him to die," he asserted, adding that "there was a death certificate made [out], and they were just waiting to put in a time. I don't know if it's in the files or not, but I saw it right there, plain as day, on the desk" (p. 24). Despite angry disputes between hospital staff and parents (many of which are documented in chapter 6), no parents reported contacting lawyers to help them exert their rights in the NICU.

Even though parents are not very skilled at using the law as a tool, physicians are intensely aware of the shadow cast by the law in the NICU and often feel the pressure of the state. Zussman (1992) has argued that ethical questions in intensive care are often superseded by legal questions—physicians ask not "Is it moral?" but "Is it legal?" The argument is that physicians practice legally defensible medicine rather than good medicine or ethical medicine. One of the social workers at Suburban described what she called a "generalized fear" (2012SW, p. 12) of the law that seemed to pervade medical practice in the NICU, especially in the wake of the Baby Doe Regulations and the subsequent legislation. And when the physicians we interviewed described how the law shaped their practice, they tended to focus on malpractice suits. The law, as they saw it, was a tool used by parents against them, not one that also helped them do their jobs. One physician who had recently weathered a malpractice suit commented: "Working here, you have to accept that you are going to get sued. Because when bad things happen, people look for it" (2002MD, p. 26).

And in our interviews with parents, they, too, noted how legalistic concerns seemed to shape the practice of medicine in the NICU. One mother recalled how the consent process before her son's surgery had been shaped by staff members' concern with avoiding blame: "The reality of what could happen is then presented to you by somebody, you know, a resident or whomever the designated bringer-of-bad-news is. They come and bring you a paper to sign which says he could die in this process, and he could get this, and he could have that, and so everything that could possibly go wrong was covered in this piece of paper, so as to make you aware of the fact that anything could go wrong, and they're not responsible, and it scares the hell out of you" (1028F, p. 30). Another mother cited physicians' fears of lawsuits in explaining why she had difficulty getting "straight answers": "Doctors don't like to give me straight answers, I guess, because they were scared of lawsuits. With so many lawsuits against them, I guess they have to be very careful as far as what to say" (2033F, pp. 6–7). The number of lawsuits may, in fact, be relatively low, but because lawsuits are memorable events, the frequency of such suits is probably overestimated.[25] Whatever their frequency, the fact of lawsuits has nevertheless strongly helped shape activities in the NICU.

What we find here, then, is that the use of tools (such as the law) requires both motivation and competence and that participants will likely vary in how motivated and competent they are to employ them. Repeat players will, furthermore, have advantages over novices even if both are

25. The "availability effect" has been amply documented by psychologists. See, e.g., Tversky and Kahneman (1974).

equally motivated to intervene in the activities of the other. Such experienced participants will be more likely to have developed routines to make using their tools easier and to have customized some tools to suit their needs. No tool works well under all circumstances, and so we would expect the tools participants use to vary with their situations. We would expect co-workers or business units in large organizations to manage interdependence differently from what we have described here. The law is the tool that allows parents to intervene authoritatively in the activities of nurses and physicians, but physicians, for instance, intervene in the activities of nurses without calling in state agents or going to courts of law. And parents enlist the support of kin as much by getting them committed to the child as by stressing that they are obliged to help. Which tools work well will depend on the nature of the situation; effective agents must be skilled at using a variety of tools and must know how to choose the tool that best suits the job.

In sum, then, in the NICU both the hospital and the parents have ultimate responsibilities for their patients and their children, respectively. While these responsibilities are in some senses distinct—with the hospital providing medical care that the parents cannot—they also overlap considerably and have the potential to create great conflict. Some of this conflict can be traced to the different scopes of participants' responsibilities: the hospital's responsibility ends quite abruptly at discharge, but the family's continues (and even intensifies) after discharge. Part of the role of the state, as we have described in this chapter, is to determine when each party has the right to intervene. Chapters 5 and 6 take up the questions of how first the NICU and then the parents attempt to shape the behavior of the other. Here, we have demonstrated that the state plays an important role in defining some of the rights and obligations of each of the participants, acting as a referee when conflicts elude resolution, and in some instances providing the tools to take responsibility by granting the limited authority to intervene in the activities of the other. In the next section, we examine how perspectives and jurisdictions shift as the main participants move beyond the boundaries of the NICU after discharge home.

Limited Liability: State and Professional Intervention in the Home

If all goes well, and the NICU patient is discharged home, the obligations of the three main participants shift dramatically. Where once the parents and the NICU staff had an overlapping direct responsibility, now the parents stand alone in their obligation to care for their child. Although other health-care workers may continue to share responsibility for the medical welfare of the child if the child's health remains precarious, it is the parents who now must play the role of case manager, seeking services from the appropriate experts. The state retains its long-term interest in the health and welfare of its young citizens (though with the 1996 "welfare reform" legislation, this no longer includes a guarantee of financial support for its most-impoverished young citizens) but will monitor this with varying degrees of intensity.[26] In a few cases, state child-welfare workers will be alerted by the NICU staff, and patients will be assigned case workers, who will follow up and help make determinations about the parents' fitness. But such continued involvement by the state is relatively rare. Only eight cases at City and two at Suburban were referred to the state child-welfare agency according to the year's worth of medical records we reviewed.[27] Many more parents apply for medical or financial aid, and these parents will have to undergo such scrutiny as is required to demonstrate their eligibility to receive benefits (recall from Table 2.1 that medical records indicate that about 41% at City and 18% at Suburban were without insurance).

Most parents, however, do not apply for welfare or Medicaid and so are not subject to even this milder form of surveillance and evaluation by the state. A different form of surveillance occurs far more often in the form of visiting nurses, who monitor the infant's progress following discharge (medical records indicate that 57% at City and 42% at Suburban had visiting nurses arranged at discharge). The visiting nurses may be requested by hospitals or required by insurers to make evaluations of the health and well-being of the child and the safety and adequacy of the home environment. These visits provide the opportunity for parents to ask questions and receive extra training but also open the door for further intervention if any serious inadequacies are detected by the visiting nurse. While they are not always paid or employed by the state, visiting nurses in fact function as state agents insofar as they are required by law to report cases of suspected neglect or abuse. After a baby's discharge, then, the social control

26. Luker (1996) argues that efforts to control teen fertility by restricting welfare payments are doomed to failure.

27. These numbers undoubtedly understate the numbers of families who received scrutiny from the state child-welfare agency, however. Some parents of NICU infants already had a caseworker assigned to them, so an additional referral was unnecessary. Of course, referrals could come from other sources as well, and while we don't have evidence about this, some referrals were likely made following discharge home.

system that was so intense while the child was hospitalized becomes suddenly quite weak for the vast majority of parents. Hospital staff members and representatives of the state lose much of their capacity to intervene. Parents are sent home with their infants and whatever training they have received from the NICU. But just as in all schools, only some of what is taught by the NICU ends up being useful after graduation, and some of what parents need to know is not included in the curriculum.

Just as schools aspire to "train children for life," so NICUs try to prepare parents to take their children home. Both institutions wish to equip key participants for a more independent existence when they leave the institution. But just as the school is a social system with many participants and goals, so is the NICU. It, like schools and other hospital units, must attend to the interests of multiple clients and cannot legitimately sacrifice the interests of one student or patient to another. Nurses often complain when parents act as though they were unaware that nurses must care for other patients as well. And, just as a school is a work setting for some (teachers, administrators, counselors, custodians, cafeteria workers), so is an NICU. Nurses, physicians, therapists, and social workers want to do their work in a way that reduces emotional burnout, increases the chances of advancement in a career, and the like.

The goal of "training for life" or "preparing for parenting beyond the NICU" then often is sacrificed or deferred in the interest of smooth day-to-day operation of the school or NICU. Though the NICU articulates the goal of equipping parents to care for their children after discharge, particularly in the early phases of an infant's hospitalization, NICU actions do not always match its words. Not surprisingly, NICUs find it more convenient to deal with relatively compliant parents who follow the rules and accept rather passively the role assigned them by unit personnel. But this is not ideal preparation for postdischarge parenting. Unquestioning or passive parents do not learn what they need to know to care for an NICU graduate. As discharge approaches, the NICU stance changes, and parents are expected to become more active participants. Such a change in stance may not completely compensate for the earlier policy. Parents may already have learned to believe that "doctor knows best" and may not have mastered all the details of their child's medical problems. Furthermore, the main textbook on the child's care, the medical record, does not automatically follow the child home. Though medical records often follow a child from one hospital or clinic to another, they cannot entirely fill the gap if a parent must take a child to an emergency room, for instance, or needs to have a more thorough understanding of the medical situation in order to make day-to-day decisions.

The NICU view of the appropriate division of labor between families and hospital staff thus contains a contradiction—parents are supposed to entrust their child to the expertise of the medical staff during the child's hospitalization but also are supposed to be the primary caretakers and act as advocates or case managers coordinating the activities of care providers, therapists, teachers, and even medical workers once the infant leaves the unit. This is a tall order, and not surprisingly, hospital staff members sometimes find themselves grudgingly admitting that parents whom they regard as "difficult" or as "nuisances" will make excellent parents precisely because they persist in making sure their children receive excellent care even when that annoys, insults, irritates, or inconveniences other people. The "best" parents are not necessarily the "nicest." Indeed, loyalty to exceptionally "nice" parents does not necessarily even predict that such parents always will be told about serious errors, as we learned from our observations.

If parents are sent home ill equipped to care for their children, however, the hospital may be found liable. But this concern about liability tends to be occupationally segregated. The discharge planners in both of the NICUs we studied have responsibility for ensuring that any medical equipment that will be needed at discharge has been ordered, supplementary nursing care has been arranged, and parents have been trained and given the resources they will need to care for their child adequately. The job requires that discharge planners take a long-range view in order to limit liability. Although they are the ones who coordinate discharge home, they are not the ones who interact with parents daily in the unit and train them in the skills they will need after leaving the NICU. Discharge planners may hope that parents will be trained to be "responsible," but they often settle for less. They arrange for visiting nurses to "police" parents, sending them out "to check on compliance and to check on the treatment regime" (2010DP, p. 3). Intervening further requires more evidence: "You can't call in [state child-protective services] for something you *think* is going to happen. You have to have more evidence. So if you do everything in the hospital possible and document teaching discussion, and then you get the extra support in the home and that person is observing something, that person has more data then to go ahead and say, 'This isn't appropriate,' or 'This isn't safe. We need to do something'" (2010DP, p. 10). In the end, however, the

NICU has "very little control over" what happens after discharge home (2010DP, p. 9).

Parenting a former NICU patient largely takes place both above the threshold of state concern and beyond the influence of the NICU. Though the state is involved deeply in some parents' lives, most parents must meet their obligations without any further enticements from or prodding by the state. The state demands that parents take responsibility for their children, but then limits its demand to the most rudimentary caretaking. But taking responsibility, as it is commonly understood and as we use it in this book, means something more. From this perspective, then, the state gives parents the obligation to take responsibility but provides few tools for them to do so. With good reason, the state is less able to invade the privacy of the home than to enter the relatively public space of the NICU, and so legal tools become less relevant once a patient is discharged home. A mother who is frustrated by her husband's unwillingness to share the burden of caring for their very needy daughter will find the state unsympathetic (except perhaps in divorce court). As long as the young citizen is not being neglected or abused, the state is relatively unconcerned with who makes what contributions in the household.[28] A father who works, but does not do his share of his daughter's care, is hardly a candidate for neglect or abuse. Parents must employ other tools and call on other resources where the state's jurisdiction ends.

Further, some pieces of the legal apparatus are entirely missing. While we are not urging that parents be tested for competence or required to enroll in continuing education classes, we nevertheless find it noteworthy that there is no evolving and enforceable "standard of care" in the home. Both tort law and regulatory law put some pressure on health-care providers to keep abreast of new developments, to follow protocols for procedures and medications, and to abide by the rules disseminated by insurers. Regular reviews by quality-assurance panels and certification bodies, as well as pressure from hospital risk managers and in-house legal counsel, keep health-care providers on their toes. One can legitimately argue that many of these pressures have counterproductive results and have led to the

28. The state is, by comparison, much more concerned with the division of labor in an organization like the NICU. State licensing for the various professions determines who will be held accountable for what part of the division of labor. Though not all aspects of the division of labor are of concern to the state, of course, certain procedures (like surgery) may only be performed by licensed physicians, not by nurses or therapists.

promulgation of many mindless rules, though it's not obvious what the net effect is.

Some pressure to be a good parent comes from schoolteachers and school social workers, coaches, family friends, and relatives, of course. And many of the parents we interviewed reported learning about parenting from childbirth educators, parenting books and magazines, and pamphlets handed out by pediatricians, as well as receiving instruction from their own parents. But because there are so few analogs to professional training and certification, we expect much more variation among parents than among health-care providers. The state has little capacity either to ensure that parents meet some minimum standard or to encourage advances in the technology of parenting. We find here that tools that work well in one setting may not be so useful in others. While the law, for instance, gives parents a way to intervene authoritatively in the actions of the medical staff—and so, we argue, to take responsibility—this same tool works less well to create rights to intervene in families once a child is discharged home. Though the state continues to provide parents with some important rights of participation in their ongoing interactions with medical personnel after their child's initial discharge home, these interactions are episodic for the vast majority of parents. The rest of the time, parents often do not have the law on their side as they negotiate their interdependence with others whose labor, commitment, or resources they might wish to enlist. And the law does little to support quality control in the profession of parenting. The law is a powerful tool, but not a universal one. Parents (and other organizational participants) must not only have the motivation and the competence to use a tool but must also know when a different tool is required to get the job done.

In the next chapter, we look closely at how the NICU intervenes in the behavior of parents. Here, we note that the NICU has two distinct, but related, concerns about parents' competence: first, as organizational members, and second, as the ones who must care for their patients following discharge home. Though, as we have argued here, the NICU's ability to intervene in the activities of parents is undergirded by the authority of the state, the NICU must also regulate aspects of parental behavior with which the state is unconcerned, for instance ensuring for their own purposes that parents are good organizational participants as well as adequate parents. The NICU has an obligation to produce "responsible" parents, but what it means to be responsible depends on the context. The NICU's definition of responsible is organizationally driven, determined as much by organizational pressures and constraints as by a notion of what the NICU graduates really need. Though the people who work in the NICU are not unconcerned with their patients' futures, organizational pressures make the standard for adequate parenting both lower and more flexible than we might suspect.

FIVE

The Social Control of Parenting in the NICU

As a baby approaches discharge from the NICU, staff members become increasingly concerned with whether the baby's family is willing and able to take over. They are concerned with whether the parents (and especially the mothers) have the skills to provide rudimentary therapies, administer routinely required medications, and discern when the baby needs more expert medical care. But they are also concerned with the commitment of the parents to reorganize their lives to meet the needs of the child. The NICU diagnoses and treats not only the medical problems of the patients, then, but also the social control problems presented by their parents. Much of the social control machinery of the NICU is thus designed to determine which parents are "appropriate" and which are not, to bring "inappropriate" parents up to a minimal level of competence and commitment whenever possible, and to draw on the authority of the state to make other arrangements for the baby's discharge if the parents' behavior cannot be reshaped. Though the hospital staff members are the main social control agents in this case, the legitimacy of the intervention into parenting by the hospital staff is built on the foundation of the legal regulation of parenting through the establishment of minimum standards of acceptable parental behavior (below which parents will be charged with abuse or neglect) and routines for referring particularly inadequate parents to appropriate state agencies.

As we will describe in this chapter, the evaluation of parents is a dominant feature of the social organization of the NICU. As part of this process of evaluation, the labels "appropriate" and "inappropriate" are routinely applied. Such labels appear in notes on the patient and his or her family (the "nursing notes" and the "patient progress notes" written by physicians and other hospital workers), but they are especially prominent in staff con-

A version of this chapter was previously published by the authors as "Interdependence and Reintegrative Social Control: Labeling and Reforming 'Inappropriate' Parents in Neonatal Intensive Care Units," *American Sociological Review* 60, no. 5 (1995):635–54.

versations and in meetings about patients—"rounds," in which physicians discuss patients; "report," in which nurses turn over patients to the nurses on the next shift and summarize their cases to the charge nurse; "social service rounds," "interdisciplinary rounds," or "discharge planning rounds," in which a variety of professionals discuss the group of patients one by one; and "patient care" meetings, or "staffings," called to discuss problematic cases.[1]

When parents are inappropriate, the social control machinery of the NICU is set in motion, and attempts are made to resocialize parents or, in the extreme, to marginalize them by removing the child from the parents' custody. Inappropriate parents may still end up taking their babies home, but their infants may stay in the hospital longer (e.g., because the staff does not believe that parents can manage complex care routines), the child may go to a foster home temporarily (e.g., while a mother goes through a drug-treatment program or finds adequate housing), or the family may receive state-supported services (e.g., visits from a visiting nurse or "homemaker" services to teach parenting skills while helping with the housework).[2]

There are also less extreme consequences of not being labeled a "good" parent. For example, those who are not considered good parents are less likely to be consulted about their preferences, and their suggestions about what might help their child are treated with less respect. Nurses are less likely to coordinate with them so that they can feed or bathe the baby. They are less likely to hear about minor as well as major events in their child's medical course. And their attempts to care for the child are more likely to be viewed as interference.

Much of the normative order of the NICU that shapes the roles of parents is governed by formal rules and routines. Many parents find these routines sensible and are motivated to follow them not only to gain access to their babies but also because they understand that the rules are designed to protect the patients (e.g., from infection). These formal procedural rules are quite accessible to parents, but many other elements of the normative order of the NICU are less so: no sign explains that "you must bond with your baby." Although it is evident whether a parent has scrubbed and gowned, it is less clear whether a parent has "bonded." This less formal,

1. Guillemin and Holmstrom (1986, esp. pp. 76–77) discuss social service rounds at "Northeast Pediatric," the hospital whose NICU they studied.

2. Guillemin and Holmstrom (1986, esp. p. 182) also discuss staff members' evaluations of families and their attempts to provide supports through referrals to protective services, visiting nurses, and the like.

less accessible part of the normative order is where parents stumble across the boundary between appropriate and inappropriate and where the social control machinery is set in motion.

Many of the rules that govern NICU life derive much of their force from external bodies. This is as true for posted rules about gowning or hand washing as for the more inchoate rules about how parents should interact with their babies. Although violations of formal rules and routines lead to consequences for the NICU or the hospital, violations of the less accessible rules lead to consequences for the parents. Hospital accreditation depends on careful attention to rules handed down by such organizations as the American Hospital Association. Because these instructions address medical matters, which vary relatively little from hospital to hospital, they may be expressed in formal rules. The less accessible rules about parental behavior are important because negative assessments of parents may lead to delays in an infant's discharge or to involvement with the child-welfare agency. But because these rules are about parenting rather than medicine, they are less clearly articulated and much more likely to vary from one setting to another.

Norms about interaction with the infant and preparation for discharge are based partly on everyday notions of what constitutes adequate parenting (and so vary, as we will discuss, with other parental traits), partly on professional assessments of what kind of parental behavior is required for child development, and partly on laws about neglect and abuse of children. Rates of maternal drug use and neglect (in the NICU this means not visiting or telephoning the NICU, or not being available to give consent for medical procedures) vary from hospital to hospital, and the explicitness of norms about visiting and preparing for the baby's discharge vary correspondingly. As staff concern about the adequacy of parenting rises, norms are more likely to be spelled out either in checklists, formal rules, or individualized contracts between the parent and the staff.

Although the social control system of the NICU is tethered to the laws of the state and implicitly (and sometimes explicitly) employs the state-based threat of removing the child from its parents' custody, the NICU must also regulate aspects of parental behavior with which the state is unconcerned. The less formal, less accessible part of the NICU normative order thus mainly governs parental behavior that is either above the state-specified minimum standard or is deviant in ways that inconvenience NICU staff members but do not jeopardize the welfare of the child. State law (e.g., about child neglect and abuse, maternal drug use during pregnancy, and requirements for financial support) and federal law (mainly about medical care for disabled people) nevertheless provide an important foundation for social control in the NICU.

This chapter, then, is fundamentally about learning and teaching how to parent, and about the evaluation of parenting skills. Alice Rossi (1968) observed that there is not much anticipatory socialization to parenthood. There is even less for an unanticipated transition to parenting a critically ill infant. In our research, we learned how nurses, physicians, social workers, therapists, and other hospital staff help define the role of "parent of sick newborn," educate parents about the norms associated with that role, and reward or punish parents for their responses. Labeling parents appropriate or inappropriate is a central part of this socialization, because labels tell staff members how much and what kind of instruction parents need and whether they are worth the investment.

Ordinarily child care goes on in private and without any particular instruction in how it ought to be carried out, and many people believe that wide variations should be tolerated because parents should be free to raise their children as they see fit. But the issue of how child care ought to be carried out cannot be ignored in the crisis situation of the NICU. When infants are critically ill, the range of behavior that constitutes "good-enough parenting" shrinks. By examining such a crisis situation, we can learn how parental behavior is assessed and how meanings are assigned to it. What we learn here tells us a great deal about the process of assigning meanings more generally—about the importance of first impressions, about the effect of background expectations in influencing labels, about how organizational uses of labels and meanings make labels more malleable than one might expect if they reflected only stereotypes, about the negotiation of labels between various assessors, and about the relative power of various assessors to alter, remove, or firmly affix labels.

More important, however, we learn what is accomplished by the assignment of labels. We argue that it is an important part of a quasi-legal system that collects and sifts evidence, administers sanctions, and even develops new "legislation," all the while keeping an eye on the demands being made on the meager teaching and resocialization resources of the NICU. Labels are part of a process of deciding whether something has to be done (Kitsuse 1972; Emerson and Messinger 1977), and negative labels mark people for exclusion or for remedial attention. Labels are applied differently in systems that can evict deviants than in ones that must reform them. Groups that must reintegrate a high proportion of reformed deviants must apply labels more judiciously and selectively. We argue that because of the inability of NICUs to control their borders and because of the interdependence between medical care providers and parents, most social control in the NICU is reintegrative rather than disintegrative (Braithwaite 1989).

The organizational setting of the NICU offers us a first glimpse of the obligations of parenting a sick child. What it means to take responsibility is defined in part by the parents themselves, along with a healthy dose of intervention from the NICU staff. The advantage of studying responsibility here is that the standards are relatively unambiguous (even if it takes parents some time to discover them). As we will describe below, parents are expected to visit, show appropriate concern, ask appropriate questions, and master the skills necessary to take their infants home. These minimum standards of parental responsibility are constructed by the organization because the organization has an obligation to ensure that its patients are discharged to homes that are equipped to care for them. Most parents exceed these minimum standards, but others must be coerced into compliance through the use of contracts that detail their obligations and threaten consequences for failure, including removal of the child from the parents' custody. "I definitely use it [the threat of a report to the child-welfare agency] as a lever sometimes," one social worker said. "It sometimes has some beneficial effects that way, to motivate people, to take things a little more seriously or consider some types of actions that maybe they wouldn't have otherwise" (2012SW, interview 3, p. 21). The threshold of compliance with these minimum standards in the NICU is not very high, as we will argue. Ironically, the NICU discourages parents from taking much more responsibility. As we will describe here and in the following chapter, parents who intervene too often or too vigorously in medical matters will be labeled "inappropriate." What is essential for the long term—taking the child's welfare seriously, setting goals, and using discretion to meet those goals—disrupts the smooth functioning of the NICU. The NICU has an obligation to produce "responsible" parents. But the hospital obligation has its limits—parents need to be sufficiently responsible that the hospital cannot be held liable, but not so responsible that they will feel compelled to oversee the NICU staff.

We begin the chapter with a discussion of the main categories of parental failure as judged by the NICU and provide illustrations of each. Although all parents can fall short in these various ways, they are not all judged by the same standards—parents are judged by standards that vary with age, gender, social class, and race and ethnicity. We consider these variations in the next section. In the third section we discuss the process by which labels are affixed to parents, noting that it entails considerable sorting, comparing, and reinterpretation; evaluation of the reputations of those attempting to affix labels; and a gradual formation of consensus about the parent being labeled. Consensus forms more easily about some kinds of labels than about others. Finally, we develop some theoretical lessons from this study of social control in NICUs, and comment on the constraints imposed on labeling by the institutional context in which the NICU is embedded, before we return to an assessment of the relationship between labeling and the production of responsibility in the NICU.

Defining the "Inappropriate" Parent

The label "inappropriate" covers a broad range of behaviors. Sometimes parents are labeled because of the quality of their relation with their child. For instance, the NICU staff deems it inappropriate to show little interest in holding or touching the baby; not to look at or talk to the baby while holding it or sitting at the bedside; to have either a "flat" affect or a very strong emotional reaction after some period of adjustment; not to visit regularly or to spend too much time in the NICU; not to telephone regularly or to telephone too often; to talk about the baby's discharge when discharge is unlikely or not to plan for discharge at all; not to learn routine baby care and simpler medical routines; and not to provide such routine care as diaper changes during visits.

Parents may also be labeled because of their relations with the staff. For example, it is inappropriate not to ask any questions of staff members or to question medical and nursing judgments too vigorously. Parents may also be labeled for an inappropriate appearance or demeanor. In our research, this included exceptionally well-dressed mothers who were unwilling to hold babies, who tend to spit up; mothers dressed in tight or revealing clothes; parents who argued, including some who got into physical fights in the unit; and parents who had consumed alcohol or other drugs before visiting. While this list is certainly not exhaustive, it does represent the broad range of behaviors that may be labeled "inappropriate" in the NICU.[3]

3. The correspondence between our observations and Guillemin and Holmstrom's (1986:176–78) bolsters our argument that definitions of appropriate and inappropriate are strongly shaped by organizational forces. Many items in our list were gleaned from an interview with one of the social workers. Others came from weekly social service or discharge planning rounds and from our observations of the daily life of the NICU. Although staff members use the words *appropriate* and *inappropriate* (and use them often), they also convey

Though nearly any extreme behavior could be labeled "inappropriate," in fact hospital personnel focus their attention on two main kinds of deviance. Parents and families may be labeled "inappropriate" either by disrupting the smooth functioning of the hospital unit or by behaving in ways that suggest they will not be able to care for the baby at discharge. A negative label thus alerts others to a staff member's doubts about the parent's ability to care for the baby or about his or her capacity to fit smoothly into the routines of the NICU. And labels may be applied either to behavior or to people (see also Braithwaite 1989). When we combine these two dimensions (evaluation of behavior vs. evaluation of person; evaluation of bureaucratic competence vs. evaluation of competence as a parent), we observe four types of inappropriate labels.[4]

We argue that the consequences of a label—the staff responses to the labeled parent—depend both on what specific parental actions and staff assessments of those actions led to the label and on whether it is applied to the whole person or only to some of the person's behavior. Typically labels are applied initially to behaviors, and then, if hospital personnel conclude that they are seeing a behavioral pattern rather than isolated instances of misbehavior, the label later becomes attached to the person.[5] But staff members are more persistent in remedial efforts when the problem is parental competence than when the problem is disruption. Table 5.1 provides a conceptual map for the rest of this section, where we discuss the links between these four categories and the consequences that flow from

---

these judgments with many other words and phrases, some quite colorful and some specific to the parents being evaluated.

4. Hospital personnel do not themselves describe their labeling practices this way. These are our analytic categories, and we have supplied category labels that capture the judgments and sentiments expressed by staff members. They make all of the pairs of distinctions we discuss (as is shown in our examples), but they do not say that they are using two dimensions and hence four separate categories. Our observations and interviews suggest instead that our typology is implicit in staff members' labeling practices.

5. The process by which parents are labeled strongly resembles the one by which patients are selected for treatment in outpatient psychiatric clinics (Garfinkel 1967:208–61). Just as patients must "survive" from one stage to the next if they are to go through the next step in the psychiatric career, so too in the NICU a negative label is first attached to behavior and only later applied to the person if that person is not in the meantime dropped from the pool of people about whom staff members are concerned by reforming, offering excuses, etc. Further, the process by which actions are interpreted is very much in line with the "documentary method" that Garfinkel (1967:76–103), following Mannheim, describes: "by waiting to see what will have happened [one] learns what it is that [one] previously saw" (77) and in this instance decides whether the problem lies in the person or only in the isolated act.

Table 5.1 NICU staff responses to parents by assessment of the problem and whether behavior or the person is labeled

	Label and Staff Response	
Problem	When Behavior Is Labeled	When Person Is Labeled
Inadequate parenting	The Remediable Parent	The Inadequate Parent
	Staff teaches parenting skills; stimulates commitment to child	Staff raises questions about whether child should be discharged to parent's care; documents parent's behavior; occasionally transfers custody
Disruption of NICU work	The Nuisance	The Pain-in-the-Neck
	Staff attempts to teach NICU rules; provides parent less information and attention.	Staff ostracizes parent; provides much less information and attention.

being placed into one category rather than another.[6] After briefly illustrating the four categories we discuss generalizations to other settings.

Four Categories of Inappropriate Parents

The remediable parent. The remediable parent is one whose behavior, especially early in the baby's hospitalization, suggests that she (or, less often, he) knows little about parenting. For example, we observed one unmarried, teenaged African-American mother at City Hospital who asked to remove her son's nasogastric feeding tube to photograph him. She complained that she wanted a "normal" picture of her baby "without all that junk in his nose." The baby's nurse scolded the mother and explained that the tube was essential for feeding and should not be removed and reinserted for trivial reasons. Though some of the mother's behavior was regarded as inappropriate, the mother herself was not classified as inappropriate because she otherwise gave considerable evidence of eagerness to learn about the child's disabilities and the care he would need at discharge. She visited frequently, cared for the baby, read books about Down's syndrome as she rocked her son, and otherwise behaved as a model mother. Because this

6. See Van Maanen's (1978) parallel analysis of police responses to affronts and challenges.

young mother responded to the staff's attempts to teach her and to encourage her commitment to her child, the initial, tentative label had little further consequence.

The inadequate parent. The inadequate parent, in contrast to the remediable parent, seems unable or unwilling to respond to staff attempts to teach parenting skills and encourage commitment. An unmarried, nineteen-year-old, African-American mother who rarely visited her premature son during his sixteen-month hospitalization at City's NICU is an example. Initially she was discussed in neutral or favorable language. Though she visited only eight times during the first six months of her son's hospitalization, her failure to visit was explained by difficulties arranging transportation from her home in a nearby state and by her responsibility for the baby's siblings. A resident's off-service note written in the child's medical chart early in his hospitalization summarizes the situation: "Mom has three-year-old twins at home and it is very difficult for her to visit often. However, she does maintain phone contact and is very involved in [her son's] care. She does not have a phone. When we need to reach her, we have to go through a neighbor's phone and sometimes it does take several days, so plan in advance for consents [for medical procedures]."

Over the months, the reports became more negative. Early favorable reports that the mother "is involved and keeps in contact by phone" were replaced by ones that she "never visits," "is very uninvolved," and "has been out of touch for a month at a time." The social worker made numerous attempts to contact the mother, including sending letters to urge her to visit and eventually sending the local police to her home with a message to contact the hospital. One year after admission, the social worker's terse conclusion appeared in the medical record: "Repeated efforts to engage mother have been unsuccessful." The mother visited three times in the last nine months of her son's hospitalization, without a single visit between his first birthday and the four months until his discharge. When he was eventually discharged to a chronic care facility in the state where his mother lived, he was dependent on oxygen and a ventilator. The child-welfare agency in his mother's home state had been contacted about the mother's lack of involvement, but the mother retained custody at the time of discharge. Several months later, the child was declared a ward of the state.

The move from remediable parent to inadequate parent in this case illustrates a typical pattern. Generally speaking, early disapproving comments on isolated actions are coupled with assessment and, often, acceptance of the parent's excuses. Staff members express hope that the parent will respond to attempts to teach parenting skills and encourage commitment. If the disapproved behavior recurs and excuses are made too frequently or come to be disbelieved, then the parent is reclassified as inadequate.

The nuisance. In contrast to the preceding labels, the label "nuisance" assesses a parent's competence as an organizational participant rather than as a parent. A nuisance is insufficiently respectful of the work routines of the NICU. When isolated instances of inconsiderate, insensitive, or disruptive behavior occur, staff members use such transgressions to teach parents how to be well-behaved organizational participants, as the following example shows. Two white, married mothers of very premature babies developed a firm friendship over the months spent at their sons' adjacent bedsides at Suburban Hospital's NICU. As they visited, they discussed their babies, pregnancies, and childbirth experiences. When one mother was not there, the other would check on the child of the absent mother and telephone her. But this practice was unacceptable to the hospital staff, and after one of the babies moved to a different section of the unit, checking on the friend's child was perceived by the staff as even more intrusive.

The "problem" was discussed among staff on the unit in terms of the "disruptiveness" of the parents' conversations to others in the unit and the inappropriateness of asking staff to breach norms of patient confidentiality with invasive inquiries. These otherwise appropriate parents were generally well liked, were clearly committed to their children, and visited the unit regularly. But the frequency of their visits only fueled the problem. Eventually, the nursing staff drafted a memo instructing parents to respect patient confidentiality and to refrain from loud and disruptive bedside conversations. The memo was taped to each patient's bed and was also added to the admission packet.

This example illustrates not only how otherwise exemplary parents can become nuisances as they disrupt the NICU but also how the NICU generates rules to manage such disruptions. The boundaries of inappropriateness are not fixed but may change over time as new rules are generated and others fall out of use. Written rules have the advantage that they can be retrieved when needed and seem to apply universally, not just to the parents causing the "disruption." No doubt parents will continue to share their experiences, but when this is "disruptive to the unit," offending parents may be reminded of the rule. Expectations often become clear only when they have been violated, and this particular violation led to clarification of an ill-articulated norm that parents should mind their own business while on the unit. But the strategy of creating new rules to manage nuisances has limitations; it is more effective in managing problems with particular behaviors than with particular persons.

The pain-in-the-neck. The pain-in-the-neck repeatedly disrupts the NICU workflow. Often pain-in-the-neck parents are simply excessively demanding, suggesting that they have little sense of staff members' overall workload. What are regarded as excessive demands may be tolerated for a time, but they may eventually lead to staff alienation. One married, middle-class, white couple, who had finally conceived with donor sperm after six years of infertility, were devastated when their infant son was diagnosed with a genetically based syndrome that resulted in low muscle tone. The prognosis varied from dismal to uncertain, and the situation was complicated when the mother also was diagnosed with a mild form of the disease.

The mother sat at her son's bedside in Suburban's NICU nearly all the time, and the father visited when he was not at work. Unwilling to believe that hospital routines were sufficient, the parents demanded almost continuous attention for their child. Even after several weeks, the parents suspiciously demanded explanations and sought a second opinion from a neurologist at another hospital. The mother was thought to have a "strange affect": she rarely smiled, focused on the "negative," and generally did not engage in the small talk that makes NICU life tolerable. The father occasionally yelled at staff members as they carried out routine procedures, and the mother complained that she was being avoided and her son neglected. The physicians, who had made a point of discussing matters frequently with the mother, were mystified. Although the nurses did not linger at the bedside after completing the infant's care, they certainly did not believe the quality of his care was being compromised. In this case, then, both parents were labeled "inappropriate," although some distinctions were made between them. And while staff sympathized with the parents, nurses and therapists were reluctant to accept the stressful assignment of caring for this child. In the end, nearly all agreed that these parents were pains-in-the-neck.[7]

Generalizing Inappropriate Categories to Other Settings

As these cases illustrate, the assignment of a parent to a particular category may be temporary. Tentative judgments are revised over time and parents

7. See Guillemin and Holmstrom (1986:177), who describe a similar case of a demanding mother who was convinced that the nurses were not attentive enough. This mother also ended up alienating staff members. Also see our discussion below of "Mrs. Croft."

reclassified.[8] As information accumulates, staff members talk more about the person's traits than about his or her behavior. In an organization with a stable population, few participants would continue to be judged primarily by their behavior, and few cases would be located in the left column of Table 5.1. But the NICU has a transient population, and the continuous stream of new entrants means that judgment is ongoing. Not all organizations are like this, of course. Our expectation is that organizations with high turnover will distinguish more carefully between judgments about behavior and judgments about people, although long-term participants may conclude that their increasingly firm judgments about particular individuals are the result of new participants "settling down" rather than of information accumulating. We believe this distinction between judgments about actions and about persons to be a common one.

We also believe the distinction between evaluations of disruptiveness and those of competence in the main business of an organization is a common feature of organizations. Which behaviors will be labeled and how and to whom labels will be applied depend on the organizational context, as Emerson (1969, 1991, 1992) and others (e.g., Waegel 1981; Gilboy 1991, 1992) demonstrate. Categorization and labeling processes are context sensitive, because they simultaneously provide markers and explanations and suggest subsequent courses of action. Classification is constrained by the resources available in a particular context and by the possible courses of action. But our evidence suggests that the argument of Emerson and others that classification and labeling systems are organization specific needs to be qualified. Insofar as all organizations try to minimize disruption and will punish participants who fail to follow organizational rules, classifications and labels applied to deviants will reflect this universal organizational problem.

While there will certainly be variation among organizations in what constitutes disruption and in organizational capacity to manage disruption, all organizations will apply negative labels to disruptive members. The "organization man" (Whyte 1956) or woman may get some limited rewards for being a team player, and because learning and following the rules bring rewards in a variety of settings, we might expect a positive cor-

8. See Hawkins (1983) on the reassessment of labels by parole boards. Emerson also sees labels as provisional: ". . . moral character is not determined permanently and irrevocably at any one time. Rather, an initial assessment holds 'until further notice' (Schutz 1962), subject to revision as circumstances and issues change while cases move through the court" (1969:100).

relation between receiving rewards in one setting and receiving them in another. At the most basic level, in quite a range of organizations, people who are prompt will be met with more goodwill than those who are habitually late. But organizations also evaluate the competence of participants in the main business, and unskilled participants will get fewer rewards than those who perform the central tasks well.[9] Because such tasks vary from organization to organization, what is being evaluated also varies, and evaluations of competence in different organizational settings will be less highly correlated. Skill in noting when a baby is having trouble breathing, for instance, is rewarded in only a few organizations.

The larger institutional context also shapes evaluations of participants' competence in the main business of the organization by specifying standards of performance in some cases and reinforcing organizational sanctions with state sanctions in extreme instances of nonperformance. The institutional environment can be expected to have a larger effect, then, when some authoritative outside body (such as a regulatory agency, a standard-setting body that makes assessments for insurers, or a professional organization) sets performance standards and when outside bodies control some rewards and punishments that depend on performance. Legal sanctions for parental incompetence do not figure importantly in the lives of most parents, though the possibility of being denied custody of one's child may haunt even "good" parents if they somehow come to be misclassified by NICU staff members.

In this section we have discussed the contrasts that underlie the four types of labels, arguing that with appropriate adjustment for empirical differences these four categories should occur in other settings as well. We have shown, then, what organizations are doing when they label participants. On the one hand, they are distinguishing labels according to how much information exists about the person being labeled—greater uncertainty makes for more tentative labeling of acts rather than more decisive labeling of whole persons. On the other hand, organizations evaluate two distinct aspects of participants' performances, their competence as members of organizations and their competence at the central tasks of the organization.

Labeling actually does much more than this, because it is a key mecha-

9. Both McCarthy and Hoge (1987) and Bowditch (1993) found that schools interpreted misconduct in the light of a student's academic record. Competence in the main business of the organization may well shape reactions to otherwise disruptive behavior in other organizations as well.

nism used by hospital staff to encourage parental responsibility. Staff have quite a sophisticated understanding of why they place so much emphasis on competence in parenting and are therefore able to couple labeling with programs to instruct and reform inadequate parents. Their analysis of why competence as organizational participants is important is less fully developed, though, and they therefore have invested much less in developing techniques for teaching these skills. As we argue in the closing sections of the book, however, responsible parenting does require that parents be skilled organizational participants who are able to function just as well in hospitals or schools as in the home. If labels are mechanisms to encourage parental responsibility, they are at the same time mechanisms to manage the organizational workload. The result, as we show below, is a compromise between getting the work done and encouraging responsible parenting, and some categories of parents therefore receive more attention than others.

Variable Standards: Stereotypes, Normal Cases, and Organizational Agendas

In the NICUs, we often heard statements about parents followed by qualifying phrases such as "given her situation" or "given everything they've been through." The elements of these qualifiers are gender, age, marital status, ethnicity or race, social class (especially educational level), employment situation, and obligations to care for other children. Inappropriate, then, really means "inappropriate for someone in your situation."

In this section, we consider how parents are sorted into categories and how this affects the judgments that are made of them. We argue that NICU personnel use standards that vary with the characteristics of the parents. Just as public defenders' strategies depend on whether a burglary is a "normal burglary" (Sudnow 1965) and child-protection workers "[incorporate] the notion of 'normal for this local culture'" (Dingwall, Eekelaar, and Murray 1983:84), so staff members' expectations and responses are shaped by their notions of how a "normal parent" from a particular social group ought to behave.[10] Any given pair of parents passes through the unit only

10. In her book on professional assessments of parental competence in the fields of child protection, adoption, divorce, and infertility treatment in Great Britain, Campion (1995) presents a different view. Campion argues that in all of these fields, assessments are rather rigidly grounded in middle-class understandings of parenthood. There is some variability from one field to another, though, because what it means to be a fit parent depends on which professions dominate the decision-making process. Legal definitions of parental fitness dominate in divorce cases, for instance, while social work definitions dominate in adop-

once, but their case is evaluated in the context of a specific NICU; cases are therefore deeply interdependent. We suggest that the behavior of staff members is influenced both by their stereotypes about particular social groups and by organizational constraints (Emerson 1983), some of which come from outside the organization. Here we disagree with Emerson (1992). While such organizational pressures as the scarcity of resources affect labeling and attempts to shape parental behavior, initial impressions still depend on quick, stereotyped reactions to parents' traits. The traits used to form the judgments in this case are drawn from familiar, readily available classification systems used in the culture at large for evaluating and ranking social groups.[11]

The pressure of organizational business—here, the ultimate dependence of staff members on parents to take their children home—forces staff members both to employ different standards for different categories of parents and to differentiate among members of categories.[12] Ironically, these pressures lead to an unusual result. Labeling theorists generally have

---

tion cases. Because there are no explicit criteria for parental fitness in any of these areas, though, decisions about fitness are idiosyncratic, because they depend on a particular professional's views on parental competence, and inflexible, because they are based on middle-class standards of parenting. Campion looks at several groups especially likely to be labeled as "unfit" parents—working mothers, nonwhites, teenagers, unmarried parents, and people who are disabled, mentally handicapped, drug addicted, or gay. She proposes a "job description" for parenting that is less biased in favor of middle-class standards, suggesting how to build in the sort of flexibility and respect for cultural variability that we argue already exists in NICU decision making (and that Dingwall, Eekelaar, and Murray [1983] suggested already existed in child-protection work in Great Britain).

11. By putting parents into categories by age, marital status, race, etc., staff members are to some degree reversing the process that we described earlier: they categorize people first (This is an unmarried mother) and then consider their actions afterward (This behavior is—or is not—up to the standard that we expect of an unmarried mother).

12. We believe that organizational time horizons are also a crucial variable here. Gilboy cites one immigration inspector's comment that "if you ignore these kinds of generalities, you become a poor inspector," and another's that "it sounds like prejudice, but it's just experience talking" (1991:585, 594). The pressure for quick decisions makes essential the reliance on generalizations about easily identified groups. But these generalizations, though sometimes related to popular stereotypes, are strongly shaped by particular organizational purposes and are typically used mainly in the first stage of a multistage sorting and labeling process. Gilboy's immigration inspectors generalize about which country's citizens alter their passports, Emerson's judges generalize about how race and poverty affect recidivism rates of juveniles, and NICU staff members generalize about which ethnic group's members twist the arms of young fathers to care for their infants. And in all three cases, additional information is collected to verify initial impressions.

But while Gilboy's primary immigration inspectors have to make quick decisions, NICU staff members can modify their views about particular families over the days, weeks, or

argued that members of disvalued groups are disproportionately likely to have negative labels attached to them (Becker 1963:12; Paternoster and Iovanni 1989:363–75; Matsueda 1992:1588). Here, although overall parents from underprivileged or disvalued groups are somewhat *more* likely to be labeled inappropriate, they are *less* likely to be labeled *for the same behavior.* Parents are only labeled and pressured to reform when they fail to reach the threshold considered "normal" for their group (see Dingwall et al. 1983).

We should note here that the NICU definition of "inappropriate" with respect to competence in parenting skills is by no means a harsh standard. Babies will not be sent home to parents who have not learned to administer required medications or simple therapies, but parents are not required to have even a rudimentary understanding of child development (so, for instance, we were cheerfully informed by one sixteen-year-old white care provider that her "nephew," who had spina bifida, was no trouble to care for because he didn't move around much [1018]) or physiology (another white couple left their very disabled son in a baby seat for long periods even though this was adversely affecting the development of his spine [1036]), let alone any notions about providing extra stimulation to overcome deficits. The standard is a minimal one, and parents will be labeled "inappropriate" only if there is well-founded doubt, shaped partly by the legal system, about whether a child is likely to be neglected or abused.

Lower Standards: No Tests or Lower Passing Grades

Though many of the articulated norms are about how parents should behave (e.g., that they should bond with the infant, visit and phone regularly,

---

months of the infant's hospitalization. Emerson's (1969) court personnel render some decisions on the spot, but the sorting of youths is a two-stage process, and some youths reappear in court many times. In the NICU, where the average patient stays about three weeks (see Table 2.1), generalizations about social groups serve mainly as a signal that additional information should be collected on organizationally relevant matters. Even in immigration inspections, though, Gilboy (1991, p. 582) argues that the inspection "unfolds" as initial impressions formed by the primary inspector are either confirmed or disconfirmed by the secondary inspector and notes that some decisions are not made on the spot but instead are postponed.

We believe, then, (1) that organizations are likely to draw on popular stereotypes but to use primarily those aspects of stereotypes that are relevant to the organization's business, (2) that over time organizations develop their own generalizations about social groups, (3) that organizations in which contact between decision makers and clients is brief will rely more heavily on generalizations about groups, and (4) that organizations are likely to have specialists whose job is to do finer screenings and to refine labels after other workers have done a coarser sort.

and exhibit a variety of emotional responses including affection, anxiety, and some anger), in fact the norms apply more stringently to mothers than to fathers. Hospital personnel often label mothers "appropriate" or "inappropriate," but fathers are much less likely to be labeled at all. Put simply, mothers are judged and sanctioned when fathers are not. Gender therefore plays a somewhat different role than other traits in the evaluation of parents, a finding that should not be surprising given the argument of chapter 1.

Parents are sometimes asked to account for inappropriate behavior, or they may volunteer excuses. But mothers are expected to have excuses in situations in which fathers need none, and more excuses are accepted for fathers than for mothers. Fathers will not be telephoned if they fail to visit a newborn, especially if the parents are not married, while mothers will always be telephoned. If a social worker is told that the father does not visit because hospitals upset him, very likely no further pressure will be applied; a mother would be expected to visit despite her discomfort with hospitals.

For some purposes parents are treated as interchangeable, and the father may be excused because the mother can substitute. Either parent can legally consent to medical procedures if the parents are married; otherwise the mother's consent is required.[13] We might then expect that married mothers would be allowed more excuses than unmarried mothers. In fact substitution of fathers for mothers only rarely occurs. Instead the mother's participation is treated as mandatory and the father's as discretionary. In one extreme case, when the mother was recovering from gallbladder surgery, staff members considered delaying the discharge of a married couple's baby rather than releasing the infant to its father. If the father appears alone, meetings with physicians are sometimes rescheduled for a time when the mother can attend as well. Such meetings would take place as planned if the mother appeared alone. A mother who fails to show up for meetings is therefore behaving inappropriately; a father who fails to appear is not.

This tendency to use different standards for different groups is interesting for two reasons. First, though the general finding is that members of

13. Legal rules about matters such as which parent can consent to medical treatment are incorporated into the routines of the NICU. These rules enter the NICU culture in a variety of ways, including through review of NICU procedures by risk managers or members of the legal department and "in-service" training sessions on legally related subjects. Of course sometimes medical people are misinformed about the law, and hospital legal departments tend to adopt risk averse interpretations.

Table 5.2 Discussions of families in "social service rounds" and "discharge planning rounds" at City and Suburban Hospitals (percentage of cases in which mothers were discussed, fathers were discussed, and no family members were discussed)

	No. Meetings	No. Families	% Mothers Discussed	% Fathers Discussed	% Families Not Discussed
City	64	1290	67.6%	40.4%	22.8%
Suburban	33	1021	29.4%	16.3%	70.0%

Note: The number of families is a total of instances in which families might have been discussed. For instance if Baby Jane Doe had been in the NICU for three full weeks, her family would be counted three times because it could have been discussed three times. A family with two or more infants in the NICU is counted once for each meeting at which it could have been discussed. A mother or father is counted as being discussed if either the parent is discussed individually (as in "the father . . . ") or a comment is made about "the parents" or "the mother and father." Fathers are rarely mentioned alone (only 6 of the 166 mentions of fathers at Suburban Hospital are discussions of fathers without comments on the mothers), while mothers are quite often discussed alone. At Suburban Hospital, there are no discussions of other family members without discussions of mothers and/or fathers. Discussions of other family members without discussions of mothers and/or fathers sometimes occur at City Hospital.

disvalued groups are more likely to be labeled negatively than members of other groups (Matsueda 1992:1588; Paternoster and Iovanni 1989:363–75; Becker 1963:12), here we find, if anything, the opposite.[14] Groups whose members would ordinarily be especially likely to be negatively labeled are not much more likely to be labeled deviant in the NICU and in some cases are quite unlikely to be labeled at all. "Everyone knows" that "kids" do not know how to care for babies, and young parents are assessed in the light of this knowledge. Because "everyone knows" that young African-American women live disorganized lives and have few resources, evaluations of them take this into account. Because expectations for men differ from expectations for women, fathers are less likely to be labeled "inappropriate" than mothers. By and large, men are simply not labeled. As Table 5.2 shows, in the interdisciplinary rounds fathers are often entirely ignored. About 40% of fathers are discussed in social service rounds at City, and only about 16% of fathers are discussed in discharge planning rounds at Suburban.

Second, because labeling is part of the process of teaching parents to care for their critically ill infants, variations in labeling lead to variations

14. Emerson (1969) tends to agree with our conclusion that social control systems are not always biased against disvalued groups. He found that the juvenile court differentiates between the "respectable" and the "disreputable" poor.

in attempts to reshape parents' behavior.[15] Differences in the labeling of mothers and fathers thus translate directly into differences in remedial efforts. If absent mothers are pressured to visit hospitalized infants and absent fathers are not, this in turn means that mothers are more likely than fathers to get information about the baby's condition and to be taught to care for a child with special needs. Even when both parents are taught, mothers are expected to learn more than fathers. Mother-child ties receive more scrutiny than father-child ties. Not being labeled inappropriate means not being punished but also not being resocialized to different behavior. Such neglect is welcomed by some fathers, but others resent assumptions that their skills and relation to the baby matter little.[16]

Similarly, a young African-American mother is less likely than an older white mother to be labeled "inappropriate" for infrequent visits. Staff members assume, perhaps with some justification, that a young, unmarried African-American mother will be assisted by her own mother (although Kaplan [1996] notes that such grandmothers are sometimes quite disapproving of their daughters' motherhood). But since this young mother is not negatively labeled, she is not pressured to visit more often and therefore has less chance to learn skills thoroughly or to glean information about child development or the management of feeding problems from a physical therapist or speech therapist as she visits her baby.

The starting point for the evaluation of what is appropriate or inappropriate is, in short, a standard oriented to older, middle-class mothers. Staff members know from their own experience what a middle-class married mother needs to care for her child adequately. They know how much help she needs from the father, when extra training is necessary, and when spe-

15. Another finding is that negative labels tend to act as self-fulfilling prophecies (Matsueda 1992; Paternoster and Iovanni 1989:375–86). Our evidence here is mixed. It suggests, we argue below, that to the extent that labels shape expectations for behavior, they do tend to act as self-fulfilling prophecies. Fathers are not expected to behave like mothers. But labels are also cues that trigger action aimed at resocializing deviants, and to this extent, they are not strictly self-fulfilling. Inappropriate young mothers are at least expected to learn to behave like appropriate young mothers.

16. Evidence for this differential treatment of mothers and fathers comes mainly from interviews with parents, though staff members also commented on fathers' reactions. One unmarried, unemployed, nineteen-year-old black father had not been contacted when the baby's mother failed to meet discharge requirements. The father was furious that he had not been informed that his disabled daughter was to go to a nursing home. Over the opposition of some nurses, he learned to care for the baby and took her to his mother's home in a housing project. One male staff member noted that the NICU is a "very female environment" (1007DP, p. 6), in which some men feel extremely uncomfortable.

cialists are needed. They are also aware that other people lead different lives and should be judged by different standards. But when nurses, doctors, or discharge planners conclude that it is unreasonable to judge a young, unmarried mother by a standard appropriate for an older married mother, they do not always ensure that the baby gets equivalent care even if that care arrives by a different route. Though they may verify that the mother lives with the grandmother before concluding that the mother's infrequent visits are not a matter of concern, they may not check how many other people require the grandmother's attention.[17] The implicit checklist for appropriate parenthood continues to be organized around middle-class mothers. Staff members' understanding of cultural differences in parenting may not lead to the use of alternate checklists to verify that "inadequate" mothers are paired with "adequate" grandmothers or partners with sufficient time, expertise, and interest to ensure that the baby gets care. Nor do staff members adjust their routines to engage, teach, and evaluate fathers, grandmothers, and other potential care givers.

But, as we discuss further below, labels are not just detached evaluations. They also affect the distribution of scarce goods, in this case triggering the expenditure of social control resources.[18] Inappropriate parents need to be brought up to the threshold. But the variable standard means that once parents reach the standard "appropriate" for "normal" parents in their category, scarce resources will likely be spent on something else. The lower the expectations for the normal parent in a given category, then, the lower the threshold to which such a parent will be raised before expenditures cease. There is of course an absolute minimum, but, as we have already noted, it is rather low.

Two processes are at work here. Standards can be low either because people are not evaluated (Heimer 1984) or because, though they are being evaluated, the "passing grade" for their group is low. In the NICU gender affects evaluation differently than other parent traits do. To overstate, gender determines whether one is tested at all, while other characteristics af-

17. For instance, nothing in the medical record suggested that when we arrived to interview one mother, we would also find the child's aunts and uncles, the grandmother, great-aunt, great-grandmother, several unrelated adult men, and a roomful of children. In this case the great-grandmother, not the grandmother, assisted with child care (1024).

18. Resources for medical care are also scarce, and negative evaluations of parents and families sometimes also influence the course of medical treatment. Guillemin and Holmstrom (1986) suggest that this was the case for "Darlene Bourne," and at both hospitals we were told that infants without intact families are not considered for heart transplants.

fect the standard to which women, who are the only ones tested, are held.[19] The low standard for fathers, then, is the result of not being "tested," while the low standard for young mothers comes about by a lowering of the "passing grade" to take account of the general incompetence of youth. Though the outcome is similar for young mothers and for fathers—expectations are low and resources are not expended to raise them to the level required of older, middle-class mothers—we argue that it comes about through different processes. Young, minority, or uneducated women are tested but held to a lower standard; men are less likely to be tested at all.

Because fathers are regarded as backups, it seems wasteful to expend resources just to provide redundancy. Realistically, the mother will be doing most of the care (so staff members respond when asked), and one should worry about her commitment and competence. The mother's response to the query "Who is going to be your backup?" then determines who will get whatever training is available for the person providing redundancy. How much redundancy is needed depends, of course, on the child's health, how much care is being provided by the mother, and whether there is funding for nursing care. Married mothers will usually not be asked about their backups, but an unmarried mother will be asked even if the father is involved. Often the backup is not the father but the maternal grandmother. From the hospital's point of view, then, fathers are nearly irrelevant backups in two-parent families, or completely irrelevant nonparticipants in single-parent families. Either way, expectations for fathers are low, and few resources are expended to equip them to care for their babies.

Disvalued Groups and Differential Standards

We have asserted that poor, nonwhite, unmarried, and very young mothers are not any more likely than richer, white, married, and older mothers to be labeled inappropriate once we take account of differences in behavior. Further, we have asserted that because of the variable standard applied to mothers in different categories, those who fall into "disvalued" groups will in fact be less likely to be negatively labeled if they misbehave (and will receive more credit if they behave well). These claims are supported both by our field observations and by simple quantitative analyses of evidence

19. Our point about testing does not apply to assessments of competence in special medical care. Both the primary and a designated secondary care provider may receive CPR (cardiopulmonary resuscitation) training, for instance, but the general skill and commitment of the secondary care provider tend not to be assessed.

from medical records and weekly interdisciplinary meetings where patients and their families are discussed.

In our fieldwork, race and ethnicity, often coupled with class, are frequently used to explain parental behavior. As we have described in chapter 2, the NICUs in our study have quite different patient populations: City Hospital serves a more ethnically and racially diverse population and treats more public aid patients than Suburban. Because of the comparative homogeneity of Suburban's NICU parents, we should expect the processes described in this chapter to appear in more muted form at Suburban than at City. But in both cases, expectations are modified by what NICU personnel know of a racial or ethnic group. For instance, alleged cultural norms about postpartum maternal seclusion were used to explain the infrequency of a Cambodian mother's visits during the first month.[20] One Hispanic couple visited their surviving premature (and now blind and mentally handicapped) twin for two years before she went home. The mother was seventeen and the father fifteen when their twins were born. Staff members accounted for the father's continued involvement by invoking his ethnicity: only a Hispanic fifteen-year-old would still be involved after two years, they repeatedly told us. Apologizing for "spouting stereotypes" as he discussed this particular case, the discharge planner assured us that in his experience the stereotype about Hispanic parents really did hold up (1007DP, p. 5).

Very young parents are likewise held to different standards than older ones. If teenage parents pay too much attention to the baby's appearance, this may be forgiven as a correlate of immaturity. Young parents get as much formal instruction but get less informal socialization to parenthood, partly because they are less likely to reciprocate with friendly banter. One nurse confided in an interview that she disliked young mothers "treating the baby as if it were a toy, and not seeing the gravity of the situation" (1006RN, p. 2). Young parents are also less likely to ask questions. To some degree, they treat hospital staff as authority figures, rather like teachers, whom they should avoid whenever possible. In a formal interview, one attending physician commented on his discomfort with very young parents whom he sometimes found "snippy" and "hostile" (2001MD, p. 18).

Unmarried parents create some discomfort for staff members. Some of this discomfort arises simply from staff disapproval of out-of-wedlock births, but staff members often are uncertain about the stability of the tie between the parents. Only through delicate inquiries—about whether the

20. When we asked one nurse how she came to know about such alleged cultural norms, she responded that "anybody who knows anything about their culture knows how they are."

parents plan to marry, whether the conception resulted from a fleeting encounter, and how to treat new "significant others" when separated parents both wish to be involved with the baby—can staff members determine whether they should treat the father as a permanent fixture of the family.

Social class shapes evaluations of parental behavior by both shaping expectations about parenting styles of people of different backgrounds and providing a range of acceptable excuses. For instance, poorer parents who cannot visit frequently either because of obligations to the infant's siblings or because of distance will be treated more tolerantly than others, because staff assume that richer families can afford to hire sitters to care for siblings, will have cars and drivers' licenses, money for a hotel or meals, and perhaps even sympathetic employers. When families lack these resources, they will be forgiven if they telephone frequently and visit regularly, if infrequently. Impoverished families may find it hard to meet even these reduced requirements.

Hospital staff have difficulty determining how much of behavior that looks disorganized or erratic (e.g., announcing by phone an intention to visit and then never appearing) can be accounted for by a shortage of resources, cultural differences, marital instability, or youth and whether any of these predict the adequacy of care a baby will receive at home. A key task for staff is to sift evidence about parental competence and to come to consensus about whether a mother (or perhaps a father) will do an adequate job.

The "Labeling Conversation"

The label ultimately attached to a parent is the result of a complex, multistranded conversation with a large number of participants and exists primarily as a part of the oral tradition of the unit. To understand how labels are affixed to NICU parents, we observed as many parts of this conversation as feasible, attending meetings and talking with and watching staff members as they worked. But while close observation yields understanding of the process by which staff members collect and sift evidence and come to conclusions about particular parents, some sacrifice in generalizability is inevitable, and we have supplemented our field observations with data from other sources. These other sources provide data on fragments of this labeling conversation.

To support our argument about the variability of standards, we need information about the characteristics of mothers (age, marital status, race or ethnicity, and social class), the mother's behavior, and the label that ultimately is attached to her. These data are available in different places. Information on age, marital status, race or ethnicity, and social class (crudely measured by whether the family has health insurance) are available in the medical record. Some information about behavior is also available in the medical record, both in nursing notes (which are written every shift) and in comments written by social workers (sometimes as a routine matter, sometimes when problems arise) and physicians (especially as off-service notes). Information about these independent and intervening variables is sometimes discussed in social service or discharge planning rounds but often is omitted or alluded to obliquely. Information about the core dependent variable, the label ultimately assigned to a mother, is available in any systematic way only in social service or discharge planning rounds. Such summary assessments only rarely appear in medical records; global summaries exist almost exclusively in the oral tradition, and inscriptions in the medical record are limited to more "objective" and defensible comments on behavior, such as whether the parents are visiting and learning to care for the baby. (Comments do include assessments of whether the parents have "bonded" with the baby or seem "emotionally invested" or "attached.") To address our argument, we therefore need to combine these conversation fragments.

Though our total number of cases in the quantitative analysis is quite small, the results lend some support to the conclusions we drew from field observations.[21] First, we find that the more disvalued statuses a mother has (dummy variables for being younger than twenty, uninsured, unmarried, and black were summed), the less likely she is to be evaluated positively in a social service meeting.[22] The correlation is −.475. This correlation fits the

21. As noted in chapter 2, at each hospital we collected evidence from the medical records of all infants admitted during a one-year period. Because medical records were available for our use only after a patient had been discharged and because we wanted to interview parents whose infants had already come home, we were constrained to collect data from the records of patients who were no longer hospitalized. Given these constraints, the time periods covered by our fieldwork and our medical records data overlap only at City Hospital and only for a two-month period. We thus have both medical records and evidence from social service rounds for two months' admissions as well as for patients admitted earlier who were not discharged before the date on which we started fieldwork. The yield is relatively small for a variety of reasons: some meetings were canceled; infants hospitalized only briefly often did not get discussed, because no meeting occurred during the baby's stay; and babies considered patients of other services (e.g., surgery) rather than of neonatology were discussed only perfunctorily in social service rounds.

22. We have coded evaluative comments (e.g., "*nice* mom" or "she's really inappropriate") on a scale from −2 to +2, assigning a 0 to instances in which the mother was men-

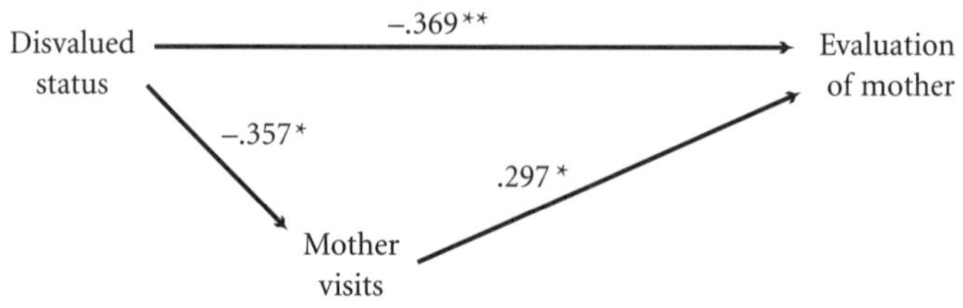

FIGURE 5.1. Path diagram showing direct effect of disvalued status on evaluation of mother, controlling for mother visits. (Standardized coefficients; forty-eight cases; adjusted R^2 = 271; *$p < .05$, two-tailed test; **$p < .01$, two-tailed test)

standard labeling argument perfectly, and so contradicts our argument. But, as we show in Figure 5.1, when we control for the mother's behavior with a measure of the proportion of days that the mother visited her hospitalized infant (drawn from the nursing notes), the direct standardized relationship between disvalued status and positive evaluation decreases to −.369.

A second measure of maternal behavior, coded from the comments of physicians and social workers, is only available for twenty-two cases.[23] These twenty-two infants were sicker and had longer hospital stays than the average City patient, and we would therefore expect staff members to be particularly concerned to evaluate the competence of their parents before sending such "involved" infants home.[24] For these families the labeling process is both more developed and more important. When we restrict our analysis to the twenty-two cases for which all data were available, the results provide some support for our argument, as we show in Figure 5.2. When we control for the proportion of days that mothers visited their infants and the physician–social work assessments of several aspects of behavior, a mother with more unfavorably ranked attributes is in fact slightly more likely to be viewed positively (with a direct standardized relationship

tioned but without any accompanying evaluation. When a mother was discussed in more than one meeting, we averaged the codes.

23. Physicians and social workers commented in the medical record on whether the mother was in contact, generally following hospital rules and routines, providing routine baby care when she visited, and learning to provide the special care her baby would require at discharge. Because comments were not made about all of these items in all cases, we averaged the behavioral assessments, producing a scale that could vary from −1 to +1.

24. The mean stay for City NICU admissions is 23.2 days, and the mean Apgar score (a scale ranging from 0 to 10, measuring the health of a newborn) at one minute of age is 5.9; for the subgroup of forty-eight infants, the corresponding means are 59.6 and 5.1; for the twenty-two infants, the means are 79.5 and 4.3.

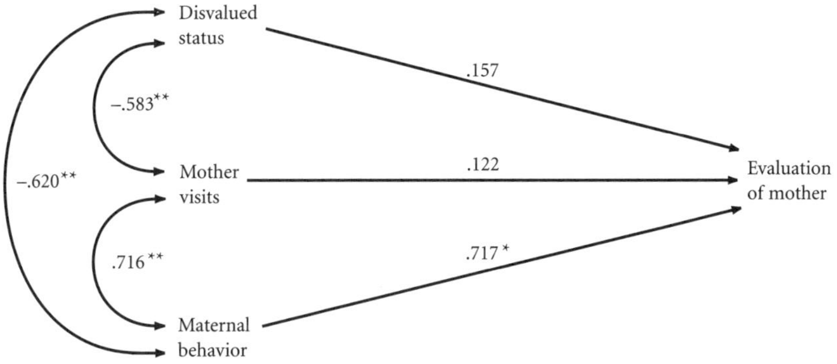

Figure 5.2. Path diagram showing direct effect of disvalued status on evaluation of mother, controlling for mother visits and maternal behavior. (Standardized coefficients; twenty-two cases; adjusted $R^2 = .438$; $^*p < .05$, two-tailed test; $^{**}p < .01$, two-tailed test)

of .157) than one with fewer disvalued attributes, though this result is not statistically significant. This result dovetails nicely with our argument that expectations for maternal behavior vary with the attributes of the mother. If less is expected of young, black, poor, or unmarried mothers, as evidence from our fieldwork suggests, then when they visit as often as older, white, richer, or married mothers, they would be evaluated more positively for these same actions. Correspondingly, if a young mother did less routine baby care or was slower to learn how to administer medications than an older mother, she would be less likely to be labeled "inappropriate" because she was doing fine for "someone in her situation." Our quantitative data also provide some support for this argument—at least in this small group of cases, lower status mothers are not any more likely to be negatively labeled than higher status mothers.[25]

The Negotiation of Labels

Much work on social control decision making assumes a degree of uniformity and consensus that is highly misleading. Our research suggests in-

25. Alternatively, staff members may devalue minority babies and accept lower standards for them. Our small case base prohibits a rigorous test of this hypothesis by, for instance, comparing age and race effects. Our observations suggest, though, that the primary nursing system would undermine tendencies to devalue minority babies. Nurses usually choose their "primaries" and become advocates for "their" babies. When mothers are absent, nurses are sometimes stronger advocates, because their standards need not be adapted to parent preferences. If anything it is minority children (and perhaps minority parents), not

stead that the construction and maintenance of the boundary between "appropriate" and "inappropriate" is a complex task, involving considerable negotiation among organizational participants. We have argued that the line between appropriate and inappropriate in the NICU is not fixed but varies with the traits of the parents and how those characteristics are thought to bear on the organization's main business. Just as Anspach (1993) finds tremendous prognostic conflict in medical decision making, so we find tremendous conflict in social control decision making. As reputations are assaulted and defended, staff members dispute what and who are really appropriate and inappropriate and how the staff should respond. Contact with parents is unequally distributed among staff members, and, as we discuss below, we observe occupationally based variations in participation in remedial efforts. Becker (1963) argues that social control requires both motivation and resources, and here occupational groups differ in how motivated they are to contribute to the social control of parents. Such variations are important because, in the diffuse social control system of the NICU, a firm consensus is essential for successful reintegration (see Braithwaite and Mugford 1994).

As readers will recall from our discussion in chapter 2, nurses have the most direct and sustained contact with both the patients and their parents. They communicate with parents about the baby's progress, interact with them while they visit, teach them both routine and special baby care, document visits and interactions, and evaluate parental competence. This kind of intense, direct contact with parents places nurses in the center of negotiations. Although physicians have some direct contact with parents, they often rely on nurses' assessments. In contrast to clinical decision making, where nurses' direct observational data are regarded as inferior to the physicians' technological data and clinical experience (Anspach 1993), nurses have a near monopoly over the kind of information that is most valued for social control decision making.

Among physicians, residents have the most routine contact with parents. But while residents rank higher than nurses in the formal hierarchy, they have little influence in social control decision making. Residents lack both clinical and social control experience, and they are not sufficiently integrated into the NICU social system to be privy to the conversation that rounds out the written record. Evaluations carry more weight when placed

minority infants, who are disvalued—staff members' much lamented myopia about the future (Anspach 1993; Guillemin and Holmstrom 1986) here leads them to think of babies as essentially devoid of future social status.

in the context of other cases, so having a reputation as a good judge depends on access to the collective memory of the NICU. Because residents have only brief rotations in the NICU, they play a peripheral role in the construction of labels. Despite this, residents are central to the maintenance of labels, as their off-service notes communicate a summary evaluation of parents to those who follow.

Social workers also play an important role in social control decision making.[26] Whereas nurses and physicians focus on the patients themselves, social workers are assigned the task of keeping families' social problems from interfering with the delivery of medical care (Heimer and Stevens 1997). Social workers talk with parents both at the baby's bedside and in the privacy of their offices. They console devastated parents, make contact with those who cannot visit in person, and encourage parents to begin planning for the future. But their work is oriented to their colleagues as much as to patients' parents. Social workers also make assessment of parents, noting how well they are coping with the early crisis and gauging their capacity to manage the care of their infants after discharge. These assessments are recorded in the patient's medical record and are also shared orally at weekly interdisciplinary meetings, where each patient's discharge status is discussed. Social workers are regarded as repositories of information about cultural variations in parenting practices, neighborhood variations in rates of illegitimacy, and racial and ethnic variations in age at first birth and number of children per family, and in both of our research sites, their judgments carried considerable weight as negotiations unfolded.

In general, we find that successful participation in social control decision making depends on both tenure in the unit and the amount and kind of direct contact with parents. Occupationally based variations among nurses, physicians, and social workers in contact with parents tend to place physicians—and especially residents, because of their short tenure—on the periphery of social control decision making. But because nurses, physicians, and social workers have different relations with parents, they are likely to come to different conclusions about them as well. Task-based occupational differences among staff in what they consider inappropriate lead to variations in consensus about labels. For example, a physician might think a parent's queries inappropriate because they question the

26. The authority of social workers varies from one NICU to another. Guillemin and Holmstrom (1986) found that social workers were often excluded from discussions and meetings and that physicians relied more on nurses' assessments of parents.

physician's competence, while the nurse and social worker might reason that the parent's questions reflect appropriate concern. Such dissensus is characteristic of organizations where evaluations are made by many participants with structurally distinct points of view.[27] Disagreements are to be expected, then, because labels have different implications for different organizational participants.[28]

Here we return to our typology of evaluations and observe that consensus varies with whether an act or a person is being labeled and whether organizational competence or competence as a parent is being evaluated. Because judgments about many individual acts are aggregated, there is usually more consensus about the evaluation of persons than about the evaluation of isolated acts. Further, our research suggests there is likely to be less consensus about whether parents are disruptive than about whether they are incompetent. Dissensus about organizational competence has two sources. Because they do different jobs, different staff members experience and evaluate parental misbehavior in quite different ways. Not surprisingly, they may then be differently motivated to reform disruptive parents. And while staff members are constrained to come to a collective, accountable decision about competence as a parent, parental disruptiveness is managed on a more ad-hoc basis and only rarely requires a collective decision.

When we add these two sources of dissensus together, we find least consensus about the nuisances, whose actions are occasionally disruptive or inconsiderate. Therc is likely to be more agreement about remediable par-

27. For example, see Gilboy (1991:592) on task-based occupational differences in assessments of travelers.

28. Readers may notice that while we have discussed how parents' demographic characteristics affect how others think of them, when we turned our gaze to staff members, we have discussed only their occupations. Wouldn't the demographic characteristics of staff members affect their interactions with parents? Might African-American nurses be less likely to hold stereotypic views about African-American parents, for instance? Might staff members communicate more easily with parents with whom they shared an ethnic or racial heritage, decreasing the extent to which staff members presented a united front and made collective assessments of parents? Such questions are hard to answer with the data we were able to collect. Given that we observed and interviewed fewer staff members than parents, that those staff members fall into several occupational categories, and that gender and racial/ethnic groups are not equally well represented in all occupational categories, we cannot speak authoritatively on these issues. Further, we believe that occupation probably dominates demographic characteristics in shaping staff assessments of parents for the sorts of reasons that Burawoy (1979) discusses. Burawoy argues that race matters relatively little once people enter the factory setting (although it has profound effects on who gets those jobs in the first place). In the NICU we would expect the most important divide to be between parents and staff members. Whatever their other characteristics, staff members face parents with the trappings of authority—they are *staff members* with authority over parents' newborns.

TABLE 5.3 Variations in consensus about labels

Consensus about dimensions

Dimension	Amount of consensus: Less	Amount of consensus: More
What is being labeled?	behavior	person
What leads to labeling?	organizational competence	competence as parent

Consensus about categories of parents

Low consensus	Moderate consensus	High consensus
"nuisance"	"remediable parent" "pain-in-the-neck"	"inadequate parent"

ents or pains-in-the-neck, although the higher consensus is produced in different ways. Staff members are moderately likely to agree about remediable parents, because it is parental competence that is being evaluated even though acts rather than persons are being labeled. In contrast, the moderate consensus about pains-in-the-neck comes from making an assessment of a person, as a reputation consolidates, rather than of isolated actions. Finally, staff members are most likely to agree about "inadequate parents," because the assessment both concerns parenting skills and is a summary judgment of the whole parent rather than of isolated acts. We summarize these conclusions in Table 5.3.

Although some disagreement about what constitutes "good-enough" parenting is still likely, our argument is that a consensus is quite likely to be generated not only because the standards are more likely to be stable across occupational groups but also because decisions about parental incompetence are more consequential—both for the parents and for the NICU staff. In essence, staff members are attempting to make predictions about the sorts of variability that we assessed after the fact in chapter 3. They want to know who will be responsible parents and, more important, who will not. Standards are especially stable and consensus especially high where the legal system impinges on the NICU. As we have noted above, rules can and do change over time, sometimes as a direct attempt by staff members to manage inappropriate behavior. But other rules are less malleable, and the solid and abiding consensus about such behaviors as drug use during pregnancy, failure to visit, and neglect of infants is reinforced by formal legal sanctions attached to these acts or omissions. The intrusion of the law, therefore, sharply curtails the capacity of the hospital staff to hold members of different groups to vastly different standards.

We have argued that a consensus is more likely to be generated under some conditions than others. We want to emphasize two features of this process. First, initial observations and evaluations of parents' behavior lead to summary conclusions that parents are either appropriate or inappropriate. During this period, both parents and staff members construct accounts for parents' allegedly untoward behavior, and identities emerge from negotiation among key participants about the credibility of such accounts (Scott and Lyman 1968). Whether an account is credible depends on the background expectancies for various categories of parents. As we have already demonstrated, different accounts are deemed credible for fathers than for mothers, and for younger, single mothers than for older, married parents. But many accounts are constructed by staff members as they negotiate about parents' identities rather than by the parents themselves. Whether an account is credible, then, also depends on how parents' identities are articulated by the NICU staff.[29] And second, because parental reputations have careers, the same behavior observed at different points in a baby's hospital stay may not have the same effect. A parent long categorized as "appropriate," will not immediately be relabeled for an "inappropriate" act. Behavior also tends to be interpreted in a manner consistent with the summary label. As Hawkins observes, "Labels of deviance are at once plastic and persistent" (1983:125). The following case from our fieldwork illustrates the difficulty of generating a consensus, and below we consider the consequences of this difficulty.

Mrs. Croft: "Concerned Mother" or "Lunatic"?

Mrs. Croft, a middle-class African-American woman in her mid-thirties, gave birth prematurely to her first child, Donna. (Mrs. Croft's relationship with the staff was unusually distant and formal. Although many parents were called by their first names, Mrs. Croft was not.) Donna was trans-

29. One nurse, for instance, assured other nurses that a mother was very involved even though she did not visit frequently, explaining that she lived at some distance, had no transportation, and had another small child. The primary nurse also posted notes, written as if from the baby, instructing staff members about parental wishes: "Mommy loves me and wants to be called every day at 10 A.M." The good press from the primary nurse very likely had some effect, particularly on other nurses who cared for the infant, but the family was still labeled "inappropriate" during social service rounds. An alternative strategy, which was used in the case of Mrs. Croft (described below), is to continue treating the family as if they have not been negatively labeled.

ported to City Hospital's NICU for complications associated with prematurity and was treated for severe seizures and other neurological problems that resulted in low muscle tone and difficulty feeding. Over the course of Donna's hospitalization, Mrs. Croft was the subject of many heated discussions, and by the time the baby was discharged, Mrs. Croft had been labeled by some a "pain-in-the-neck," by others an "inadequate" parent, and by many as both. Even her few allies conceded that she was a "nuisance."

Mrs. Croft was very attached to Donna and became so anxious about her daughter's condition that she was reluctant to go home—even to sleep. The NICU has a multipurpose "parent room" where parents are permitted to stay in extreme crises. Defining Donna's hospitalization as a crisis, Mrs. Croft took over the parent room. Clerks, nurses, and physicians resisted, insisting that the room had to be available for other parents as well. As a result, an ill-defined policy about the use of the parent room quickly became more formal. But the nearly daily need to reassert the policy with Mrs. Croft created considerable tension.

While some staff accounted for Mrs. Croft's behavior by describing her as extremely committed, others complained that she made excessive demands. Jane, Donna's primary nurse, gradually became overwhelmed by the mother's demands. As evidence, Jane complained to other nurses and one of the researchers that the mother telephoned to check on her daughter twelve times during a single night—an incident that she believed summed up this mother's demanding nature. Other nurses doubted the report. Calling to check on the baby is in itself appropriate, but calling too frequently was disruptive and was furthermore a sign of distrust. According to Jane, efforts to reshape Mrs. Croft's behavior had failed. When she continued to make excessive demands on staff time and attention, Jane began to describe Mrs. Croft as a "lunatic" who did not fully comprehend the seriousness of Donna's condition. When told that her daughter might remain in a vegetative state, Mrs. Croft claimed that she might "win the lottery" and Donna would recover fully, a response that seemed unrealistic to Jane. Increasingly exasperated, Jane explained that the mother's excessive demands affected Jane's ability to care for Donna and her other patients and in addition were evidence of Mrs. Croft's inability to take account of Donna's needs.

Not all staff agreed with Jane's assessment of Mrs. Croft. Among those who argued that Mrs. Croft was simply concerned and committed was Cathy, Donna's regular evening-shift nurse. Jane publicly ostracized Cathy for her disagreement: "She doesn't know what the hell she's doing anyway. I don't think she'd know a pulse drop herself if she saw one. She's not even an RN yet herself." By dismissing Cathy's assessment as that of a novice, Jane attempted to rally support for her own definition of the situation and to enlist other staff in marginalizing both Cathy and Mrs. Croft. Although Jane was largely successful, one clinical nurse specialist, disagreeing with the group's assessment, continued to interact with the mother as if she were behaving rationally and appropriately, listening to her concerns and frustrations with empathy.

The tension peaked in a clash over Donna's feeding protocol. In consultation with Donna's physicians, the speech therapist decided that because of a prolonged difficulty coordinating suck and swallow, Donna should be fed through the NG tube, receiving only one feeding by bottle a day. Mrs. Croft, however, disagreed. She believed that feeding Donna through the tube would delay her discharge because she would not learn how to take a bottle. Jane and the other staff explained to Mrs. Croft that the danger of pulse drops (a consequence of Donna's difficulty swallowing) had to be weighed against the delay in her learning to bottle-feed. Mrs. Croft insisted that Donna could take a bottle; Jane countered that Mrs. Croft underestimated the seriousness of the situation. Mrs. Croft yelled at Jane, charging that she was undermining her right to make decisions about Donna. When the shouting subsided, Jane had resigned from the case. Because staff members disagreed about Mrs. Croft's competence and because discharge can be delayed only when there is incontrovertible evidence that a parent will not be able to manage, Donna was eventually discharged to Mrs. Croft, who had in the meantime become estranged from her husband and was living with her own mother.

Labels about behavior and labels about people are obviously intimately related, but this example illustrates how conclusions about competence as an organizational participant may influence conclusions about competence as a parent. Sometimes staff believe that reluctance to accept hospital rules or staff members' advice has implications for the parent's ability to care for the child. Mrs. Croft's commitment to her infant was undisputed. But her refusal to accept the consensus about a feeding plan, for instance, led to questions about her ability to parent. Many staff members concluded that Mrs Croft's inability to fit into the unit or accept the baby's medical situation were indicators of her poor judgment and poor social skills, and that she would be an inadequate mother despite her commitment to the child. In this case, the mother, and not just her behavior, was judged inappropriate, and inappropriate on both grounds.

Negotiating a Consensus

In this section, we have argued that social control is an organizationally complex task involving considerable negotiation about assessments of behavior and the corresponding accounts. The boundary between appropriate and inappropriate in the NICU not only varies with the characteristics of the parents, then, but is also contestable, as the case above illustrates. Hospital staff members have a stake in labeling parents, as labels flag parents who may make trouble and alert other staff members to the need to document the inadequacy of truly incompetent parents so that they will get extensive teaching and extra assistance at home.

An important characteristic of the NICU social control system is its decentralization. Many different organizational participants interact with parents and assess their parental and organizational competence. Evaluation is decentralized, as is control over the corresponding social control resources. In the case above, staff members spent considerable time discussing and debating whether Mrs. Croft was behaving appropriately given the seriousness of her daughter's illness, her commitment to Donna, and the tension created by her own health problems and the dissolution of her relationship with Donna's father. When Jane could not enlist the support of her associate nurse on the evening shift, she eventually resigned from the case. The lack of a consensus about Mrs. Croft meant that there were few remedial efforts and that those attempts were met with contempt. When social control resources are distributed widely throughout the organization, then effective social control is difficult without a firm consensus.

Resocializing and Marginalizing Inappropriate Parents

Braithwaite (1989) argues that social control mechanisms can be designed either to marginalize or to resocialize and reintegrate the offender. He characterizes much of the response to deviance and crime in the United States as disintegrative, but we believe that the NICU is a setting in which reintegrative social control plays the dominant role.[30] The dominance of reintegrative social control mechanisms in the NICU depends on two factors: (1) the inability of social control agents to restrict entry or otherwise

30. Although Braithwaite (1989) is discussing the reintegration of former deviants, we believe that the argument applies equally well to settings such as the NICU, into which former or potential deviants are being integrated for the first time.

close organizational borders to likely deviants and (2) the interdependence between social control agents and deviants. Labeling works differently in reintegrative than in disintegrative social control. When interdependence and open borders make it difficult for social control agents to escape the results of their labeling, they are more motivated to move beyond stereotypes. It is in the variation within categories, the places where stereotypes do not fit, that agents of social control find their capacity to maneuver.

The labeling of parents in the NICU is a mechanism for identifying cases where resources are needed to bring parents up to the appropriate threshold. But such labeling is also a marginalizing mechanism, used to separate remediable from hopeless cases. Labeling identifies a problem and provides a kind of resolution, either a flow of action designed to reshape inappropriate behavior or to marginalize the inappropriate person (either by activating the state's child-welfare agency or by discouraging parental involvement), or an explanation for why things are not going as they should. Because it stimulates the "corrective cycle" (Goffman 1971), the label requires the expenditure of time, resources, and commitment.

Inappropriate behavior, whatever its cause, calls up remedial efforts. Mothers who do not visit will be phoned. Parents who come in drunk will be told to come back sober. Parents who wake sleeping babies will be informed that premature or sick babies need rest. If inappropriate behavior is not repeated, staff members conclude that the parents are learning. But if parents are indignant or slow to respond, a negative label is applied, often rather forcefully, to the person rather than the act. Inappropriate parents, then, are those who display a lot of inappropriate behavior and who do not respond to staff suggestions, explanations, or reprimands. As labels become attached to persons rather than behavior, social control agents correspondingly move from reintegrative to disintegrative social control mechanisms.

Ironically, the most inadequate parents are not the ones who are the most disruptive to the unit. Parents who simply do not visit and never make discharge plans are only episodically troublesome. Staff members look for early signs that a parent is unable or unmotivated to care for the child. In essence they are looking for information that would allow them to sort parents into the kinds of categories we used in chapter 3, although they are especially concerned with distinguishing truly irresponsible parents from all others. Parents who do not call or visit will be discussed and perhaps telephoned, with gradual escalation of pressure as discharge approaches. If a mother does not respond to pressure, the staff will may send the police with a message if there is no phone, send letters, attempt to contact the mother through relatives and friends, and eventually contact the state child-welfare agency. As staff members become convinced that the mother's failure to visit is a valid indicator of her lack of commitment to the child (because there are no meaningful accounts, such as cultural variation, health problems, or transportation difficulties, for her behavior), they invest more heavily in documenting her deficiencies and in finding alternative places to send the child at discharge. Inadequate parenting must be documented much more carefully than adequate parenting since it constitutes a core element of the legal case justifying the removal of a child from the parent's custody.[31] One social worker described how she instructs staff members to record information about parents: "If a family member, a parent, is coming in regularly very intoxicated, or appears to be high on drugs, then we'll encourage staff to document—factually, not subjective but objectively—what they see, the behaviors that are there. . . . Knowing that at some point that may be evidence that will help determine [whether the child-welfare agency intervenes]" (2012SW, interview 3, p. 21). So one function of the label "inappropriate" is to call up routines for documenting concrete instances of inadequate behavior.[32] Such cases are a small minority, of course, but they figure prominently in the lore of the unit and play an important role in creating consensus by providing clear examples of what is "really" inappropriate (see Emerson 1983 on precedents). In the NICU reintegrative mechanisms are used first and only gradually replaced by marginalizing ones. But the criteria for differentiating appropriate from inappropriate probably have higher consensus than they otherwise would because they are used to marginalize extreme deviants.

This move from reintegrative to disintegrative social control mechanisms occurs when labels are affixed because of both disruption to the unit and inadequate parenting, though of course the particular mechanisms

31. Documenting that one has tried everything else, Emerson (1969, 1981) notes, legitimates the use of a last resort strategy—such as getting the state to take custody of the child. Gilboy (1992:294) also discusses the construction of a sturdy record.

32. Though nurses have responsibility for recording phone calls to and from parents and visits from parents and other family members (some hospitals even designing special forms on which to record contact with the family), nurses vary in their diligence in recording such information. Their records of family contact can be trusted if one can determine that an especially diligent nurse constructed the record or that nurses were instructed to document all contacts so that the social worker would have solid evidence to use in discussions with the parent or with state's child-welfare workers.

and timetables differ. When efforts at resocialization fail, parents are often squeezed out, though staff members persist longer in attempts to teach adequate parenting than in attempts to reduce disruptive behavior. Nurses limit interaction with such parents, and when they do call or visit, they find the visits uncomfortable and their presence unwelcome. The inadequate parent we described earlier in the chapter had just such an experience toward the end of her son's stay in City's NICU, according to the social worker. During one of her last visits this mother was made to feel quite unwelcome by the nurses caring for her baby. When her son clung to the nurses and treated her as a stranger, the nurses did little to decrease her discomfort. When the toddler began to experience respiratory problems, they attributed this to his reaction to his mother and took him back, making it clear that they knew how to care for him even if she didn't. Because resources are limited, and socialization is resource intensive, some parents are marginalized if their response to resocialization efforts is too slow or too weak. Labeling a parent a pain-in-the-neck may not trigger actions aimed at resocialization. Instead, the label may eventually become a cue to avoid the labeled parent or to be on guard when that parent is around.

Several features of the NICU social order shape staff thinking about parents and about the costs of resocializing or marginalizing them. Fundamentally, the NICU has little if any control over its patient population.[33] Contracts with referring units oblige NICUs to accept transfers from those units or to find alternative hospitals for patients that cannot be accepted. NICUs have some control over which hospitals they enter into contracts with—all want to avoid the local county hospital, where the vast majority of patients are on public aid, for instance. But the competing pressure to keep beds full limits how often NICUs can exercise their preferences. Even if hospitals have some control over the selection of patients, they have no control over the selection of patients' parents. An attending physician may refuse the transport of a patient if the unit is full or if the patient is not sufficiently ill, but the attending cannot refuse a patient because the patient's family will be difficult to manage. Because NICUs have little capacity to screen the socially troublesome part of the clientele, namely the parents, some proportion of parents will deviate from the ideal.

What proportion of parents will be difficult to manage varies from one hospital to another. We have shown that City's parents are considerably more likely to be unmarried, less likely to have health insurance, and more

33. Roth (1972) also considers lack of control over organizational borders and clientele but does not tie these features to reintegrative or disintegrative social control.

likely to be nonwhite (see Table 2.1). We have also shown that on the average, parents who are unmarried, uninsured, and nonwhite are less likely to visit their hospitalized infants (Tables 2.3 and 2.4). NICU routines vary accordingly, with social control of parents receiving much more attention at City than at Suburban. As we noted in chapter 2, City's nursing record includes space for recording parent visits; Suburban's does not. Because Suburban's parents are more likely to be compliant, about 70% of families are never even mentioned during Suburban's discharge planning rounds. In the equivalent meetings at City, only 23% of families are never discussed (see Table 5.2). Although social control of parents is a much more prominent part of NICU life at City than at Suburban, the steps for evaluating and managing parents are nevertheless roughly equivalent in the two units, because neither may refuse admission on the grounds that an infant's parents are likely to be troublesome.

When it is not organizationally feasible to recruit an ideal clientele to replace the troublesome one, the staff can manage less-than-ideal parents in two ways: they can try to reshape parents' behavior toward the ideal, or they can marginalize troublesome parents so they need not be managed at all. Which strategy staff will use depends on how long they estimate the patient will be on the unit. With every NICU patient, the relationship between staff and parents is temporally bounded. Some NICU stays are shorter than others, but all stays are relatively brief, especially when compared with other unselected "clientele," like public school children or prisoners. A related, but not perfectly correlated, consideration is the amount of special care the baby will need at discharge. Typically, patients who have been on the unit for a long time require some measure of special care after discharge. Questions about parental competence are especially likely when the baby's well-being could be compromised by discharge home. Strategies for managing parents are adjusted to reflect estimates of the length of hospitalization and the amount of care the baby will need at home.

If a patient will only be in the unit briefly and will require no special care at discharge, then the staff will invest little in resocialization. Parents may be scolded or ignored, but very few efforts at reshaping behavior will occur. If, in contrast, staff anticipate a long hospitalization and expect that special care will be needed at discharge, then staff members will work harder to reshape behavior. In the most extreme cases, parents are asked to sign a contract detailing when and for how long they will visit the baby and what kinds of skills they must master. Only after numerous attempts to reshape behavior is the state's child-welfare agency contacted (unless maternal drug use has been documented, in which case a report is mandatory in the state where we conducted our research).[34] Because social workers need relatively solid evidence before reporting a case to the state child-welfare agency and it is easier to get the agency to take a case once the child has gone home, the social workers and discharge planner may go ahead and send the child home but put in "maximum nursing services" to protect the baby while building a case for further intervention.

Control over borders and interdependence are of course related. Hospital staff members have correspondingly little control over exit from the unit, because exit depends largely on the medical condition of the patient. Infants can be discharged to other institutions—to lower-level nurseries if they still need medical care but no longer require intensive care, or to long-term care facilities if special needs make home discharge impossible. Discharges to other units do not depend much on parent behavior. But most discharges are to the home, and these depend heavily on parents' being ready to take the infant home. Sending a patient home to an ill-prepared or unfit parent or a poorly equipped home is grounds for a legal case, as staff members are well aware. One discharge planner, for instance, described himself as "legally liable for inappropriate discharges" and regarded himself as occupying the "next level of responsibility, just above the parents" (1007DP, p. 8).

The interdependence between hospital staff and family severely limits the use of disintegrative social control mechanisms. Marginalizing troublesome parents may be a sensible short-run strategy, but it can be quite costly in the long run. The capacity of the state to absorb graduates of NICUs is rather limited, and staff members are loath to undertake the cumbersome process of documenting inadequate parenting unless no alternative exists. We stress that NICU staff members are not simply taking society's viewpoint and thinking of parents (and especially mothers) as the cheapest providers of child care. When infants cannot be discharged to their parents, the hospital accrues substantial costs. The state usually does not pay the full cost of the infant's hospitalization and pays nothing after the hospital

34. Recall that according to the medical records we viewed at the two hospitals, only eight of the parents of City Hospital infants and two of the parents of Suburban infants were reported to the state's child-welfare agency. These formal referrals may be the tip of the iceberg, though. One Suburban social worker suggested that contacts between the child-welfare workers and the NICU social workers were much more common: "Well, I'd say on the average it [reporting to the child-welfare agency] comes up maybe a couple of times a month here which, isn't a lot compared to some of the other NICUs. But it comes up" (2012SW, interview 1, p. 1).

has consumed its allotted "public aid days" for the year. "A hundred and eighty days of no payment," one staff member commented at one point, referring to the hospital stay of the infant of the "inadequate parent" discussed above. Additional days of hospitalization are thus expensive for the hospital because the hospital will not be fully reimbursed and because of the displacement of paying patients who might occupy that hospital bed. Moreover, the costs to children who may become wards of the state are certainly part of the calculation: a less-than-perfect home is often better than no home at all. The deep dependence of the NICU on parents is no doubt also increased by a cultural belief that parental ties are sacred and that the bonds between parents and their children should be preserved whenever possible.[35] In such a cultural climate, substitutes for birth parents are acceptable only by parental choice or by a demonstration that the parents are grossly and irremediably incompetent.

In the organizational context of the NICU, then, most deviant parents have to be reintegrated into the unit. Labels are part of a complex economy in which staff members negotiate about who really cannot be allowed to take a baby home, who "looks" bad but can be taught, who knows enough so that she or he may safely be ignored, and who may not need much teaching but learns quickly and so makes good use of resources. This complex negotiation depends fundamentally on the context in which it is embedded. Stereotypes about social groups shape expectations about parenting styles of group members and ultimately lead to varying standards for different groups. But though staff members may start with stereotypes, the press of organizational business forces them to move beyond stereotypes, for instance to sort bad apples into usable and rotten. State and federal laws mold staff members' behavior both by reinforcing their sense that some parents are beyond the pale and by lending force to threats that parents will be denied custody unless they reform. We have argued that the labeling process lies at the center of this complex system and have tried to show how a flexible, quasi-legal system, drawing on the authority of outside bodies, emerges to collect and evaluate evidence, draw conclusions about those charged, administer sanctions, and even develop new legislation.

Comparisons and Implications for Institutional Design

In his discussion of reintegrative shaming, Braithwaite (1989) argues that people who are less integrated into a society will be less responsive to at-

35. In their investigation of child-protection work in England, Dingwall, Eekelaar, and Murray (1983:79–102) argue that, in a liberal society, the belief in "natural love" between

tempts to shame them. He focuses on the responsiveness of those who have been labeled, but we focus instead on the obligations of those affixing the labels to reform and reintegrate deviants. The question is not how attached deviants are to the community but instead how dependent the community is on the contributions of reformed deviants. The facts considered are the same, but the emphasis is different. If, as Braithwaite contends, a person who is less attached to a community is less subject to shaming, we would agree but argue that those variables indicating a person's attachment to the community can instead be seen as indicators of a community's dependence on its members. Unemployment, for instance, can be read as an indicator that a person is not attached to any employer or as an indicator that no employer needs the person. We emphasize the latter. Societies, communities, or organizations will make more effort to reform and reintegrate deviants if they need them as community members than if such deviants are superfluous to the community. Labels will be applied differently in a community such as an NICU, which is dependent on its rehabilitated deviants, than in one which is not.

When we reverse the focus of analysis from the dependence of deviants on the community to the dependence of a community on reformed deviants, we can identify sites where Braithwaite's theory of reintegrative social control applies even in such individualistic societies as the United States. Further, by identifying strategic reasons that organizations are especially dependent on deviant participants, we see alternative mechanisms that increase the interdependence of social control agents and clients and therefore increase the motivation to reform and reintegrate deviants.

We believe that it is appropriate to think of the dependence of social control agents on their clients as a variable. We have argued that NICUs are quite dependent on their clients and that this dependence arises from a cultural belief that parents are not interchangeable with other potential care providers, from the inability of NICUs to turn away infants of potentially troublesome parents, and from the bureaucratic, legal, and financial costs of making other discharge arrangements. We turn now to a brief illustration of how NICUs might be compared with other kinds of organizations.

Comparisons across organizations are difficult. It is hardly obvious what measuring rod should be used to compare deviance among NICU

---

parents and their children supports a "rule of optimism" that requires overwhelming evidence of incompetence before the tie between parent and child may be severed.

parents with deviance in other populations such as white-collar criminals, juvenile delinquents, or high-school students. But without detailed comparisons we cannot say whether interdependence is higher or lower, or whether equally deviant acts lead to equally vigorous remedial efforts and equal attempts to reintegrate deviants. Nevertheless, in discussing techniques used to get rid of troublemakers, Bowditch (1993) strongly suggests that inner-city high schools are little concerned with reforming and reintegrating deviants but instead have well-developed techniques for excluding students who repeatedly misbehave. The dependence of schools on their clients varies, of course, and according to our argument, such variation should predict variations in attempts to reintegrate reformed rule breakers. An organization's dependence on its members can take different forms. For instance, though schools, like NICUs, must accept all comers, the functioning of a school is probably less disrupted by student incompetence than the NICU is by parental incompetence; Bowditch, for instance, found that "DuBois High" held back about a quarter of all tenth graders. A school's obligation to take all comers shifts sharply when a student reaches age seventeen. Bowditch found that administrators interpreted this to mean that they had no obligation to keep "overage" troublemakers and routinely dropped them from the school's rolls. School disciplinarians believed the goal of their office was not to solve students' problems but to protect school operations (Bowditch 1993:504). Such a view suggests that schools are not very dependent on individual students and that interdependence decreases even further when attendance ceases to be mandatory.

School dependence on clients varies with funding arrangements as well as with legal obligations to students. At one extreme are private schools, which can pick and choose among applicants. In between are public schools that must take all comers but need not compete for them. And at the other extreme are public schools in systems where voucher holders can choose which school they wish to attend.

We stress here that the effect of open borders on the treatment of members or clients depends on what role those people play in the functioning of the organization. We must be careful not to paint too rosy a picture here. Coupling the need to protect the school's operation with a perceived legal obligation to keep a student in school until age seventeen, schools developed elaborate procedures for transferring troublemakers from one school to another. We would only expect reintegration when an organization is stuck with the deviants *and* has to use them (and not someone else) to do some key task. Even in the case of NICU parents, the reform and reintegration may be relatively short term, and the NICU has no routine for being concerned with whether a teenage mother or the baby's grandmother actually cares for the child once it leaves the unit. We would argue that reforms that required organizations to take on the tasks of incorporating unemployed people, disabled people, prison releasees, or other categories of people not ordinarily sought by the organization would depend not just on making the organization expand its borders to include such people but also on creating a deeper interdependence by making such people uniquely responsible for key functions in the organization. The more open the border, the more uniquely assigned the task, and the more important the task to the functioning of the organization, then the more likely an organization is to make sustained efforts to diagnose and correct deviant activity.

Conclusion: Social Control and Responsibility

In this chapter, we have described one side of social control in the NICU—when and how staff members evaluate and attempt to shape the behavior of parents. Here, we have argued that the NICU uses minimum standards that vary with the characteristics of the parents. Both the NICU and the parents are responsible for the care of critically ill infants. But although the NICU staff has a deep responsibility for managing the medical care of the hospitalized infant, the NICU has a rather limited responsibility for what happens after discharge. Of course the NICU staff must be confident that the baby is healthy enough to be sent home. Beyond that, though, the NICU's responsibility is fundamentally shaped by its interest in limiting its culpability for sending infants to homes that are not equipped to care for them. The NICU does little to encourage the fuller commitment of parents and occasionally even discourages parents from intervening in what staff regard as inappropriate ways, as the case of Mrs. Croft illustrates nicely. Preparation for discharge is focused more on teaching skills than on fostering commitment.

Does this elaborate social control system then contribute anything to the process of encouraging parents to take responsibility for their critically ill infants? We have argued in chapter 3 that flexible adjustment to the child's needs is a fundamental part of taking responsibility and that such flexibility is required of both parents and professional health-care providers. We argue here that in addition to identifying and correcting the most egregious instances of irresponsible behavior, the chief contribution of the

NICU social control system is to highlight the importance of flexible adjustment to the needs of individual children.

Requirements for flexibility are built into routines in different ways for the medical professionals and for parents. In medicine, physicians, nurses, and other health-care providers are expected to choose among a menu of options for treatment and to follow treatment and medication protocols exactly unless they have some carefully worked-out reason for deviation. Although this sounds like a prescription for inflexibility, flexibility is engineered into the system with at least three different mechanisms: routine discussion of cases with colleagues in medical rounds or nursing report, consultations with colleagues in nearby fields, and periodic modifications of protocols. Physicians may be expected to provide care that is consistent with established standards, but courts of law will not accept a defense that a physician's practice meets the standard of care unless the appropriate standard is being used.

Parents are similarly expected to respond flexibly to the particular needs of their critically ill infants. But how is such flexibility designed into hospital routines in such a way that medical care providers can be sure that they are sending children home to parents who will tailor care to the needs of the child? Parents are not trained professionals who keep abreast of the latest developments in their field through continuing education classes. Because NICU parents are no more likely than any other parents to have gone through a standardized curriculum in preparation for parenthood, we might expect to find more variability in the practice of parenthood than in the practice of medicine. Our interview evidence suggests that some parents read pregnancy and parenting books, and others do not, and that mothers are considerably more likely than fathers to read about these topics.

If hospital staff members cannot assume that parents have been adequately prepared by learning the core routines and rules of thumb about when alternative routines should be employed, how do staff members ensure that parents have either basic parenting skills or the capacity to adapt normal routines to meet their child's special needs? Although the NICU has no integrated parenting curriculum (and may not be the appropriate site for such a curriculum), the rudiments of training for parenthood are present and, more important, are customized so that parents learn how to care for their own child. The foundation is laid when parents are given information about their child's medical condition, but the core of this curriculum is preparation for discharge, documented in the child's medical record in the discharge checklist.[36] These days all new parents are required to undergo a bit of training whether the child has been in an NICU or an ordinary newborn nursery, but for NICU parents discharge training often extends well beyond verification that the parents know how to feed the baby, change diapers, and care for the umbilical cord stump or the circumcision wound. In the NICU, radically individualized discharge training programs and checklists go some way toward ensuring that parents are aware of the special needs of their child and equipped to feed through a nasogastric tube, suction secretions, perform physical therapy routines, change the dressing around the tracheostomy and check the ventilator, or perform infant CPR as needed.

Perhaps most important, though, preparation for discharge conveys the message that each NICU patient has unique needs. One child may have follow-up appointments with a physical therapist, while a second will need to be seen by a cardiologist and a third by an orthopedic surgeon. A child with a cleft palate may need to be fed with a special nipple, and another will need special high-calorie formula. Some parents may need to perform daily checks on the shunt that drains excess fluid from the ventricles of the child's brain to the abdomen, while others will be trained to administer medications on a rigid schedule. Discharge instruction thus sets parents on a path of flexible adjustment both by showing them what kinds of adjustments are necessary in the period just after discharge and by constructing ties with professionals who can help them determine what adjustments will be appropriate at subsequent stages. Of course, a good deal of the adjusting we have been discussing is as much adjustment by staff as by parents. But in tailoring treatments to individual infants and working out discharge plans jointly with parents, staff model flexible adjustment for parents and help them figure out what responsibility means when it is parents who must do most of the adjusting.

36. How the information is given may affect parents' capacity to use the information. Maynard (1996) argues that when physicians (and other tellers of bad news) "forecast" the news rather than either stall or tell the news too bluntly, the resulting collaboration between the deliverer and recipient of the news to some degree mitigates tendencies to misapprehend the situation (e.g., by denying or blaming). Forecasting helps recipients to "realize" the bad news and starts them on the path of managing the practical problems associated with their fundamentally altered world. If NICU care providers do a good job of telling the bad news, then, they can minimize parents' feelings of anomie and associated feelings of anger, hurt, hostility, and indignation, and get parents started on the job of constructing a (different) future with their child.

The social control system we have described in this chapter is focused mainly on identifying and reforming inadequate parents, on establishing compliance with minimum standards. But although the focus is on the establishment of a floor, we stress that this is an unusual kind of floor in two respects. Because many NICU graduates go home needing some special care, NICU parents are expected to have a few skills that other parents may lack. The floor is thus marginally higher for NICU parents than parents of ordinary newborns.

More important, though, expectations vary with the needs of the child. Social control typically focuses on ensuring compliance with fixed standards; here social control instead focuses on compliance with individualized standards. Insofar as rules and sanctions instruct people about their obligations, this social control system teaches parents that what they have to do varies with their child's circumstances. In stressing that the routines and skills are child specific, the social control system highlights the core of the NICU normative system. Deviance, shirking, and responsibility are all measured by a peculiar yardstick here. For each level of compliance or noncompliance, the special needs of the child are factored in. An ordinary baby would not need to see a pediatrician at the first sign of a common cold; a baby who has been on a ventilator is much more likely to develop serious respiratory problems and may require medical attention. Whether or not it is neglectful not to take an infant to a pediatrician thus depends on the child's medical history. In emphasizing flexible adjustment to individual circumstances, the NICU social control system inculcates the standard by which parents should guide their behavior and shows inadequate parents what they should aspire to. There is no sharp discontinuity here—irresponsibility, shirking, and responsibility are simply different levels of compliance with a radically individualized standard. The articulation of the principle of flexible adjustment at the low end may well increase the likelihood that nonconforming parents will catch on that hospital staff members are not simply heavy-handed authority figures insisting that things be done their way, and thus may smooth the way for simple compliance to grow into responsibility.

We turn next to the other side of social control in the NICU—when and how the parents evaluate and attempt to shape the behavior of NICU staff members. Although one might expect social control *by* parents to be the mirror image of social control *of* parents, in fact parents use quite different tools to encourage responsible behavior in hospital staff members than staff members use to encourage responsibility in parents. To evaluate, label, and press for reform requires resources that parents lack. As laypeople attempting to regulate the behavior of professionals, parents often lack the expertise to evaluate staff behavior, although their expertise grows over the period of the baby's hospital stay. Because they operate as isolated individuals rather than as members of a team, parents have little capacity to label staff members. Because they are outsiders who control few important sanctions, they have little capacity to insist on reform.

Nevertheless, we find that most parents believe that they have some obligation to ensure that medical care providers behave responsibly, for instance believing that they should intervene if they thought that a staff member had made a mistake. Even when parents intervene often and effectively, though, they employ different tactics and different sanctions from those used by staff members. Parents vary a good deal in how they conceive their role in the NICU and their relation to the staff and in their ability to act as effective advocates for their children. They face formidable obstacles as they attempt to evaluate and intervene in the care their infants receive. In chapter 6, we categorize the parents we interviewed according to how much they trusted the medical staff who cared for their infants and explain why parents differ in how much they trust hospital staff and how variations in levels of trust affect the likelihood of parent intervention. We find, for instance, that parents whose infants require long hospitalizations learn a great deal about how to evaluate and intervene in the activities of the staff and, in this way, start to assume responsibility for the care their infants receive long before discharge home. For many parents, these early experiences in the hospital provide advance training in how to be a parent outside the home. Parenting is not confined to the home (an argument to which we return in chapter 8), but it is not easy to tell where parental obligations end and those of nurses and physicians (or, later, teachers or coaches) begin. In the NICU, parents learn how to negotiate a division of labor with those who share some responsibilities for their children. Parents who spend more time in the NICU are of course more likely to learn the skills of parenting on someone else's turf than are parents who visit less.

Nurses and doctors who take on the responsibility of caring for precarious newborns may give excellent care to their small charges while simultaneously undermining parents' feelings of competence and control and their capacity to accept responsibility at discharge. It is a delicate matter to strike the right balance between present and future. More parental involvement may make for less efficiency in the NICU in the short run but better care for the baby in the long run. But tipping the balance too far in the direction of parental involvement can also lead to unacceptable sacrifices in quality of care. When, then, does it make sense to allow people—parents in this instance—to make mistakes from which they will learn and which will show them how very much their child depends on their competence and attentiveness as well as on their affection?

NICU social control provides important support for parental acceptance of responsibility. But as we have seen in this chapter, NICU social control efforts are much more directed at shaping the behavior of mothers than of fathers, apply tougher standards to some parents than to others, and are as much shaped by the goals of avoiding disruption of organizational business and blame from the state as by the goal of ensuring that parents are ready and able to accept responsibility for precarious newborns. Parental responsibility is sustained by forces other than NICU social control, of course, but we should inquire into whether and when the NICU social control system ultimately supports or undermines parental responsibility.

SIX

Novice Managers of Expert Labor: Parents as Agents of Social Control in the NICU

"YOU HAVE TO REALIZE . . . there's not much you can do at all. I mean, you couldn't take the baby out of there and do better at home" (2012M, p. 17), one father commented, quickly summarizing the dilemma parents face. "You're totally at their mercy" (2017F, p. 79), a mother remarked. On the one hand, parents are deeply dependent on the NICU staff because they themselves lack medical expertise. "We don't know what's supposed to be going on; they do" (2013M, p. 41), one father commented. "I'm not an expert" (2015F, p. 73), one mother acknowledged. "They were the professionals" (1005F, p. 26), who "went to school for all this stuff" (2037F, p. 23). On the other hand, parents are intensely aware of variations in staff competence and commitment and of value differences between themselves and the staff. When a physician offered suggestions about how to inform an older sibling about a newborn's condition, one father curtly responded, "Thank you, but we really don't need your advice in this" (1028F, p. 22 [mother reporting father's words]). The same physician gave offense by suggesting that the parents "forget" their baby (1028F, p. 23). Echoing the sentiments of many parents, one mother noted that they have more at stake than the medical staff: "It's not their kid on that surgery table under a knife" (1001M, p. 27 [mother interjecting comment]). Another father (1025M), who ultimately concluded that the City Hospital staff "had it together" (p. 10), felt it only prudent to assess staff performance: "I watched. I watched all the time I was there. I watched every move he [the physician] made. I think everybody should watch them. I mean, like, doctors [are] going to jail for giving the wrong medicine [the father stated that the mother's first obstetrician had served a jail term]. You know, some of them [are] hooked on the medicine there—you know, taking pills and stuff. You have to know what's happening" (p. 9). Parents also routinely commented on mistakes that staff members made.

Although none of the parents could be described as facing their infant's hospitalization with equanimity, they coped with their dependence on medical staff in quite different ways. One ordinarily skeptical mother felt it wise (and fair) to trust her child's physicians: "Like I tell my children, when you go to the doctor, you go there for the doctor to help you. So you go along with whatever the doctor wants. . . . I put my faith in the doctors, and what the doctors say is necessary, I'll go along with that" (1002F, pp. 30, 34). Some parents' views on their own role changed as they became more familiar with NICU procedures and better versed in the details of their child's medical condition. One mother, for instance, was indignant that staff members continued to consider her a novice: "My child has been in the hospital for three months—like I'm not going to know something about this" (2025F, p. 6). Many parents felt that the only reasonable course of action was to acknowledge their vulnerability and distrust and to monitor their child's medical care as best they could. One father had the grace to handle the situation with humor. "I'm going to be your worst pest" (1008M, p. 36), he informed the staff. For many others, though, the situation was too tense for jokes, and they instead talked about needing to keep tabs on the staff, seeking second opinions, and feeling that they couldn't leave the NICU because they then wouldn't know what was going on.

When critically ill infants are patients in an NICU, they are unequivocally the responsibility of the medical staff. When they leave the unit, these same infants are unequivocally the responsibility of their parents. Some parents feel from the beginning that the infant patients are really their responsibility. Others only gradually begin to feel that they at least share responsibility for the baby. By the time of discharge, all of the parents have to believe that the child is their responsibility—or else they will not be permitted to take the baby home. Over the course of babies' hospital stays, then, several changes take place. Most simply, the proportion of parents who feel that the child's welfare is their responsibility rises, with corresponding shifts in parents' sense of competence and in their views on how responsibility should be divided between them and the staff. As they come to understand their child's medical condition and the social organization of intensive-care medicine, parents are transformed from anxious, but somewhat passive, bystanders to active participants who gradually assume managerial functions. At the heart of this remarkable transformation are the puzzles explored in this chapter. We know little about how the transformation occurs and even less about why it occurs earlier for some parents than for others.

In chapter 5, we argued that the social control of parents is a dominant feature of the NICU. Yet staff members are not the only participants making judgments and attempting to reshape what they regard as inappropriate behavior. Research on social control often treats the objects of social control as just that—objects. They may be resistant rather than compliant, of course, as Scott (1985) points out, but our argument here is less about whether parents resist or comply than about how they try to reshape staff members' behavior. Here we find that the objects of social control may also function as agents of social control. But although NICU parents are both objects and agents of social control, the social control resources at their disposal are not nearly so vast as those controlled by staff members. In describing the social control of parents by NICU staff, we described how inappropriate behavior, whatever its cause, trips social control "machinery" aimed at evaluating and reforming deviants. There is, however, no corresponding machinery at the disposal of parents who attempt to make evaluations of staff performance or to reform what they regard as inappropriate behavior. Instead, most parents have to start from scratch and fashion their tools as needed. In short, social control *of* parents is very different from social control *by* parents, and parents face formidable barriers that limit their effectiveness as social control agents.

Parents enter the NICU as outsiders, as laypeople in a sea of experts. As we have taken pains to demonstrate in previous chapters, the role of "parent of critically ill infant" is largely defined by NICU routines and the pressing organizational business of treating critically ill patients. Rather than be permitted to work out their own roles as they see fit, mothers and fathers are told how to parent their babies. NICU instructions about when parents can visit the unit, and when and whether they can touch, feed, and hold their infants, suggest to them that parenting is subordinate to medical care. Actions speak louder than words here, and although they are repeatedly told that they play a crucial role in their child's life, parents quickly get the idea that parenting is not right now as important as doctoring and nursing. Disputes with staff members about such matters as feeding can lead swiftly to the label of poor organizational participant and even to a fairly firm label of hopelessly "inappropriate." As the staff members themselves are quick to note, parents do not have expert knowledge about the appropriate course of treatment for their child or about what constitutes appropriate doctoring or nursing.

In the previous chapter, we viewed such disputes mainly from the perspective of the hospital and its staff. In this chapter, we will examine parental interventions not as disruptions of NICU routines or as indicators of parental competence but as parents' attempts to ensure that hospital staff members do their jobs in the way the parents believe is appropriate. We would regard it as irresponsible if parents entrusted their child to a babysitter, day-care center, or teacher without checking on the reputations and monitoring the performance of those to whom they entrusted their child. Should something go wrong in the NICU, we would similarly wonder whether parents had neglected their obligation to verify that their child was in good hands. Recognizing their ignorance of medicine, parents nevertheless typically feel some pressure to sift and sort information to the best of their ability, to watch for indications that their child is being neglected, and to make sure that no gross errors have been committed. Despite their discomfort with the role, parents become agents of social control because that is what they believe is required of responsible parents.

Parents certainly vary in the extent to which they define it as their responsibility to ensure that their baby is receiving adequate care. Mrs. Croft's case is an illustrative but exceptional one in this regard. While most parents do not dispute the treatment decisions of the medical professionals in the NICU, they are intensely aware that their newborn is in the hands of strangers who may or may not be competent and who may or may not have their baby's best interests in mind. To ease their anxiety in the first days, they may ask detailed questions about medical decisions, ensuring that all possibilities have been considered; they may also track more routine care, such as whether the baby is fed regularly, has his or her diaper changed frequently, or has clean dressings on surgical wounds. This early attentiveness to staff members and their routines often leads to increased confidence in the hospital staff. However, if parents conclude that NICU routines are inadequate or that staff members vary in competence, early observations may instead lead parents to become increasingly watchful.

While the role of parent is largely defined by the organization and its protocols, parents do retain some capacity to decide for themselves how actively to monitor and when to intervene. The involvement of parents is framed both by their legal rights as parents, especially as embodied in consent procedures, and by the organization's dependence on them to take their babies home at discharge. All organizations are fundamentally dependent on those who "consume" their "products." But here the NICU's dependence on parents is coupled with a requirement to verify that parents are competent and committed before permitting them to take the NICU's product home. In essence, then, by protecting parents' rights to participate in treatment decisions and providing incentives for NICUs to involve them in both decision making and the more routine aspects of infant care, the law provides the wedge that allows parents to become social control agents. Beyond these minimal levels of participation that are protected by the law and buttressed by the organization's dependence on parents, parents have to define for themselves what their roles should be, learning enough about NICUs to intervene effectively, and finding allies among NICU staff and in the legal system as needed.

Collecting and evaluating information about how their infants are doing, exploring treatment options, and evaluating the quality of care all present a challenge to parents precisely because they are outsiders. We begin the chapter with a brief description of the organizational and knowledge barriers parents face as they try to oversee and intervene in the activities of the staff. As regulators, parents face the usual disabilities: they are outsiders, less expert than those they are attempting to regulate. In addition, though, they are relatively weak outsiders—they have few resources, and no clout. Parents also face an unusual regulatory task—their attention is concentrated on a particular case rather than on an overall process.

We draw on the insights of agency theory, which is concerned with how principals can motivate agents to take their particular interests into account, to help explain why the social control of NICU medical experts by parents is so difficult. Because many of the basic assumptions of agency theory are violated in this setting, the main social control mechanism posited by agency theory, the contract, is insufficient. In the NICU, the parents are intermediaries between the infants and the staff. However, the parents are relatively weak agents of social control and have few effective formal sanctions at their disposal. Parents therefore must negotiate with the staff and use informal sanctions to get what they want.

But before parents can intervene in the activities of the staff, they must conceive it as their role to monitor and evaluate the care their infants receive. We therefore explore variations in how parents define their roles. Drawing on our interviews with parents from City and Suburban Hospitals' NICUs, we array parents' conceptions of their roles along a continuum, ranging from faith to contingent trust to distrust. At one extreme are parents who have faith and who feel no obligation to oversee the care their infants are receiving. Recognizing their own lack of expertise, they reason that the medical staff knows far more than they about what should be done. Parents who trust contingently, in contrast, feel some obligation to visit and to test staff competence by making careful observations, asking questions, and even perhaps reading the medical chart. For such parents, collecting observations and weighing the evidence often result in increased trust. At the other extreme, however, are parents who distrust. These parents are the most active overseers of the care their infants receive, and are quite likely to think it necessary to intervene.

Clearly, not every parent responds to the critical illness of an infant in the same way. Our task is to move beyond a simple categorization of parental responses to an explanation of why some parents have so much faith in the NICU team while others are distrusting supervisors who note every possible false move. Using Gerson's (1985 and 1993) work as a model, we offer a developmental explanation of these differences among parents. We show that though parents arrive at the NICU with varying inclinations to trust or distrust health-care providers, they also respond rather strongly to their experiences in the NICU. Even quite trusting parents are shaken by graphic evidence that their child may not survive and begin to wonder whether some blame should be laid at the feet of the health-care team.

Parents not only have different orientations to their roles in the unit, but they also are differently endowed with the kinds of resources that make social control possible. It is easier to be skeptical about the care a child is receiving when one has an educational background that makes it possible to comprehend medical pamphlets and medical journal articles. Similarly, having funds to hire babysitters makes it possible to spend time in the NICU overseeing one child's medical team when there are other children at home. But social control is not a simple story about parents' resources. In this sense, our story is not just about constraints. Of the parents we interviewed, those who assumed the least active roles on the unit all had (or started with) relatively few resources, but not every parent with few resources assumed a passive role. Some of the parents with the fewest resources were also the most actively involved social control agents in the NICU. As they learned about their deficiencies, these ingenious and committed parents devised ways to acquire or substitute for the resources they lacked.

We conclude the chapter by noting that it makes a difference where and when parents try to intervene. Though they recognize that parents bear the ultimate responsibility for the welfare of their babies and so have a right to be concerned with the quality of the care they receive, health-care providers do not always welcome parental intervention. We make a rough distinction between the core and the periphery of medical care, and argue that parents will face more resistance if they attempt to intervene in the core than if their efforts are concentrated on the periphery of medical care. But exactly where the boundary between core and periphery lies is of course ambiguous, and the inevitable result is some pushing and shoving over where one party's responsibilities end and the other's begin.

Organizational and Knowledge Barriers: The Parents' View of the NICU Revisited

We have made this observation previously, but it bears repeating: Parents do not plan to have sick babies, but the staff does plan to treat sick babies. This simple observation underscores the asymmetry between parents and hospital staff. Although both are brought to the NICU by the critical illness of an infant, parents and staff have very different relationships to this central fact. The parents' crisis is the staff's daily business (to paraphrase Hughes 1981:54, 88). Parents are "one shotters" and staff are repeat players; parents would not want it any other way. If the hospital has a deep dependence on parents for a successful discharge home, as we argued in the previous chapter, then the parents have an even deeper dependence on the hospital for the medical care that makes that discharge possible.

Parents face substantial organizational and knowledge barriers when they take on the central activities of social control: monitoring, evaluating, and intervening in the activities of the staff. Having an infant hospitalized means being separated from that infant. Even though parents have nearly unlimited access to their infants in the NICU, many parents are simply unable to keep a vigilant bedside watch because of travel time, illness, employment, or other family obligations. Previously, we addressed this problem from the point of view of the hospital: not visiting may signal to staff members that parents are not sufficiently committed, that they will be unprepared, or unable, to take their infant home. But here we stress that those parents who are unable—for whatever reason—to overcome the physical distance that separates them from their infant will be unable to monitor or influence the activities of the staff. As organization theorists point out, decisions are much influenced by the structure of participation (Cohen, March, and Olsen 1972; March and Olsen 1976). Participation rights are important of course, but it also matters who just happens to be there when a decision is being made.

Distance itself is perhaps the most important barrier faced by parents. We have estimated that the average travel time for our sample of City Hospital families was eighty-three minutes, with two families facing a travel time of about four hours and two others living about fifteen minutes from the hospital. The Suburban families in our sample lived somewhat closer, with an average travel time of about fifty-four minutes. Two Suburban families traveled about two hours to visit their babies, while one family traveled only about twenty-three minutes.[1] Of the parents we interviewed, 30% mentioned distance as an impediment to visiting their hospitalized infants; in addition, 20% complained of other difficulties with transportation (e.g., not having access to a car). The effects of distance, travel times, and transportation difficulties are also magnified for families who have other children, and 12% of the parents we interviewed mentioned that the need to arrange child care for older siblings made visiting the hospitalized infant difficult.[2]

Although both mothers and fathers are affected by distance from their hospitalized child, the biggest effect occurs at somewhat different periods during the baby's hospitalization. Mothers are disproportionately inconvenienced by distance in the first days of the baby's hospitalization, when they may be recovering from the birth in a different hospital. Among the parents we interviewed, 33% mentioned illness or recovery from childbirth as impediments to visiting the hospitalized infant. Later, distance appears to pose a greater impediment to fathers, who must fit hospital visits around their work schedules once the initial crisis is over. Nine percent of our respondents commented on how work obligations interfered with visiting the baby. In the early period, the crisis often warrants time off work. Fathers may be able to arrange time off work for the first few days of their newborn's hospitalization but typically must return to work after that. Great physical distance may thus make visiting difficult for mothers during the crucial first days and for fathers only if the infant remains hospitalized for an extended period.[3] Not all mothers are able to overcome the barrier of physical distance, of course. But in general, since mothers are more likely to visit than fathers, they are also more likely to engage in the central

1. With a few exceptions (in which parents explicitly said that they used public transportation), we have calculated how long it would take parents to travel by car, adjusting for city vs. highway driving and parking time. When parents did not live together, we have averaged their estimates (which were within a minute or two of one another in any case) to produce a single estimate of parental travel time for each child.

2. We discuss here only the impediments to visiting mentioned most frequently in our interviews (with eighty-five parents; we excluded the mother who was incarcerated when her baby was born). On the average parents mentioned one impediment to visiting their hospitalized child (mean = 1.1), with a range from 0 to 5 difficulties mentioned. In addition to the impediments we discuss in the text, 10% of parents also mentioned the emotional strain of visiting the NICU as a reason they visited infrequently.

3. Anspach (1993) argues that mothers are especially disadvantaged in life-and-death decisions that occur very early in the infant's hospitalization. They are often unable to visit the NICU and participate fully in the decisions about their infant's care but must live with the consequences of these decisions.

activities of social control. Mothers, then, are not only more likely to be the subjects of social control, but they are also more likely to be the agents of social control.

We want to emphasize the importance of visiting, but it would be a mistake to assume that parents cannot influence what happens in their absence. Parents who visit often are more likely to have their requests honored even when they go home at night. Parents who never visit will have difficulty exerting influence, because visiting has a double effect: it allows parents to monitor activities but also to gain expertise. As parents learn more about their child's illness, course of treatment, and hospital routines and procedures, they are better equipped as social control agents in at least two ways. First, they are able to monitor the staff's activities more meaningfully having gained some knowledge of what is normal and routine and what is not. Of equal importance, however, parents who demonstrate expertise in their child's condition and care will have more influence than those who do not. Those who visit have more opportunity to demonstrate their expertise than those who do not.

In addition to distance, parents also must confront the obstacles created by the organizational structure. Parents' participation rights are limited, although less limited than many parents imagine, as clever and persistent parents eventually learn. Many parents visit the unit regularly, sit at their infant's bedside, and watch what is being done. But visiting gives them only a partial view of the unit and its activities, because many activities do not take place at the bedside and even those that do are difficult to interpret, especially at the beginning of an infant's hospitalization. Except during rounds, few physicians will be found at the bedside. And although nurses can be found there, they routinely discuss only day-to-day progress, referring parents to the physician for the more weighty issues of diagnosis, prognosis, and treatment alternatives. The rotation of physicians confounds parents' attempts to monitor, evaluate, and intervene even further. Parents routinely complain that just as they get to know one physician, another has stepped in to take over the case.

The parents' partial view from the bedside may be enhanced by information that is dutifully recorded in the infant's medical chart. The nurses' notes for the day are typically kept at the bedside, but the doctors' orders and progress notes are kept on a cart at the front desk. But if they are to use the information in their child's chart to monitor and evaluate the activities of staff members, parents first must know that they have a right to see the chart. Not surprisingly, staff members do not advertise this right to parents. Instead, the right must be claimed. As the staff members are quick to argue, the information recorded in the chart is often incomprehensible to parents and other laypeople without expert translation.

Even if comprehensible, however, the information that appears in the chart has limited utility to parents for the purposes of intervention. In part, this is because the medical chart is an artifact of the child's medical history; it is a place mainly for recording what has already been done. Further, a layperson may find it difficult to identify key decision points and to discern the range of alternatives that might have been pursued but were not. "Do Not Resuscitate" orders are one of a handful of notable exceptions to this rule. The consultation with the parents about DNR orders and the ensuing decision are painstakingly documented. In general, though, decisions that are not conceived as matters of life and death appear as artifacts of activities: feedings were advanced, the nasogastric tube was removed, or the oxygen was decreased. Although information is recorded faithfully in the chart, it appears in a form that makes it difficult for the layperson to see decisions rather than simply "continued progress" or "continued deterioration." When decision points are obscure, intervention is nearly impossible.

Finally, it should be noted that the information in the chart has been recorded with full knowledge that the medical record is only a semi-private document—with potential audiences including the parents and even the courts.[4] One social worker said that in writing notes in the chart, she was always mindful of how they would sound when read by the parents at home on a Sunday afternoon and crafted her comments to avoid gratuitous pain. All three social workers had testified in court and had had their chartings used for a variety of legal purposes, including malpractice suits and legal proceedings to declare the infant a ward of the state. Hospital risk managers occasionally conducted training seminars for physicians and other staff members, giving advice about such matters as how to write records to minimize the chance of suits and to make them easier to defend. Under the best of circumstances, then, information recorded in the chart provides only a partial view of the NICU and its activities and so offers only a partial solution to the problem of monitoring and evaluating the staff's activities.

Furthermore, since most parents have no expertise in treating critically ill infants, they depend on the experts to treat their newborns and to give

4. See Heimer and Stevens (1997) for an analysis of social work entries in medical records.

them information about how their infants are doing, what should be expected, and whether anything else might be tried. Most parents lack access to the diagnostic tools, information about the range of treatment alternatives, knowledge of the likely outcomes, and perhaps most important, access to alternative sources for this vital information. Because the infant is not just sick, but critically ill, seeking supplementary sources of information is often infeasible. Treatment decisions must be made too quickly to allow much time for consultations and second opinions. And even when time would permit, second opinions and consultations are difficult to acquire. Parents cannot simply take their hospitalized critically ill infants from one doctor to another. In rare cases, parents may be able to arrange a consultation with a physician from another hospital, but this is by no means routine. Because much of the information needed for evaluation is produced by the very people who are the subjects of evaluation, then, parents find it very difficult to assess staff performance.

Of course, parents vary in their dependence on the NICU and its staff for crucial pieces of information. A very small proportion of NICU parents has some medical expertise, or has access to close friends or relatives who will lend their expertise, and is therefore less dependent on the staff. We take up these variations in more detail below, but here we should note that variations in capacity to monitor and influence the activities of medical staff are to some degree class based. Those with fewer resources will have more difficulty than those who are better endowed in overcoming the organizational barriers and knowledge deficits that impede intervention.

The laws of informed consent were designed to help mitigate the effects of these tremendous barriers for all parents, regardless of class. However, while the laws of informed consent supply an important minimum standard for the parents' participation in treatment decisions, they offer no panacea (Anspach 1993; Zussman 1992). Consent procedures sometimes appear to be designed to fulfill the requirement that a consent form be signed, not to ensure that parents are full and active participants in treatment decisions. Furthermore, even if consent procedures encouraged meaningful participation by parents on some treatment decisions, not every treatment decision requires parental consent. For instance, once a patient has been placed on a mechanical ventilator, additional consent is not required either to change the rate of mechanical respirations or the oxygen level. How rapidly the patient is weaned from the ventilator, and conversely how quickly the oxygen level is dialed up, are both consequential decisions, but ones to be made by the physicians in the course of managing the case.

Managing a critically ill infant is a minute-by-minute, hour-by-hour, day-by-day activity. Decisions can be—and are—made at any time of day or night. Even with informed consent, parents may be unaware of many treatment decisions, other treatment options, and the consequences of choosing one option over another.

Parents face impressive obstacles, then, as they try to monitor and evaluate the care their infants receive. As compared with the NICU staff, parents are very impoverished social control agents. However, they do have a combination of informal sanctions—both positive and negative—at their disposal. One of the most powerful negative sanctions at the parents' disposal highlights the double-edged nature of social control in the NICU. Behavior regarded by the staff as inappropriate or disruptive may be deployed to punish the staff. Parents can make staff members' work lives difficult by not cooperating, by insisting that things be done their way, or by refusing to fit smoothly into the routine. Parents may also use other negative sanctions, including threats. Sometimes "inappropriate" demands are followed by threats—to transfer the baby, to contact a lawyer, to go to a higher authority in the hospital if a demand is not met. Such threats are ordinarily used only as a last resort when all else has failed. Although threats are sometimes successful, parents must use them judiciously. Because of the double-edged nature of social control, such threats may result in the parents being firmly labeled "inappropriate," ultimately serving only to alienate the staff from the parents and the infant.

Many parents never have to use threats. Instead, they exert influence through the use of positive sanctions. The most powerful incentives are controlled by the organization, not the parents. It is the hospital that employs the physicians, nurses, and technicians, and it is the hospital that retains control over financial and career incentives. However, parents can provide some incentives. Just as disrupting the staff's work acts as a negative sanction, so making that work more pleasant, rewarding, or enjoyable acts as a positive sanction. Some of what parents provide is material—cookies, flowers, a holiday gift. But parents also provide nonmaterial rewards—praise, a note expressing gratitude for a job well done, and the like. Such incentives make the staff feel that what they do is worthwhile, and these incentives add up.

A nurse at Suburban Hospital explains how seemingly small gestures can have big effects. Here, the nurse describes why a parent whose son was very ill was well liked by the nurses and other staff: "You didn't get the feeling that she was watching you like a hawk expecting you to do something wrong. She was . . . friendly. She would ask you how you were doing, too. She wasn't just completely focused on the baby. I mean, she'd come in and talk about the traffic on her way here or whatever. I mean, she was just friendly. And I'll tell you something. She got to hold Thomas whenever she wanted to, even when he was on the vent" (2009RN, p. 6). Of course, we must acknowledge the limits of "kissing up" to doctors and nurses as a mechanism of social control. But we also must recognize that parents who are appropriate, are well liked, engage the staff in friendly conversation, show signs of commitment to their baby, and show respect for the staff are more likely to be consulted and to have their wishes respected. Such parents are exerting social control, albeit of a different kind from that described above, and staff will be willing to go the "extra mile" for these parents and their infants.

Although organizational and knowledge barriers profoundly impede the parents' capacity to monitor, evaluate, and influence the activities of the NICU staff, and the laws of informed consent are not much help in overcoming these impediments, the situation of parents is not unique. Others attempting to influence the medical care of infants have encountered similar obstacles (see, e.g., Heimer 1996a). NICU routines are designed to get work done efficiently and safely, not to maximize the participation of outsiders. Anyone wishing to shape the course of events in an NICU, whether he or she wishes to affect the fate of a single child or to reform the routines themselves, must first learn the lay of the land. Many outsiders imagine that the difficulty is that they know too little about medicine. While that is undoubtedly true, it is equally important that they know too little about the NICU as an organization. Both of these are problems encountered equally by regulators, reformers, and anxious parents. What parents have going for them is a zeal and persistence unmatched in most regulatory bodies.

Supervising the Experts: Principals and Their Agents in the NICU

We have argued that parents in the NICU are dependent on the staff—not only for the skills that will be used in treating their infants but also for the information that is crucial in assessing staff performance. Such deep dependence is not unique to this setting, according to social scientists, but rather is an example of the general class of relationships where one party (referred to as the agent) is a specialist who provides a service to another party (referred to as the principal) who is not. Social scientists, especially economists, have written extensively about principal-agent relations, arguing that such relations are simultaneously robust and fragile forms of association (see the essays collected in Pratt and Zeckhauser 1991, particularly the introduction by Pratt and Zeckhauser and the essay by Arrow; Bergen, Dutta, and Walker 1992; Coleman 1990; Fama 1980; Fama and Jensen 1983; Monsma 1993; Petersen 1993; Sobel 1993). Principal-agent relations are robust because principals are able to draw on skills and expertise that extend beyond their own. The principal need not be an expert in medicine to receive treatment, an expert in tort law to receive representation in a civil court case, or an expert in financial markets to invest in a mutual fund. The principal can instead hire an agent, or expert, to act on his or her behalf—to prescribe medicine, to resolve a legal dispute, or to maximize returns to mutual fund investors. But principal-agent relations are fragile as well. The central irony here is that what makes principal-agent relations valuable—that the agent has skill and expertise the principal lacks—is precisely what renders them vulnerable. Principals may not be competent to select agents and are often unable to monitor the behavior of agents because of obstacles such as distance, organizational structure, secrecy, and lack of expertise (Shapiro 1987). Because the principal cannot control the activities of the agent, agency relations entail some degree of uncertainty. The challenge from the principal's point of view, then, is to ensure that the agent acts primarily with the principal's best interest in mind.

In the standard version of agency theory, assumptions are made about the preferences of the principal, the choice of an agent, and the use of a contract to control the activities of the agent (Heimer 1990). According to agency theorists, the principal has a set of preferences (typically expressed as wants or goals) which cannot easily be met without the help of an agent who has specialized knowledge, skills, or contacts that the principal lacks. In choosing an agent to reach these goals, the principal must collect information about whether the agent is technically skilled and likely to honor the fiduciary obligation. The principal must also design a contract to induce the agent to act on the principal's behalf in achieving these goals. The contract must be a sophisticated instrument, because the agency relation involves both hidden action (the agent carries out activities the principal cannot directly observe) and hidden information (the agent has information that the principal lacks and can choose whether to use this information to benefit the principal) (Arrow 1991).

Although NICU parents confront the two core problems discussed by agency theory—hidden information and hidden actions—many of the standard assumptions about the social control of agency relations are violated in this case. First, agency theory assumes that the principal's preferences are unproblematic. But in this case, the preferences of the parent principals are inchoate and may change over time as the infant's condition changes and as the parents become more knowledgeable about the consequences of one course of treatment versus another. Their preferences cannot, therefore, be fully specified in advance of the action the agent is supposed to take on the principal's behalf. Many parents, for instance, articulate a very general preference to have "everything done." Early in the infant's treatment, the parents are especially unlikely to understand what "everything" means. Some parents discover only much later that they have preferences they were unable to articulate. In a case we will describe in more detail below, one mother developed a strong preference to breastfeed on demand only when her son's condition failed to improve while he was being bottle-fed on a four-hour schedule (1026). Another mother pressed to have her son's surgery performed first thing on a Tuesday morning, because she thought the surgeon would be more rested after a day off (1028). Preferences such as these only develop over the course of the infant's hospitalization, as parents become more knowledgeable.

Not only are parents' preferences unclear to them in advance and difficult to articulate, they are also shaped in large part by the very agents who are supposed to be acting with those preferences in mind.[5] One attending physician at Suburban Hospital was acutely aware of his role in helping parents develop, or discover, their preferences: "So you're really a guide for them and then they make it [the decision about treatment]. What happens is you help them come to at least a decision they are comfortable with, and then you have to maintain communication. . . . You are really going through a process of sorting out their values. . . . They don't even know what they [their values and preferences] are. . . . They do have values—they [just] don't know what they are. . . . They have never thought of them in those terms, so they have to figure out what decisions they want and what they would mean, and then get a chance to think out how am I going to feel about that versus this. That takes a lot of work. They may change their mind" (2003MD, pp. 8–9).

Agency theory also assumes that principals have the time, skill, and

5. Zussman (1992) makes a similar point about adult intensive care units.

knowledge to collect information about potential agents and the capacity to hire and fire agents. In this case, most parents have no warning that their infants will require hospitalization and so have no time for due diligence in selecting either a physician or a hospital. One mother, whose experience is not uncommon, had a relatively uneventful pregnancy, went into labor expecting to deliver a healthy baby, and delivered her full-term son vaginally. It wasn't until after the baby was transferred from the hospital where he was born to City Hospital and had surgery that his shocked mother felt she really understood the situation. "I didn't really understand what the problem was until after I got over to [City Hospital]. They told me then at the [local] hospital that he couldn't pass his own bowels, that they might have to do surgery on him. So they shipped him to [City] in an ambulance, and [they were] putting all these tubes in him and everything. I was so scared. . . . I thought my baby wasn't going to live" (1025F, p. 4).

As another mother explains, nobody expects to have a sick baby: "I mean, they talk about the normal childbirth, that's why you have this class [Lamaze]. Everybody is expecting in this class to have a normal child" (2040F, p. 3). Just a few days after attending her first Lamaze class, this first-time mother discovered that her amniotic sac was leaking. She delivered seven weeks early and, like many other parents we interviewed, felt she hardly got to see her new baby before he was whisked away: "I saw my son for like five minutes . . . and that was it and then it's bye-bye and he's gone" (2040F, p. 10). In general, parents have little time to prepare for the birth of a critically ill infant.

Furthermore, parents have precious little control over the disposition of their infants. As we have explained, neonatal intensive care resources are distributed in regional networks. The contracts between hospitals that ensure the smooth transfer of a patient from one hospital to the next are arranged independent of any particular infant's hospitalization. Some of our parents were able to press for transfers to one hospital rather than another. For instance, the woman whose son was born seven weeks early pressed for a transfer to Suburban Hospital, because it was closer to her home than an alternative hospital with an NICU. However, most transfers occur without consideration of parents' preferences. And although we have evidence that some parents successfully pushed for transfers to the units we studied, we of course have no idea how many other parents unsuccessfully pressed for transfers.

Finally, agency theory assumes that it is the principal who designs the contract to induce appropriate behavior from the agent.[6] In this case, however, principals do not form unique contracts. Instead, parents are members of a class of principals entering into contracts with a strong agent that has designed a standard contract that applies to all parents. Because the principals here are novices, and the agents are expert repeat players, it is the agents that design the contract that defines the terms of their relationship. This contract is designed in advance of any particular parent's arrival on the scene, is as much a response to legal and medical requirements as to the needs of parents, and is embedded in the routines of the NICU. For instance, the consent form that parents are asked to sign is a standard document designed by the hospital, not by the parents. Parents may sometimes modify the consent form, for instance crossing out clauses giving blanket consent for blood transfusions, but they do not design their own consent form, let alone write a contract specifying the conditions under which they are hiring the doctor or the hospital staff to act as their agents in providing medical care for their child.

Because the standard assumptions of agency theory do not fit our case very well, we conclude that the standard social control measure posited by agency theory—designing a contract to induce the agent to behave in appropriate ways—is unlikely to be an effective mechanism of control. If designing a unique contract to induce appropriate behavior is infeasible, principals may employ other strategies to cope with the uncertainties created by agency relations: they may avoid or limit their participation in agency relationships; they may reduce their exposure to an agent by spreading the risk, either over time or over agents; or they may embed their agency relations in social networks (Shapiro 1987).

However, none of these solutions to the problem of misaligned interests is perfect. Principals vary in the extent to which they can limit participation, reduce exposure, or embed the agency relationship in personal networks. In neonatal intensive care, as in most emergency medical situations, limiting participation in the agency relation is simply not feasible. Parents' rights to refuse medical treatment—that is to refuse to enlist the services of an agent—for their children are legally limited. Under some conditions

6. Coleman (1990:146–49) discusses two alternative forms of agency relations, "independent contractor" and "servant" agency, which differ in the extent to which the principal has authority over the agent. Although most of the literature on agency focuses on servant agency, the hospital staff members we discuss here more closely resemble independent contractors, at least in the sense that contracts are not designed by the principals (parents and their infants) and principals have very little authority over agents.

(mainly when the treatment is necessary to save the child's life) the law gives the staff the right to treat an infant, even over the parents' objections. Parents may sometimes be permitted to refuse or to terminate life-saving treatment when it is futile and merely prolongs dying. That staff, not parents, make many of the judgment calls about treatment demonstrates rather clearly that parents do not negotiate unique contracts with medical care providers, but rather step into prefabricated standard contracts.[7] If parents refuse medical treatment, the parents' wishes are subsumed under the contract between the medical staff and the state. The state grants physicians a great deal of discretion, but physicians who fail to provide life-saving medical treatment, even over parental objections, can be charged with medical neglect and lose their licenses. Charges of medical neglect are rare. But their rarity also reflects the mutual influence of law and medicine and demonstrates how deeply the state's requirements have been incorporated into the routines of the hospital (Heimer 1996a). Hospitals now have standard procedures for acquiring a court order that grants temporary custody of an infant to the physician when the parents refuse what is regarded as necessary, life-saving intervention. Although this, too, is a rare occurrence, the hospital is well equipped to take the necessary steps to fulfill its contract with the state, even over parents' objections.[8]

Limiting participation in agency relations, then, is not always feasible, because it inevitably restricts access to the benefits controlled by the agents—receiving treatment for an illness, advice about a contract dispute, dividends from mutual fund investments, and so on. However, for parents of critically ill babies, the penalty can be especially severe. In addition to foregoing the benefits of participation, if the parents try to limit their exposure by limiting participation in agency relationships, they may lose cus-

7. In disagreements with staff, parents are more likely to prevail if they wish to continue treatment while the staff encourages a limitation of treatment. If the parents want to discontinue or limit treatment when the staff does not concur that treatment is futile, parents will have much more difficulty enforcing their wishes. See Stinson and Stinson's (1983) moving account of their struggle to convince the medical staff that continued treatment for their son, Andrew, was futile. Not all decisions about whether to continue treatment are retained by the staff, however. Occasionally desperate parents take matters into their own hands, and usually such parents are treated sympathetically by the legal system. One father who had opposed life-saving treatment for his very premature son disconnected the child from the ventilator within hours after his birth. Although he was indicted and brought to trial on a charge of manslaughter, he was acquitted (*New York Times* 1995; Frey 1995, p. 24).

8. Recall the case of the Jehovah's Witnesses discussed in chapter 4. In that case, after hours of tense negotiations that included extended family members and church representatives, the physicians decided they had no choice but to seek court intervention.

tody of their infant. That is, in the extreme, the parents may be stripped of their role as principals.

This possibility of stripping parents of their role as principals arises only because parents are, in fact, intermediaries between the infant patients and the hospital staff. Because the infant patients are unable to express their preferences, the parents become the natural repositories of what little information there is about their infants' interests and are expected to act as representatives for their infants. The parents have a dual role in a chain of agency relations: they are agents with respect to their infants, and principals with respect to the hospital and its staff. But as principals, parents are expected to act primarily on behalf of their children, not to pursue their own independent interests.

As much of the ethics literature recognizes, though, the ambiguity of the infants' preferences exacerbates the potential conflicts of interest between infants and parents, on the one hand, and between infants and staff members, on the other. Because the infant is incapable of expressing preferences and has, in fact, never had preferences to express, questions may be raised about the legitimacy of both parents and physicians as representatives of those interests.[9] As agents, both parents and physicians have other preferences that may clash with the interests of infant patients. For example, the parents have a competing interest in preserving the family resources for other family members, and the hospital and the staff have a competing interest in pushing the frontiers of medical science. The infamous Baby Doe cases raised questions about the need for guardians to ensure that the infant's rights, especially to life, are protected.[10] Such cases have highlighted the precariousness of the parents' role as agent-principals.

Although medical staff and parents may have interests that conflict with those of the critically ill baby, such conflicts are in fact a more significant impediment for parents as agents than for medical care givers as agents. In the NICU, the staff must act as agents. That is their job, and they are morally and legally obligated to do so. And because medical staff cannot do their work without knowing what is in the patient's best interest, infants will be treated as principals and will have preferences and rights imputed to them. Any conflict of interest between medical staff members and pa-

9. See Anspach (1993, chapter 2), for a fuller discussion of the NICU ethics literature.

10. See chapter 4 for a fuller discussion of the Baby Doe cases and the resulting legislation.

tients is muted by the routinization of medical work.[11] Deep questioning about whether babies really profit from NICU care or how to think about the future of some hopelessly damaged child are buried under the press of business as usual. But for parents there is no "business as usual" in having a critically ill baby, and the parental role as intermediary is therefore ill defined, less thoroughly institutionalized, and relatively exposed to outside scrutiny and challenge. No family bureaucracy is in place to defend parents' legitimacy as agent-principals acting on behalf of their children and their families, to reassure parents that what they are doing is right and proper, or to stamp parents' actions with the authority that would be conferred by previous generations of parents doing exactly the same thing.[12] In the absence of pressures encouraging uniformity, it is here that we find the important variations. First, parents themselves differ in the extent to which they see it as their role to act as agent-principals. Further, others vary in the extent to which they accept parents as legitimate agent-principals.

Because both the parents and the staff are in some senses suspect representatives of the babies' interests, several "guardians," in Shapiro's (1987) language, have been assigned to watch over the care they receive. These guardians, like the guardians in other circumstances, offer a mix of "normative prescriptions, socialization, institutional arrangements, structural constraints, networks of interdependence, and sanctions to ensure that the abuse of trust does not become either too tempting or too easy" (1987:636). The regulation of agency relations often depends on standards that are enforced through various carrots and sticks. Here, laws, ethical prescriptions, and organizational guidelines and rules of procedure are enforced through some combination of organizational and institutional arrangements, internal and external quality control review, regulatory agencies, and courts of law. However, as Shapiro notes, the guardians offer no panacea either. Normative prescriptions may be ignored. Socialization may

11. See Chambliss (1996) for superb discussions of how the routinization of medical work takes place and how routinization and the division of labor among medical professionals shape thinking about ethical questions.

12. In theory, this role could be played by parent-support groups. And while many NICUs do have parent-support groups, the meetings of such groups are attended almost exclusively by parents of NICU graduates. Apparently it is only after the crisis has passed that parents have sufficient time and energy even to seek advice and solace from others in similar situations. Support groups do provide substantial encouragement for social control efforts, then, but typically only for families whose babies have already left the NICU.

be incomplete. Institutional arrangements may not provide sufficiently strong incentives. Structural constraints and networks of interdependence may be weak. And sanctions may have no teeth. Perhaps most crucially, the safeguards controlling agents and making them look trustworthy can be simulated. Physicians can appoint cooperative ethicists and dominate the ancillary professionals who have the most contact with patients. They can present principals with a limited range of choices, as Zussman (1992) and Anspach (1993) show, and also formulate choices in arcane language that principals cannot understand. They can also make it seem as if they were informing and consulting their patients by trotting out the standard, very general consent form that is signed before treatment begins.

Regulation is intended to shore up agency relations by decreasing the principal's vulnerability to the agent through such mechanisms as setting standards and applying sanctions. But principals may instead find themselves protected by a net whose holes are simply too large to prevent injury—little comfort to a parent who is consumed by grief over the critical illness of an infant.

Unlike the principals of agency theory, parents have virtually no formal sanctions at their disposal. They cannot really hire or fire staff members (although more than one parent spoke of "firing" a physician, and several told us that they requested that particular nurses not care for their baby); they cannot give promotions, pay raises, or even financial bonuses. There are in fact formal norms that prevent client economic sanctioning of physicians, and prevent insurance coverage for treatments not recommended by a physician selected or approved by the insurer. Without formal sanctions, parents must devise other ways to reward and punish the staff.[13] Rather than offer such contractually based incentives as money and promotions, they must offer gifts; rather than command, they must negotiate with the staff in order to influence their activities. Social control by parents is less formal and less uniform than the social control envisaged by agency theorists (or accomplished by the staff), but its effect may nevertheless be quite substantial. As one nurse notes: "The way parents treat you really makes a

13. Monsma (1993), analyzing another example in which the principals were unable to control agents through contracts (relations between Argentine landowners and ranch managers in the early 1800s), shows how patronage and contracts worked together to make agency relations possible. Patronage both allowed principals to monitor and enforce contractual obligations (which were not easily enforceable under a weak state) and to supplement the rewards offered through contracts.

difference in the attitude you have about coming to work. It's really a big job around here, just dealing with the parents" (2009RN, p. 9).

NICU parents are sufficiently weak principals, though, that they lack even the sanction of last resort, the ability to exit. While most consumers can vote with their feet, parents cannot simply remove their critically ill infants from the hospital. They can, however, threaten to bring a lawsuit against the hospital and its physicians, and such threats are often used when all other means of influence have been exhausted. By their very nature these lawsuits are retrospective, though, taking account of what has already been done, assessing whether it deviated from standard practice, and deciding whether compensation is warranted. Because of this retrospective focus, malpractice suits cannot influence the course of treatment as it unfolds, which is, of course, parents' primary goal.[14]

In order to monitor, evaluate, and influence the activities of the staff, parents must call on other resources. Parents' success as social control agents will depend on how much time they spend on the unit; how much they know about medicine, the hospital, and its procedures; and the amounts and kinds of resources they are able to marshal to support their position. Parents have very different pools of resources on which to draw, a point to which we will return below. Because parents tend not to pool their social control resources (as staff members do) and cannot call on the resources of an organization to supplement their individual efforts (as staff members can), parents who are well endowed have a tremendous advantage over those who are impoverished. But parents' success as agents of social control also depends deeply on whether they are able to convince staff of the legitimacy of their interventions. As we argue below, staff members will be most receptive to parental intervention that does not interfere with core technical matters.

A crucial intervening factor here is the extent to which social control is a collective enterprise. While staff members share the responsibility for monitoring and evaluating the parents—together making up a diffuse, but effective, social control system—the parents stand alone in their efforts.

14. Other researchers (e.g., Freidson 1989:171) have argued that the rise in malpractice lawsuits has had an aggregate effect on the practice of medicine, for instance, increasing the number of diagnostic tests ordered by physicians and increasing the overall cost of health care. Although malpractice suits undoubtedly have some net effect on how medicine is practiced, that does not mean that they are an effective mechanism for social control at the individual level. *Threatening* to sue is another matter, of course, and we have argued that this is one sanction of last resort for parents in the NICU.

The unit provides the nurses with such infrastructural support as forms for documenting their interactions with and observations of the parents; no infrastructural support is provided for parent monitoring of staff activities. Monitoring, evaluating, and reforming parents are routine activities for the NICU staff; monitoring, evaluating, and reforming NICU staff members are not routine activities for parents. And while parents are encouraged to visit the unit, the information packet they receive does not instruct them to keep a watchful eye to ensure that their preferences are being honored in the practice of medicine. Parents are not even instructed that they should have preferences. Parents, then, must initiate the acts of monitoring, evaluating, and reforming the staff, and they must do so as individuals working without institutional support. Each family must reinvent appropriate "technology," deciding what needs to be recorded, devising "coding sheets," and finding ways to make unobtrusive observations. Not surprisingly, then, we find much more variation among parents than among staff in how they view and execute their roles as agents of social control. At the crudest level, some parents simply do not act as social control agents; in contrast, every parent is monitored and evaluated by the staff.

But this radical individualization of parental social control has implications beyond matters of infrastructural support. Parents must decide for themselves what is appropriate and what is not, a difficult matter for those who are intensely aware of their lack of expertise. Consensus about what is appropriate doctoring or nursing is therefore quite low, and parents are likely to have widely differing reactions to the same event. With no community of peers to set or enforce standards, parents vacillate between speaking up and remaining silent. As one father commented, "You sort of vacillate [between] feeling like you as parent should intervene, and feeling like you don't want to bother them with this stupid question" (2025M, p. 9).

Finally, the collectivization of social control has implications for how resources are used. Parents have limited resources for engaging in social control activities. As we argued in chapter 5, the NICU also has limited resources for engaging in social control. But the shortage of social control resources has a different effect on parental attempts at social control than on those of staff members, because social control by the staff is a team effort. To economize on resources, NICU staff members "triage" parents, separating those who can be reformed from those who are beyond hope. Parents, working as isolated individuals or couples, cannot as easily engage in triage. Often they have too little information to decide where social control efforts should be concentrated, and they have little capacity to redistribute or pool resources.[15] As a result, the distribution of parental social control depends much more on which parents are resource rich and which ones are impoverished rather than on which staff members could be reformed with appropriate parental intervention.

In the next section, we ask what accounts for the variation we observe in the extent to which parents conceive themselves as social control agents in the NICU. When do parents see themselves as intermediaries in the agency chain linking infants as principals and staff members as agents? Without any "job description" to guide their thinking about their role in the NICU, parents vary a good deal in whether they conceive it as their job to monitor the activities of the NICU staff and to intervene in those activities.

To Trust or Not to Trust: How Parents Define Their Roles

Although scholars have noted a general decline in the American public's trust in professionals (e.g., Barber 1983), when one looks closer, this sweeping generalization masks considerable variation. And while this variation may not be important to our understanding of aggregate changes, it is crucial in understanding parents' definitions of their roles in the NICU. Parents' orientations toward medical professionals can be arrayed along a continuum, with parents who have faith in medical care providers at one extreme and parents who distrust located at the other extreme. Between these two extremes we find the majority of parents who trust contingently.

Parents Who Have Faith

A small group of the parents we interviewed expressed unfailing faith in the unit and its staff. Typically, such parents explained their position by noting that since they had no expertise in critical care medicine, they were not qualified to oversee the activities of the staff. These parents usually described their infant's fate as being out of their hands—because it was in God's hands, or the doctors' hands, or both.[16] Such parents only fulfill their

15. In chapter 5, we discussed one exceptional instance of cooperative social control by two mothers, who ended up being regarded as nuisances. Staff members did all they could to discourage such joint monitoring, nipping in the bud any possibility that parents would develop routines and forms to facilitate their own and others' social control efforts.

16. Of course, for some parents having faith in God is incompatible with having faith in the medical professionals. For Christian Scientists, for example, having faith in God means not seeking medical intervention and therefore makes moot any questions about the trustworthiness of physicians (Frohock 1992).

role as agents in the most limited sense—for example, by signing consent forms—because they simply do not recognize an agency chain in which they have a role. Though these parents may visit the unit, it is not because they feel a need to oversee their infant's care.

Paul and Rose have a large, very religious family. When they learned their daughter was critically ill, they prayed for her recovery. "It was out of our hands," Paul commented, describing how his daughter's life was "in his [the doctor's] hands, in God's hands" (1011M, p. 10). Tess was born full-term but suffered from severe respiratory distress from meconium aspiration. Meconium is the dark green mucilaginous substance that accumulates in the intestines of the fetus. Serious respiratory problems occur when meconium is excreted into the amniotic fluid and inhaled by the baby. She was first transported from the small community hospital where she was born to a larger hospital where she was placed on a ventilator. When Tess's condition continued to deteriorate, she was transported by helicopter over 100 miles to City Hospital and placed on an ECMO machine to give the lungs a chance to heal. Paul and Rose had never visited the hospital or met the physicians who would be caring for Tess. However, they felt no urgent need to oversee their daughter's care. They were comforted by the doctors' telephone calls and never doubted the staff would do all they could. Rose, in fact, recalled her reluctance to visit, in words that suggest more resignation than faith: "I didn't want to go down, because I didn't want to get attached to her, because I thought, you know, if she would die or something I didn't want, I didn't want to be attached. I just didn't" (1011F, p. 5).[17] Paul and Rose eventually visited and took Tess home from the hospital when she was well. Both parents were very happy with the outcome, believing Tess would never have recovered without the skillful care she received. But they also firmly believed that the outcome was not in their hands.

Most of the parents who have faith in the health professionals do not base their faith on religion, however. Instead they simply feel that it would be inappropriate to second-guess the NICU staff, whose expertise makes them better judges of what should be done. One mother describes her orientation this way: "Well, they just sounded like they knew what they were talking about. In medical terms, I'm pretty confident with the doctors" (1012F, p. 24). Another young mother recounts how she left the staff to determine what was needed: "They just kind of did what they needed.

17. We have labeled this category "faith," but in some cases it is difficult to distinguish from "resignation," a point we return to later.

They called me like in the morning and told me, 'Well, we're going to do this today. Is it okay?' you know, and I'd say 'Just do it, whatever it takes'" (2011F, p. 25). Rather than approach the staff with questions, this mother "always waited until they came to me" (p. 22). When asked, she says she never felt she had to "oversee" the staff. One father who did not visit his son during the hospitalization explains that his son's outcome depended less on what he did than on what others did: "It's not so much what we do. It's what the doctors do" (1018M, p. 34). These parents are relatively inactive participants in the agency chain. Having recognized that they are not experts, they resign themselves to a limited role.

Parents Who Distrust

At the other extreme are those parents who distrust all or some significant portion of the NICU staff. Some parents enter the unit with an already established sense of distrust; others come to distrust the staff during the course of their baby's hospitalization, following the discovery of a medical mistake or because of numerous setbacks in the baby's hospital course. Other parents become distrustful because of difficulty diagnosing and treating the baby's illness, or because they believe their wishes about treatment are not being respected.

Whatever the cause of distrust, such parents tend to engage in rigorous surveillance of the NICU and its staff. Worried about what might be done in their absence, they sit at the bedside in a near-constant vigil: "You get to a point where you don't trust them anymore, where you think if you're not going to be there that they might do something that will cause a lot of harm or damage" (2040M, p. 23). These parents often have an adversarial relationship with the staff. They believe it is their responsibility to make sure everything goes as it should. Taking their role in the agency chain seriously, such parents feel that no one else could replace them. It is they, in particular, who must keep watch, because no one else will look out for their infant's interests as a parent does. In essence, they attempt to limit the agency relations that others have with their infants by limiting either the number of agents (e.g., not allowing a particular nurse or physician to care for their infant) or the scope of other agents' authority (e.g., demanding to be consulted in routine matters such as dialing up or down the amount of oxygen a patient receives).

Charlotte and Bruce's profound sense of distrust followed a medical mistake at Suburban Hospital: their daughter was given an overdose of medication. Charlotte describes how she "lost complete trust" (2024F,

p. 32) when she discovered the mistake and from then on took a very active role in monitoring the staff and intervening in their activities. She sat at Ellie's bedside around the clock, participated in her care as much as possible, read the medical chart, and watched the staff "like a hawk" (p. 41). Bruce was supportive of her need to be at Ellie's bedside, but as their daughter's hospitalization stretched to weeks and months, her bedside vigil put a strain on the marriage.

Their trust was further undermined after a meeting with the doctors who were responsible for Ellie's care. All were visibly tense, according to Charlotte. Ellie had been doing poorly and had recently suffered a series of cardiorespiratory arrests, the most recent requiring heroic resuscitation efforts. Ellie had been saved, but her doctors now suggested there was evidence of severe brain damage. All in attendance, including the neonatologist and neurologist, believed further heroic treatment was futile. All were in agreement, that is, except Ellie's parents. Bruce describes this meeting as a turning point, when he and Charlotte decided "these people [NICU staff] really don't know what they're talking about. . . . We know more than they do about our child" (2024M, pp. 45–46). Both he and Charlotte became convinced that they had to become advocates for Ellie. They felt it was more than their right—it was their obligation—to make suggestions to the staff about the care their daughter was receiving. They read their daughter's medical chart, sought opinions from physicians outside the unit, and oversaw every treatment decision. By the end of Ellie's hospitalization, Charlotte had done everything she could to limit the number and authority of other agents. She rented a room in the hospital (an expense not covered by insurance) and cared for Ellie herself.

Parents Who Trust Contingently

The vast majority of parents fall into an intermediate category—they have contingent trust in the NICU and its staff. Such parents neither feel that everything is out of their hands nor that they must keep a vigilant bedside watch. They neither abdicate their role in the agency chain nor attempt to limit competition from other agents. Just as staff members begin by judging individual actions and only later draw conclusions about parents as persons, so parents also are likely to revise their conclusions as time passes. These parents trust the NICU and its staff, but their trust is contingent on weighing new evidence as it accumulates. One father summarizes the orientation of contingent trust well: "I was confident out there because I was watching with my own eyes how they were taking care" (2022M, p. 8).

The difference between faith and trust, then, is that although faith is blind, trust is not. And the difference between distrust and contingent trust lies in how closely parents surveil. Parents who distrust expend vast resources on surveillance. Parents who trust contingently expend some resources collecting and weighing evidence to determine whether their trust is well placed, but without allowing surveillance to become an all-consuming mission. Many parents who have contingent trust educate themselves about their infant's condition and otherwise look for independent sources of information to verify what they are being told by the NICU staff. But they do not go so far as to treat staff members as adversaries. Parents who trust contingently are differentiated from distrusting parents by degree, not kind.

To put it another way, faith, contingent trust, and distrust entail different conceptions of the team responsible for caring for the critically ill child. The key question is who is a member of the team and who is not. Parents who have faith do not conceive themselves to be members of the team. Instead, the team is composed exclusively of health-care providers. Parents who trust contingently believe that they too are members of their baby's team. Doctors and nurses have important roles to play, but parents have an assigned role as well. Within this view of parents as members of the baby's team there is considerable variation. Some parents believe that their role is relatively minor and that they are distinctly subordinate to physicians, but other parents see themselves as having a somewhat larger role. But the point is that parents who trust contingently balance respect for medical expertise with a healthy understanding that everyone is fallible. They act as advocates for their children in matters that are important to them but feel comfortable leaving some details to other team members. Parents who distrust conceive roles more hierarchically, placing themselves at the top of the hierarchy. They are the bosses, not members of a team. As the ones ultimately responsible for their child's welfare, it is their job to oversee the work of the health-care team. In effect, the parents function as general contractors; they have adopted an "entrepreneurial role" (Darling 1979). At this point, their child needs the services of an NICU team, and so that is what they have hired. But an NICU team is in principle no different from a team of teachers, a nanny, or a coach. Should they believe that the health-care team—or any other team, for that matter—is not doing a good job, it is the parents' job to replace an incompetent health-care team with a competent one.

Parents' orientations are not static, though. Parents who arrive at the

NICU full of faith need not continue to have faith in their medical team, just as parents who are skeptical or distrustful may come to respect and trust their child's team.

The Developmental Approach: Changing Orientations and Redefining Roles

Kathleen Gerson's work about how women and men make choices about work, career, and parenthood serves as a model for our analysis of how parents decide how actively to supervise their child's medical treatment. Gerson (1985, 1993) argues that people's choices must be understood as the product of both their socialization, or expectations about what kind of lives they will lead, and the opportunities and constraints they face along the way. Hers is a developmental approach to understanding women's and men's roles in late twentieth-century America, where people must strike a balance between work and family obligations but where there is considerable variation in how that balance is struck.

We draw two crucial insights from Gerson's work, the first empirical and the second theoretical. First, it is women who face the "hard choices" described in Gerson's work. As much as women's and men's roles have changed in the last half of the twentieth century, women still shoulder a disproportionate share of responsibility for domestic labor. Men can more easily choose simply to avoid domesticity or to escape domestic burdens if they find them too onerous. This fundamental empirical fact extends beyond routine domestic responsibilities to extraordinary ones, as our discussion of life beyond the NICU will demonstrate in chapter 7. But Gerson also offers an explanation that emphasizes the agency of the men and women she interviewed and shows how choice and constraint are balanced in their lives. Gerson, for instance, recognizes that women are socialized to accept some roles as appropriate and to reject others. She also recognizes that women face structural constraints on their advancement in the world of paid employment. However, this is only the beginning of the story, not the end. Women respond thoughtfully and intelligently to their expectations, adjusting their strategies as they meet obstacles or unexpected opportunities along the way.

In the world of the NICU, we similarly find that parents' choices about how they define their roles are the products not only of the beliefs, values, and previous experiences that they bring with them to the NICU, but also of their particular experiences while their infants are hospitalized. We therefore take a developmental approach to how parents define their roles in the NICU. Most parents come to the unit expecting that they will have no need to monitor closely the care their infants are receiving. After all, the NICU is a high-tech unit where skilled professionals practice state-of-the-art medicine. Some parents, especially those whose children experience relatively long or complicated medical courses, come to reevaluate this orientation.

Most parents of critically ill babies have an orientation of contingent trust, and many distrusting parents trusted the hospital staff at the beginning of their ordeal. However, for some parents, that trust is undermined over the course of the infant's hospitalization (see Charlotte and Bruce's case [2024], above). For other parents, an overwhelming sense of uncertainty is what undermines their trust in the doctors, and even in medicine more generally.

Jason's parents were discussed in chapter 3 as people who had taken a lot of responsibility for a child with ongoing serious medical problems. Their case suggests important connections between skepticism and responsibility—when parents feel that they cannot rely on physicians, they may become especially vigorous representatives of their children's interests. Jason, who was born with anomalies of the bladder and urinary tract, had been hospitalized several times since his initial crisis because of recurring urinary tract infections. He had several operations but still was not able to urinate through his penis at the time of our interviews with his parents. His parents felt that a great deal of uncertainty lingered about whether he would ever have good bladder control and a normal sex life. When Jason was born, neither Cindy nor John had reason to distrust doctors or medicine in general, but their frustration grew, as John explains, when they could not seem to get any "straight answers" (1001M, p. 3).

Parents often have difficulty accepting the uncertainty surrounding their infant's care, sometimes blaming the physicians who seem unable or unwilling to resolve it: "Doctors will never give you a straight answer even if they know it. You know, and they'll, they can confuse you worse than anybody else on the face of the earth" (1001F, p. 29). Parents (and other laypeople) cannot easily distinguish between uncertainty that reflects the limits of a particular doctor and uncertainty that is inherent in the situation and reflects the limits of medical practice more generally. In either case, parents often come to distrust the physicians, because they cannot tell them what they desperately want to know: What will the future hold for my child? And by extension, What will the future hold for me? Pressure for predictions about the future is so common that one attending physician had a well-rehearsed response: "I always make the point about predicting is very difficult and there's not an absolute. I'll point to this quote I cut out one time, that it's difficult to make predictions, particularly about the future, to point out that we cannot predict. That's one thing that parents want from us, but we cannot absolutely predict that" (2002MD, p. 11).[18]

Not all changes in orientation are in the direction of distrust. Sometimes distrust is replaced by a renewed sense of trust. Kate and Pat grew to distrust the doctors at two different hospitals before their son, Sam, was transferred to City Hospital, and his problems with apnea (a cessation of breathing for longer than twenty seconds) and bradycardia (a slowing of the heart rate that often occurs just after the onset of apnea) were resolved. Sam was born prematurely but required mechanical ventilation only during the first hour after his birth. For a twenty-nine-week gestation infant, he was doing very well. However, he had repeated spells of apnea and bradycardia. The doctors at the hospital where Sam was born told Kate and Pat that the spells would resolve as Sam matured and gained weight. But as Sam grew, the spells continued, and his parents became very concerned. The doctors suggested Sam's apnea might instead be caused by an airway obstruction, but no obstruction was found. The uncertainty exasperated Sam's parents as the weeks of his hospitalization stretched into months. Kate began to wonder whether his treatment plan was appropriate. When Kate suggested that Sam's health might improve if she were allowed to breast-feed him on demand, Sam's physician disagreed and refused to allow her to try. An argument ensued, and the doctor asked the social worker to intervene. After a brief stay in another hospital, Sam was eventually transferred to City's NICU. At City, Sam was given a transfusion for anemia, allowed to feed on demand, and even to breast-feed. His condition improved dramatically, and he was discharged home within a week.

Kate and Pat had become convinced that they needed to monitor their

18. In addition to their understandable reluctance to make firm predictions, the neonatologists we talked with were also reluctant to discuss statistics with parents. They suggested that there was little point in telling a couple that their child had a 30% chance of developing cerebral palsy, for instance, when the child would either have cerebral palsy or not. As the child grew, its experience would be either 0% or 100%. In this sense, they argued, the likelihood (30%) was not a good estimate of the child's experience and so would be misleading. It is worth noting that this position on the use of statistics is somewhat at variance with geneticists', genetic counselors', and statisticians' views on probability. One might expect that neonatologists would have a somewhat distinctive ideology about probability given the realities of their work.

son's care closely because his condition failed to improve and the doctors were unable to provide a satisfactory explanation. Kate collected information on her own, read what she could find, and tried to educate herself about her son's condition. Here, the uncertainty about when Sam would be discharged, coupled with her frustration that the physicians disregarded her suggestions, undermined her sense of trust. As she described her experience, her anger was apparent: "They would not listen to any of our suggestions at all. . . . A lot of people think doctors are gods. I don't. People think doctors are powerful and that you shouldn't challenge doctors. And I'm not like that. I'm pretty outspoken and I wasn't afraid to speak my mind" (1026F, pp. 7–8). When her son's condition improved after his transfer to City's NICU, Kate felt vindicated: "Suddenly to be treated like an adult again, like a responsible person with opinions that might matter and with input and with, 'Hey, this lady knows the kid better than anybody else'" (1026F, p. 10). She was relieved to feel she could finally trust the care her son was receiving.

Whether or not parents trust that their children are receiving the best possible care clearly depends on how well their infants are progressing. Quick recoveries tend to build trust (or prevent trust from being undermined in the first place). But trust does not depend solely on the outcome. Sometimes even when the outcome is less than miraculous, parents who are distrusting will experience a change in orientation. Anne's mother, Nancy, describes herself as very distrusting of medical professionals. At birth Anne was diagnosed with a tracheoesophageal fistula (TEF), a passage connecting the trachea and the esophagus. Such an abnormality causes respiratory difficulty because air flows into the esophagus and stomach instead of the lungs and because saliva and the contents of the stomach may enter the lungs via the fistula. When the baby was just two days old, she had surgery to correct the TEF. When she continued to have trouble breathing, she underwent a second surgery two days later to correct an obstructed nasal passage. After her recovery, Anne was discharged from the hospital but was re-admitted the same day because her mother noted that she was again breathing with difficulty. She underwent another surgery to widen her nasal passages and was hospitalized for about four weeks before she was transferred to City's NICU.

By the time Anne was admitted to City, Nancy had become quite distrusting. She describes an incident at the referring hospital that helped undermine her trust. While visiting, Nancy noticed that her daughter was breathing with even more difficulty than usual. But when she spoke to

Anne's doctor, the doctor responded by saying that Nancy would just have to get used to Anne's condition. Nancy later learned that the wrong nasal stent (a device to keep the nasal airway open) had been inserted in Anne's nasal passages. Rather than make it easier for Anne to breathe, the too-long stent actually obstructed her airway. Another incident further eroded Nancy's trust. Nancy recalls her outrage when a nurse seemed to blame Anne's problems on Nancy's disposition: "She thought that was because I was a nervous mother, Anne wasn't breathing right" (1031F, p. 25). Nancy explains that she "just didn't trust them" because of incidents like these (p. 25).

Nancy pushed for Anne's transfer to City Hospital. She became firmly convinced that it was her responsibility to make sure her daughter was receiving the appropriate care: "Sometimes you think a doctor knows it all and then, you know, the doctor and the nurses, they don't" (p. 35). Anne eventually had to have a tracheostomy (a surgically created opening that allows the infant to breathe through the trachea rather than the nose or mouth), because she was "turning blue all the time" (p. 5). Unlike Sam (whose case is described above), Anne did not experience a miraculous recovery at City. Nevertheless, the staff at City earned Nancy's trust. Nancy visited often, carefully observed Anne's treatment, and was reassured that her child was receiving the best possible care. At the time of our interview, Anne was prone to frequent bouts of pneumonia, and Nancy insisted that City was the only hospital where she would allow Anne to be treated if she was "really sick."

In sum, trust and distrust are not simply immutable personal attributes, like gender or race, that parents bring with them to the NICU. Parents monitor the care their infants receive and make evaluations, adjusting their responses as new evidence accumulates. Figure 6.1 depicts the relationship between orientations. Parents who have faith do not feel an obligation to test staff competence and oversee the care their infants are receiving. Because they do not invest in assessing the performance of staff, they are less likely than other parents to get information that would make them change their stance. Usually, though, monitoring and evaluating staff activities increases the confidence of parents. When parents detect no mistakes, feel that they are receiving adequate information, and are convinced that everything possible is being done, their trust rises and they may feel that their intervention is unnecessary. But for some parents early oversight leads to decreased confidence and more intensive monitoring. Trust is eroded

PARENTS' ORIENTATION

FAITH
Passive Role
No Obligation to "Test" Staff
Very Little Monitoring, Evaluating

TRUST/DISTRUST
Active Role
"Testing" Staff Competence
Monitoring and Evaluating Infant's Care

CONTINGENT TRUST
Increased Confidence
Less Intensive Monitoring
Fewer Efforts to Intervene

DISTRUST
Decreased Confidence
More Intensive Monitoring
Greater Efforts to Intervene

FIGURE 6.1. Alternative orientations of NICU parents: faith, contingent trust, and distrust

when parents detect mistakes, feel a sense of overwhelming uncertainty, or believe that more could be done for their child.

Because parents do not have uniform experiences, they do not have uniform responses to the hospitalization of an infant. Some parents have enough resources so that they can visit often and collect a lot of evidence, have medical expertise to help them make evaluations, and have access to additional sources of information. Others do not. And in some cases, recoveries are swift, while in others, parents are frustrated by setbacks and delays. Being responsible—that is, being a good agent for the child—requires different things in different situations. When they arrive at the door of the NICU, some parents are already well equipped to act as social control agents. Such an orientation makes it easier for these parents to collect and process information about the NICU and its staff and to respond quickly should they uncover any evidence of error, poor judgment, or inattentiveness. But many parents who had not previously anticipated having to challenge medical experts are able to rise to the occasion when the welfare of their baby is at stake. They quickly learn that their job as parents begins in the NICU, not after they take their baby home.

Who Trusts and Distrusts: Resources and Roles

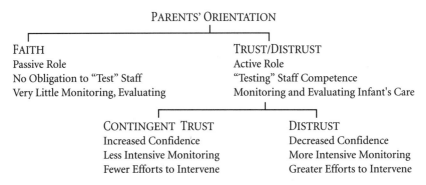

While we emphasize that parents exercise some choice about how actively to oversee, monitor, and evaluate their infant's treatment, we must acknowledge that their choices are often constrained. We find that the parents who take the least active roles often are those who face the most serious constraints and have the fewest resources (including such things as information and emotional support, as well as financial resources). At one extreme are those parents who simply cannot visit. One young mother, who was still recovering from childbirth while her son was briefly hospitalized at City, reported that she was happy to receive phone calls from the nurses and felt comforted because "they called every time they did something to him and told me what was happening" (1014F, p. 13). However, she could not actively oversee her son's medical care because she was physically separated from him. In the most extreme instance of physical separation, another couple was unable to visit their infant for the duration of his hospitalization because both parents were incarcerated. Although the mother maintained phone contact with the unit, her ability to monitor the staff was severely limited. Parents who are physically separated from their children often have passive roles by default.

In general, parents who have faith in the medical staff tend to have relatively low educational levels and very limited resources.[19] They are likely to have trouble with basics, like transportation to and from the hospital and arranging child care for older children. As Table 6.1 shows,[20] these parents are much less likely to visit their infants in the unit (mothers in this category visit just 7.9% of the days their infants are hospitalized, and fathers visit just 4.8%),[21] are much less likely to have insurance (only 12.5% of these parents are insured), and have on average 2.4 other children at home

19. We mentioned above that "faith" and "resignation" may sometimes be indistinguishable. In other words, parents who could not visit often or at all, were poorly educated, or had no medical expertise may have felt they had no choice but to leave everything in the doctors' and nurses' hands. Our emphasis on constraints here should make this clear. Though the connotation of resignation is more negative, the result is the same: the parents do not monitor, evaluate, or try to intervene in the care their infants receive. In this context faith should be thought of as more faith in physicians than in oneself.

20. In this table we provide means for some variables which almost certainly play a causal role (e.g., number of other children, length of hospital stay, and payment method, our crude indicator of social class) and for one variable (parental visits per day of hospitalization) that is both cause and effect of parental orientation. Because we have not percentaged the table to present the proportion of parents with each orientation in each category of the independent variables, readers are cautioned to read the table carefully.

21. Some of the differences between categories in percentage of days parents visited are accounted for by the length of hospitalization. Mothers, and to a lesser degree fathers, have difficulty visiting during the first days of the baby's hospital stay. The statistics on visitation will be more distorted by the early incapacity to visit when the baby is hospitalized only briefly than when the baby's hospital stay is lengthier.

TABLE 6.1 Profiles of parents with orientations of faith, contingent trust, and distrust in two NICUs, ca. 1990

	Faith (N = 8)	Contingent Trust (N = 32)	Distrust (N = 9)
Mean length of stay (in days)	19.6	38.5	89.9
Mean parental visits (percentage)[a]			
Mother	7.9	18.1	31.2
Father	4.8	13.2	12.9
Method of payment (percentage)			
Insured	12.5	71.9	66.7
Public aid/uninsured/unknown	87.5	28.1	33.3
Mean Number of Other Children	2.4	1.1	1

Note: These data were taken from the medical records of the infants whose parents were subsequently interviewed. Parents were coded by case, rather than by interview, so the Ns here correspond to the number of cases in each category, not the number of parents interviewed. When both parents were interviewed, they were coded according to the most active and interventionist parent's responses. Though we noted some differences between mothers' and fathers' views, respondents held remarkably similar orientations to their infants' hospitalization. The most striking difference between mothers and fathers is not in their orientation but in how actively involved they were in the activities of social control. As we argue in this chapter, even when parents held the same view, mothers were much more likely to be the ones monitoring and intervening in the activities of the staff.

[a]Because lengths of stay vary, parental visits were computed by dividing the number of days on which a parent visit was recorded in the medical record by the length of the infant's hospitalization (in days). This yields the percentage of days on which a parent visited the infant in the NICU.

to care for. Several are young, single mothers; many are poorly educated. Although they do not determine parents' definitions of their roles, these constraints surely shape them.

While this first group of parents assumes a relatively inactive role in their infant's hospitalization (i.e., not visiting and not making observations), most parents feel an obligation to visit. Parents who visit regularly have an opportunity to make observations and to evaluate the staff—in short, to "test" staff competence. Parents who tested staff members usually ended up trusting them more, but this was not invariably the case. All of the middle-class parents we interviewed felt an obligation to visit and, to a greater or lesser degree, test staff competence. This suggests that middle-class conceptions of parenting require parents to visit their hospitalized offspring. But it also suggests that middle-class parents have the resources to visit and to make evaluations. However, among those who became the fiercest advocates for their children were parents with very few resources and relatively low educational levels.

Each case in the NICU is unique. Because no two infants have the same medical course, no two sets of parents have the same experience. Despite this, we found striking similarities in parents' descriptions of why they felt they could trust their child's team. A common theme in the statements of the more trusting parents was their satisfaction with the information they received. When parents felt that doctors and nurses were supplying all the information they needed, they were likely to feel they could trust the care their infants were receiving. Physicians seemed to understand the importance of information in building trust. All of the physicians we interviewed rated communicating with parents a crucial responsibility requiring great skill. One attending physician with fifteen years of experience described the importance and difficulty of communicating information to parents: "The most difficult part in medicine is not medicine, but how to communicate what you are doing with the other laypeople. . . . A little thing which means nothing, you can blow it up and make it look big, or you can brush it off and explain to them in easy terminology so they don't have to worry about it. A lot of times I have frantic parents coming in. You sit down with them, talk with them, understand, and they go out smiling, and everything's fine. People do not know how to communicate, especially the residents" (2004MD, p. 7). Communication is crucial to building trust, but miscommunication can spell disaster.

In addition to being satisfied with the information flow, many of the more trusting parents reported that they had no reason to distrust the staff because their infants seemed to be doing so well. When their children were progressing satisfactorily, parents were likely to be reassured and to conclude that careful monitoring and intervention were unnecessary. Many of these parents also evaluated the doctors and nurses positively, saying that they were "good" or "nice." Of course, we cannot say for sure whether trust fosters positive evaluations or vice versa. Are parents likely to develop trust when they feel they are given adequate information? Or, conversely, are more trusting parents more likely to feel the information they receive is adequate? For our purposes, the important point is that when parents are pleased with their infant's progress, are convinced that everything possible is being done, and are satisfied with the amount and kind of information they receive, they are much less likely to step up their efforts to monitor the activities in the unit and much less likely to intervene.

When infants have complicated or lengthy medical courses, however, their parents are more likely to feel their trust has been undermined and that intervention is necessary. As Table 6.1 shows, the parents who distrust the staff tend to be the ones whose infants have had especially long hospitalizations: 89.9 days on average, compared with 38.5 days for those whose parents contingently trust the medical staff and only 19.6 for those whose parents have faith in the staff. Long and complicated hospitalizations can by themselves erode trust, as parents begin to question why their infants have not yet recovered. But there is another process at work here, as well. During long hospitalizations, parents have the opportunity to learn hospital routines, to become familiar with the infant's medical care, and even to develop some expertise in that care. As they become more expert in making observations and evaluations, parents also become more likely to notice mistakes. The longer the hospitalization, then, the more opportunity parents have to develop their skills as social control agents.

Regardless of parents' definitions of their roles, the parents we interviewed stated overwhelmingly that they would intervene if they thought the doctors or nurses were doing something wrong. To be effective social control agents, however, parents need the ability to monitor and evaluate the activities of the staff and the resources to influence them. For some parents, that is a lot to ask.

Principals Who Would Be Agents: Small Hurdle or Steep Ascent?

In agency relations, principals are often unable to monitor the behavior of agents, because of impediments such as distance, organizational structure, secrecy, and lack of expertise. NICU parents are no exception in this regard, and it usually is difficult for them to monitor, evaluate, and intervene in the activities of the staff. Although some parents enter the NICU armed with the kind of knowledge and expertise they need as social control agents, many others do not. To meet the challenge, these less-equipped parents must ascend a very steep learning curve.

Although the NICU does not discriminate—putting up more obstacles for some parents than for others—variations among parents in education, work experience, medical knowledge, and other resources affect whether parents will experience these organizational and knowledge barriers as small hurdles or as insurmountable obstacles. Parents who have sufficient resources to visit often, a lot of experience as organizational participants, knowledge of medical organizations, and some medical expertise will have less difficulty than those parents who do not. In general young, poor and unemployed parents have more difficulty acting as social control agents than older, professional ones. But parents who enter the NICU without medical expertise or competence as organizational participants can overcome these deficits during the course of their infant's hospitalization.

Above, we used Jason's case to illustrate how distrust can develop when parents are faced with overwhelming uncertainty. Here, the case illustrates the "steep ascent." When Jason was born, Cindy (1001) already had another child at home. Her experience as a parent of a healthy child had not prepared her, however, for what she would face with Jason. His abdominal deformity is relatively rare. And like many parents, she had never even heard of it before his birth. She struggled to understand the implications of his problems and had difficulty comprehending what the surgical repair would entail. Cindy spent a great deal of time with Jason when he was hospitalized at City's NICU. When asked, she says she visited a lot because she felt he needed her, not because she had to watch over the hospital staff. But she did feel some obligation to collect information herself and to oversee his medical care. In order to understand what was wrong with Jason and to be a better advocate for him, she even went to the medical library in search of articles about her son's condition.

Cindy's story is unremarkable until we look more closely. Unmarried, uneducated, young, and poor, Cindy felt the doctors had little respect for her. Undaunted, she continued to ask questions when she failed to understand something and to make suggestions when she felt it was appropriate. When unsatisfied with the answers she was given, she looked elsewhere. Her trip to the medical library served two purposes: to educate her, but also to give her more legitimacy in the eyes of the medical staff. In order to become an advocate for her son, she had to visit frequently, ask questions, be an astute observer and an eager student, and adjust her strategy when she was not satisfied with the results. The skills she had when her son was admitted to the NICU had not prepared her to evaluate the care he was receiving, so she took steps to augment those skills over the course of his hospitalization.

Cindy's story is remarkable, then, in two ways: not every parent has such large obstacles to overcome, and not many overcome them. Going to the medical library is not so unusual if a parent has a college degree. But few parents who lack a high school degree research their infant's condition independently. What made a difference for Cindy is that she felt an obligation to visit and that she was able to amass the resources to allow her to visit often. Once she began visiting, she could make observations of the care Jason was receiving, speak to his physicians and nurses, and learn about his condition and his care. Visiting the hospital regularly is difficult for many parents—especially when they have few resources and other children at home. Cindy could not have managed without a room in the nearby hostel for parents of sick children and without her sister's help with child care.

In sharp contrast to Cindy are those parents who enter the NICU already well equipped to evaluate the care their infants are receiving and to act as social control agents. Parents like Charles (1005) have college educations and careers in large organizations. Though Charles lacked any significant medical expertise, his education and work experience had taught him how to collect and evaluate information. He was very meticulous. Right from the beginning, he took copious notes, read the nurses' notes at the bedside, asked detailed questions, and learned as much as he could about his daughter's condition, her equipment, and her prognosis. Charles had an additional resource, as well. His brother-in-law is a physician. While most NICU parents cannot consult a physician for a second opinion, Charles could. His brother-in-law visited the unit at Charles's request and proved to be a great help. Charles thought the staff was very receptive to his requests for information and felt he had all the information he needed. He was very well equipped to evaluate the care his daughter was receiving and never felt the frustration of parents like Cindy.

Being a social control agent in the NICU, then, is not just about resources. Middle-class parents like Charles are not the only ones who attempt to monitor, evaluate, and intervene in their infants' care. Other parents, like Cindy, have far fewer resources, but nevertheless manage the steep ascent. We stress here that being a social control agent required something different from these two sets of parents. Parents who enter the NICU with many resources need only refine their skills as collectors and evaluators of evidence to suit this particular setting. Charles knew virtually nothing about neonatal intensive care before his daughter's birth. But as a middle manager in a large organization, he was skilled at collecting and evaluating information and was a savvy organizational participant who could transfer these skills to a new setting. Such parents are more likely to know their rights and are more likely to know how to assert those rights from the very beginning. In contrast, parents who lack resources must build requisite skills virtually from scratch. Cindy did not take detailed notes about her son's condition or read the nurses' notes right from the beginning. She learned over time to ask questions, to ask them again, and finally, to look elsewhere when she was not satisfied. But this takes both time and extraordinary commitment. We find, then, that parents who have very few resources are likely to become effective social control agents only when their infants are so sick that the parents have sufficient time to acquire relevant skills and orientations. Paradoxically, then, parents with the fewest resources are more likely to become social control agents in the NICU when their infants require the most resources.

Periphery versus Technical Core: Variations in the Resistance of Health-Care Providers

In describing the multitude of obstacles parents face when they try to monitor, evaluate, and intervene in the medical care their infants receive, we have thus far focused on the technical core of neonatal intensive care, the area where the asymmetry between parents and staff most favors the staff and most disadvantages the parents. But the obstacles parents face decrease as they move from the center to the periphery of activities in the NICU, and their ability to act as social control agents correspondingly increases. Success in social control depends not only on who is trying to exert pressure but also on where they are trying to exert it.

In an interview, a young attending physician describes his view of the parents' role this way: "I think it's our decision to make the choice on what type of care to deliver and then to explain that to the parents and involve them in what our thinking is and why we're doing what we're doing, and keep them informed in terms of what we think is going on. In terms of the medical decisions for the infants themselves, I think parents have very little role just 'cause it's real hard to bring them up to speed" (1002MD, p. 1). Although this physician is especially parent oriented, even listing communicating with parents as one of his main responsibilities, he expresses a view that is common among staff members. The parents are not experts in medical matters, and they are not expected to be involved in most medical decisions.[22]

22. Of course, DNR (do not resuscitate) orders, decisions about experimental treatment, and decisions to discontinue treatment represent some notable exceptions to the rule. These decisions must involve parents, because they require the parents' consent. Here, the effort must be made to bring the parents "up to speed." However, as our informants indicated, and as Anspach (1993) concludes, parents are often persuaded to accept decisions already made by the experts. This same attending physician informed us that the physicians at City would not pursue a DNR order, for instance, without the parents' consent, but that when they discuss their position with the parents, they rarely have difficulty convincing

Although parents and medical staff do not use the language of "periphery" and "technical core" (a language introduced into sociology primarily by Thompson [1967]), they do distinguish between the two. Defined by the technical core, the periphery is simply composed of everything that falls outside it. The boundary between the core and periphery is often quite fuzzy—with physicians and staff arguing that parents lack the ability to understand the full complexity of the medical problem and parents arguing that the staff refuses to respect their wishes. The medical staff tend to define the technical core more expansively, and parents tend to define it more restrictively.[23] The important point, however, is that the medical staff, and not the parents, have the last word about where the periphery ends and the core begins.

Many of parents' preferences about how their infants should be treated fit smoothly into NICU routines—for instance, that the infants be kept warm, that they be fed (or given intravenous nutrition), that their diapers be changed, and that they be given the best possible medical care. Other preferences, however, are not accommodated within the established routines. Such preferences fall into two main categories: parenting preferences and medical preferences. The first set of preferences are ones that parents, as parents, are expected to have and that will be honored on that basis alone. For instance, some parents bring clothes from home to dress the baby, request that tapes of their voices be played in their absence, ask to hang mobiles above the baby's crib to stimulate development, and the like. Parents, as parents, have legitimacy on such peripheral issues; no special certification of expertise is required.

As long as dressing the baby in a certain manner does not interfere with the medical care or playing a tape does not interfere with the infant's sleep, the NICU staff is likely to accommodate the parents. However, as we move closer to the technical core, the staff is less likely to accept the legitimacy

them of their expert conclusions: "In that type of a decision, first thing we do, if an attending thinks that [a DNR order is appropriate] by himself, we'll run it over amongst us as a group. And if we decide as a group it's the right thing to do, then we bring in the family, primary nurse, social worker, resident and sit down and talk and say where we think things are and where the family is. Some families, you know it's a moot point, why even bring it up. But for some families, they can come to a decision, and we try to make it seem like it's a group decision, and we think it's in the best medical interest of the kid" (1002MD, p. 21).

23. Zussman (1992) similarly observes that many decisions have both technical and moral aspects but that ICU physicians have some tendency to see decisions as purely technical. In this way, he argues, physicians protect their discretion while still respecting patients' and families' rights to participate in medical decision making.

of parents' claims as parents. Here, the staff demands expertise, not just in parenting but also in medical care. Recall that Sam's mother, Kate (1026), was convinced that her son's health would improve if he were allowed to feed on demand rather than on a fixed schedule. Kate's suggestions were disregarded as a novice's attempts to intervene. This conflict and others like it show us a great deal. First, we learn that parents' preferences are not automatically incorporated into the routines of the staff. Second, we learn that what may usually be considered a routine matter of parenting—feeding—may be shifted to the technical core in the NICU. And finally, we learn that it is the staff who decide whether or not a parent's claim is legitimate.

In general, then, when the staff can shift a matter from the periphery to the technical core, they are able to retain control. In the process, parents may end up feeling that their capacity to make decisions—even seemingly routine decisions—has been stripped away. Parents, in fact, find such strong resistance at the technical core that they often ask for their infants to be transferred when their disagreements with the treatment make them desperate. When parents are not permitted "voice," and "loyalty" is not an option because the stakes are too high, they choose the third option discussed by Hirschman (1970)—"exit." A few parents, however, are able to demonstrate competence in matters at the heart of the technical core by repeatedly showing that they understand their child's condition as well as, if not better than, the medical staff.

Sue and Will, whose daughter Tiffany (1009) was discussed in chapter 1, attempted to intervene in medical matters more than once. They first attempted to influence medical decisions when they pressed the doctors for alternatives to a tracheostomy and arranged for Tiffany's transfer to City Hospital, where a pediatric surgeon hoped to make a surgical repair to her damaged trachea that would make the tracheostomy unnecessary. Although the surgery was unsuccessful, and Tiffany underwent the tracheotomy, Sue and Will learned valuable lessons about their capacity to intervene on their daughter's behalf.

Before Tiffany was transferred back to the referring hospital, Sue was taught the procedures for Tiffany's tracheostomy care by the nurses at City's NICU. Sue mastered Tiffany's "trach" care routine and was shocked to discover that the trach care at the referring hospital seemed sloppy by comparison. This led to Sue's second attempt to intervene in the technical core, which met with immense resistance and was ultimately unsuccessful.

Sue complained to the nurses first, describing in detail how she wanted Tiffany's trach care performed. When the quality of care did not improve, she complained to the "superintendent" of the hospital. When there was still no improvement, she simply took over that aspect of her daughter's care herself. Convinced that Tiffany was receiving substandard care, Sue requested a transfer to a university-affiliated hospital in the area. Tiffany's enraged doctor tried to dissuade her, even asking whether Sue wanted her daughter to die. She succeeded in getting the transfer and was much happier with the quality of care, though she remarked: "I still have to make sure that things get done. It gets lost in the shuffle, I guess, somewhere" (1009F, p. 36).

Grace and Roger, who were discussed in chapter 3 as a couple taking a great deal of responsibility for a child who continued to have major medical problems, also felt fierce resistance when they tried to intervene near the technical core. Grace and Roger provide a useful example of the flexible adjustment that is required to meet obligations in extreme circumstances. Their daughter, Tammy (2016), was born with multiple congenital anomalies that required a series of surgical repairs and resulted in many complications, including repeated bladder infections, difficulty in feeding, and dehydration. Tammy was initially treated at Suburban Hospital but was subsequently admitted to City for one of the many operations she would endure. During one rehospitalization at City, Tammy became dangerously dehydrated after a resident had discontinued her IV the night before her surgery was scheduled to take place. Grace and Roger were at her bedside during the night and noticed that she appeared quite ill, but according to them, they were unable to convince the resident to restart her IV fluids. When the attending physician saw Tammy before surgery in the morning, he was startled by her condition. He canceled the surgery and ordered her IV reconnected immediately. Grace thinks Tammy nearly died because of that mistake, and she vowed she would never let anything like that happen again.

Grace was transformed by the experience: "We are not going to take any more crap. No more. We will listen to our doctors. If we don't like it, we are going to tell them like it is, and that's it" (2016F, p. 35). Roger describes how their understanding of their roles changed after this event: "We pretty much knew then that if she was going to get the care that we wanted her to have, we were going to be the ones doing it, and seeing that she gets it" (2016M, p. 13). In their repeated interactions with hospitals, doctors, and nurses, they would feel the necessity to intervene again. But as they gained expertise in Tammy's care, they became more convinced of their own abilities and less likely to back down in a disagreement.

Later, Tammy had to be readmitted to City Hospital again because of severe dehydration. And Grace became fiercely protective of her, leaving her bedside only when her primary nurse was on duty. The doctor had decided to feed Tammy through the nasogastric tube, since her intake of formula and calories was not adequate when she was bottle-fed. When Grace learned of this plan, she resisted, saying she knew her daughter could eat from the bottle if only the nurses took enough time with her. Her assessment was that many of the nurses were "burned out" and could not be trusted to take adequate time to bottle-feed Tammy. She decided her only choice was to feed Tammy herself: "I was always there. I always took care of my kid" (2016F, p. 35).

Because she was "always there," Grace learned quite a lot about Tammy's care. When she noticed Tammy's IV setting seemed to be wrong, she brought it to the attention of the resident who was caring for her. Rather than simply check the IV, the resident quipped: "What do you know?" But Grace did know. She had been watching carefully. She had been learning. And she was right. What is perhaps most telling is that the attending physician gave the resident the option of either apologizing or being removed from the case. The resident chose not to apologize. This was not the last confrontation Grace would have with doctors when she disagreed with them. Another doctor at Suburban Hospital became so angry with her when she resisted having an NG tube inserted again that he threw a fit, calling her an "unfit mother" and hurling a chair across the room.

Parental consent is required for surgery and other discrete interventions. But parental consent is not required for many other equally consequential interventions that fit seamlessly into NICU routines. Parental consent is required for a tracheotomy, the surgical procedure to create an opening in the trachea, for instance, but once a patient has tracheostomy parents are not routinely consulted about how the trach care is performed.[24] Similarly, parents are not routinely consulted about IV settings or feeding protocols. Such care is within the technical purview of the physicians and nurses. These are matters about which parents are certainly expected to be concerned but not about which they are likely to be consulted.

24. In general, an *-ostomy* is a surgically created opening, and an *-otomy* is the surgical procedure in which the opening is created.

And when parents attempt to exert control at the technical core, they are likely to get a strong response.

The cynical might conclude that physicians are more interested in protecting their authority than in treating patients. When recalling parents who distrusted them, some staff responded with moral outrage. When asked to describe the "ideal" parent, a nurse at Suburban with more than twenty years of experience noted that parent distrust made her work particularly difficult: "Okay, the big thing is a parent who trusts you, that you are going to give their baby good care. Because that's, I think, one of the most difficult parents to work with is one who doesn't trust us, for whatever reason. It is *very* difficult" (2006RN, p. 24). An attending physician at Suburban recognized the tensions involved but attributed the insecurities about authority to parents: "It does work out better for everyone involved if there is a trusting relationship. But some people you can't do that with. That's not part of their repertoire for a lot of different reasons, whether they have psychiatric problems, they have some basic trust issues, whether there's issues of relating to authority or issues of turf. You know, there are so many different ways. You have to know where your limitations are as a professional in impacting these kinds of things within whatever system you have" (2003MD, p. 16).

The less cynical might conclude that since most parents lack technical expertise, their suggestions may be disregarded as well-intentioned, but largely useless, opinions. In an environment of strained resources, it is simply more economical to dismiss parents' suggestions than to evaluate the parents' level of expertise. Parents who wish to be active participants in their infant's hospitalization simply demand more physician and nursing resources than those who do not. Time that could be spent treating the infants must be expended explaining the treatment to the parents. As one nurse at Suburban with fifteen years of NICU experience put it: "Taking care of these babies is a piece of cake. It's dealing with the parents that's the hardest part sometimes" (2008RN, p. 19).

It is not surprising that parents have such difficulty when they attempt to intervene at the technical core. Anspach (1993) has argued that even among staff members, not all knowledge claims are treated equally. The legitimacy of the knowledge claims of various participants closely parallels the hierarchy of authority, with the clinical experience of the attending physician coming out on top. If the knowledge claims of nurses and residents are suspect in some circumstances, then parents' knowledge claims are even more suspect. Parents who attempt to intervene at the technical core will be much more successful if they can enlist the help of other medical experts who will plead their case and lend them some legitimacy in the process.

The main conclusion of recent sociological research in intensive care settings is that doctors have retained a great deal of autonomy, despite recent advances in patients' rights (see Staffen 1994). Our evidence certainly does not contradict this claim. However, we also have evidence that parents are able to intervene at the technical core under some circumstances. The most effective and forceful advocates are often those parents who have had to endure the greatest tragedies—prolonged and repeated hospitalizations. These parents become experts in their own children's conditions and care because they have the opportunity—if we dare call it that—to learn how to evaluate and intervene in that care. Although it may be easier for parents, and other laypeople, to intervene at the periphery of medicine than at the technical core, some of our parents pressed for transfers, "fired" doctors, refused treatment that seemed futile, asked for second opinions, and otherwise intervened at the heart of the technical core. What is interesting is not that it was difficult for them to do so or that they faced resistance. This, as we have pointed out, is to be expected. What is interesting here is that even the parents with the fewest resources will define it as their role to confront these obstacles when their children need them to do so. Heroic parents, it turns out, are not necessarily well endowed. They are simply ordinary people with extraordinary problems.

Although staff resistance to parental intervention is understandable, such intervention is crucial to the patient's welfare in the long run if not in the short term. Time spent giving explanations to parents is not time wasted; accommodations that encourage parent involvement are sensible investments. Parents who become involved in overseeing their child's care in the hospital are more likely to be able to manage the care of an NICU graduate once their child goes home. Just as schoolchildren, gradually taking more responsibility for their education, come into conflict with their teachers and their parents about what decisions they are and are not ready to make for themselves, so NICU parents, taking over many (but not all) of the tasks and decisions that were once in the domain the hospital staff, come into conflict with the hospital staff about where they can and cannot intrude. Just as parents of adolescents find themselves tempted to do things for their children rather than putting up with the hassles of correcting mistakes and accommodating unstable preferences, so NICU staff may find themselves wishing that they could proceed without parental "help." It may seem to staff that it would be easier to have full control of the baby's care up until the moment of discharge, and then to make a clean break. Responsible parents have to take over from the staff, and everyone knows that. But that doesn't mean that the transition will always be comfortable or that staff members will always welcome the intervention of parents.

Conclusion

Both parents and health-care professionals are, formally speaking, agents of the baby. One might expect, then, that the two groups would adopt parallel strategies in pursuing the baby's interests. Yet this appears not to be the case. Parents talk about what is in the baby's interests, their responsibility for the baby's well-being, and what they can do to shape the actions of others (such as nurses and doctors) in desired ways. Although agency theory at least fits parents' image of their role, it does not seem to fit the self-images or activities of health-care professionals. Instead, the activities of NICU staff are strongly shaped ("scripted") by medical protocols. Occasionally health-care professionals do seem to see themselves as the baby's agents, for instance when they disagree with parents over treatment and must decide whether to take temporary custody of the child.

These differences between parental and staff roles show up especially in attempts to reshape the other party's behavior. As agents of social control, hospital staff members employ the tools described by labeling theorists—they categorize parents as competent or incompetent, appropriate or inappropriate, nice or unpleasant, and use these labels as guides for interaction with parents. Such strategies are of little use to parents. Because no one else's reactions to the staff members are affected by a parent's negative assessment, affixing a negative label to some physician or nurse thus has little practical consequence. As outsiders to the hospital organization, parents must therefore rely on other tools. And although they conceive of themselves as agent-principals or even as principals, they cannot deploy most of the tools discussed by agency theorists. They cannot design contracts, directly compensate health-care providers, or easily transfer their child to the care of a different neonatologist or nurse. These observations led us to a series of questions about what social control tools are available and how the tools people employ vary with their conceptions of their obligations (to do a job, to pursue someone's interests).

In their structurally weak position as outsiders, parents are not well positioned to intervene in such a carefully designed organization as the

NICU. They are largely ignorant about the core technology. They cannot draw on any infrastructural support and must act as isolated individuals without the assistance or succor of co-workers. And they have outside obligations that keep them away from the NICU part of the time. But whether parents remain weak agents of social control, or become forceful advocates depends on a number of variables: whether they conceive it as their role to monitor, evaluate, and intervene in the activities of the NICU staff; whether they have or acquire the resources to overcome the obstacles they confront; and whether they seek to intervene on the periphery or at the core of medical practice.

Social control *by* parents is intimately related to the social control *of* parents. Parents may believe that everything is out of their hands or that they have a key role overseeing their child's medical team. At either of these extremes, the NICU's social control machinery is likely to be set in motion. On the one hand, repeated objections to routines and disagreements with medical experts may be read as a symptom of poor judgment and a prognosis of inadequate parenting. On the other hand, staff may worry that the parents who have complete faith have not demonstrated the capacity to take over the infant's care. Although it may reduce disputes and economize on staff time, the NICU must not go too far in discouraging parents from taking their role in the agency chain seriously, for it is the capacity to act as an agent on the infant's behalf that is necessary in the long run.

Although the sociological literature on the professions often cites trust as an essential component of professional autonomy (e.g., Freidson 1988), the response of the staff when not trusted reflects more than a violation of their sense of themselves as professionals. Distrust not only violates the professional's identity, it also creates more work. Distrusting parents make extra demands on unit resources by requiring that staff members demonstrate their trustworthiness and provide reassuring evidence. Distrust is, in short, resource intensive. Distrusting parents who try too hard to control staff behavior will find that they are themselves subject to social control as staff attempt to rein them in.

It would be easy to overstate the uniqueness of our case. Here, we have an agency chain with highly motivated intermediaries who have a unique relation to the infant-principals, the principals have very little ability to exit, and they have many opportunities to monitor at least some of the activities of the agent through face-to-face contact. Furthermore, not all agency relations deal with such weighty issues as life and death. Nonetheless, we believe we learn something fundamental by looking at agency relations "on the ground," in a situation in which principals' preferences are inchoate and agents, rather than principals, design the contract.

It is not a revelation that agency relations are vulnerable. But what we learn here is about variations in the extent to which principals engage in social control of their agents. It is clearly in the interests of the agents to make monitoring seem unnecessary. Credentials, licensing, quality control, peer review, and the like all signal to the principal that monitoring is already being carried out by people or organizations more qualified than the lay principal to judge the soundness of the services being provided. Some principals do not engage in social control, then, because they simply believe it's unnecessary. It's somebody else's problem. Others fail to engage in social control because they lack the resources to do so. Resources don't tell the whole story, though. Although those with more resources are more likely to engage in some "testing" of the competence of their agents, even resource-poor principals will find (or make) the resources to engage in social control if they believe that something is amiss. The longer or more complicated the transaction, the more likely the principal is to engage in social control, because the principal has the opportunity to learn over time and to detect mistakes.

A comparison with a formally parallel principal-agent relationship at the other end of the spectrum illustrates exactly what is required to make inexpert principals become responsible supervisors of expert labor. Although the relation between investor and mutual fund manager is formally parallel to that between parent and staff, social control by investors never reaches the intensity of social control by parents no matter how long and complicated the transaction. Other features of the relation between investor and mutual fund manager may help account for these differences. The principal and the fund manager never have face-to-face contact. If the principal is not happy with the return on investment, money can be moved relatively easily from one fund to another, and, furthermore, the outcome is easily measured (and is not the life or death of one's child). In addition, though, mutual fund investors are less likely to be held accountable by others for the fate of their investments and are not expected to take over the work of the mutual fund manager at some point in the future. The "responsible" mutual fund investor simply monitors the performance of the fund, a task which is nowadays easily done from a home computer, and requires no face-to-face contact. If disappointed with the performance of a fund, the principal, or investor, "intervenes" by simply moving the investment to another fund. Because mobility is easy, this principal does not attempt to change the behavior of the fund manager by advising a different investment strategy. Not every mutual fund investor pulls money out of a losing fund. Such investors may not monitor the performance of their funds closely, or they may simply leave decisions about investments to investment advisors, or other intermediaries. Under these circumstances, we might hesitate to call investor interventions social control.

What the principals who intervene seem to share is a sense of unique responsibility for a consequential outcome. Often that sense of responsibility is reinforced by institutional protections. A right to intervene, however precariously protected, is in part a signal that intervention is sometimes expected. And a requirement to assume complete responsibility at some point in the future gives inexpert principals (or agent-principals) both a stake in current activity and an incentive to get involved. We believe the social control of agents to be a prevalent feature of principal-agent relations, but we also believe that social control will take quite different forms depending on the features of the relationship. When principals have a unique sense of responsibility for an outcome that they believe is consequential, they are more likely to engage in social control than when they believe that the outcome is trivial and is simply—or fully—out of their hands.

But how does social control, whether by parents or by staff members, contribute to responsibility? Responsible caretaking, whether done by parents or by health-care professionals, requires the coordinated efforts of numerous people. Parents of critically ill infants cannot do their job without enlisting the help of doctors and nurses, and health-care professionals likewise depend on parents. It should have come as no surprise to readers, then, to encounter some of the parents discussed in chapter 3 as sterling examples of responsible parenting in this chapter on the social control of hospital staff members. Both responsible parents and responsible staff members must monitor the performance of their counterparts, ensuring that they neither break rules nor shirk. Ideally they do this in a way that reminds others of the importance of adapting to the needs of the child in question.

Deviance, shirking, and responsibility are not just isolated points on a continuum of levels of compliance with obligation, then. Instead, as we have shown in chapters 5 and 6, they come together in two ways. They come together, first, when those who have accepted a responsibility recognize that their success depends on the contributions of other people who may not take their own obligations quite so seriously. Taking responsibility then requires adjusting for the inadequacies of others' performances. The hospital staff members, whose role as social control agents was the focus of chapter 5, have difficulty meeting their obligations to young patients without the help of parents, whether those parents accept responsibility or not, and the parents, whose parallel role received our scrutiny in this chapter, cannot meet their obligations to their newborns without the assistance of staff members, whether those staff members are skilled and committed or unskilled and apathetic.

Responsible parents must adjust for deficiencies in the performance of staff members. They do this, for instance, by seeking second opinions when they have doubts about a physician's judgment or requesting that a particular nurse not care for their child if they believe that she has cut corners in the past. Responsible staff members adjust for the deficiencies of parents by substituting their own labor in the short run and the labor of other care providers in the long run. When the baby is well enough, parents typically begin to provide part of their child's care. But if parents do not arrive to feed a baby, administer medications, change dressings, or perform minor tasks with medical equipment, staff members do the chores in their place. If parents do not begin to care for their child reliably and competently while it is still hospitalized, responsible staff members eventually press for the replacement of parents by other care providers such as foster parents or the staff of a long-term care facility. People who accept responsibility must assess whether others have a responsible orientation to their part of the work or are instead inclined to break rules and cut corners. Accepting ultimate responsibility means compensating for others who do not take responsibility.

As agents of social control, parents and staff members must do more than just monitor others' performances and compensate when others do not act responsibly. Because they have only limited capacities to do each others' tasks—parents cannot become physicians, and physicians cannot permanently take custody and act as parents—both groups also try to induce responsible behavior in others. Staff members try to show parents that the core concern is whether they are adjusting sufficiently to the unusual needs of their particular child. Parents in turn stress that staff members should treat their baby as an individual with a unique combination of medical problems rather than provide it with standardized care. Responsibility and social control come together in a second way as each group tries to move the other in the direction of responsible behavior by employing social control methods that highlight the importance of flexible adjustment to particular circumstances. In this context, social control is not just about policing the boundary between deviance and conformity but is also about pointed reminders that perfunctory compliance is insufficient. For these parents, the best ain't hardly good enough.

SEVEN

Beyond the NICU: Variations in the Acceptance of Long-Term Responsibility

LIFE IN A NEONATAL INTENSIVE CARE UNIT is highly regimented. Work is subdivided and tasks are assigned to carefully trained and supervised people. Given the number of discrete operations performed each day and the number of people performing those operations, one might expect frequent confusion about who should be doing what. Yet such confusion only rarely occurs. Responsibilities are clearly assigned so that everyone knows (or can find out) who is caring for which child, who is doing which chores, and even whose job it is to ensure that tasks are done correctly. The structured nature of NICU life arises partly from a careful division of labor but also from careful selection of some of the key participants. Neither the workers nor the patients are randomly selected. Instead variability in both groups is reduced by screening (for both groups) and training (for workers). Competence as a nurse, neonatologist, respiratory therapist, or other health-care worker and commitment to performing the task well are prerequisites for being hired to work in an NICU. Further, the limited stake of the workers probably increases the predictability of their performance. Though NICU work is often physically hard, intellectually demanding, and emotionally draining, nevertheless the physicians, social workers, nurses, and therapists do get to go home at the end of the workday and are to some degree able to leave the work behind. Though they may sometimes agonize over patients or worry about relations with co-workers, nevertheless what the NICU asks of them (their labor for a fixed number of hours a week) and gives in return (a good paycheck) is relatively predictable.

It may seem odd to claim that NICU life is predictable and orderly given that the tiny patients are there for around-the-clock monitoring precisely because their needs and responses are unpredictable. In saying that NICU life is predictable and orderly, we are not saying that is naturally so. The orderliness and predictability of the NICU are important social achievements. We mention the predictability of NICU life here because we wish to contrast the NICU with the homes to which infants go when they are discharged from the hospital. Infants' homes are more variable than NICUs on three dimensions. First, parents vary more than hospital staff in their preparation and willingness to care for a sick baby. NICU staff have all undergone rigorous training and have chosen to spend at least a portion of their lives caring for sick babies. Parents may or may not have chosen to have a baby, but certainly would not have chosen to have a sick one (though a few did learn about their baby's condition prenatally and declined to abort, and all could have relinquished their babies for adoption). Generally, parents have less training in child development and in the rudiments of medical care than hospital staff, though of course they are required to learn to care for their own child, including such skills as administering medications, changing colostomies, or assessing the functioning of a shunt, if the child will require such care at home. As care providers for sick babies, parents are thus a more variable group than are hospital staff members.

The social control system of an NICU is also less variable than that of the home. In the NICU a clear hierarchy governs and supervises the activity of the staff. This supervision is facilitated by the production and review of the medical record, a series of documents in which workers record what they have done and which are used to coordinate the activities of the group caring for a single infant. In addition to facilitating coordination, though, such written records facilitate social control by making it possible for workers to check each other's work even if they were not present when that work was performed. The presence of many workers also means that there are limits on the extent to which one can fail to do his or her job by either neglecting or abusing the child. Social control by co-workers need not be as obtrusive when there are alarms to signal an emergency or merely that an IV needs to be changed or a monitor lead repositioned. The social control infrastructure makes control less costly—it is easy to collect information about whether a nurse is lax about changing IVs, for instance—and therefore probably more consistent.

The social control systems of homes vary a good bit, with intensive "supervision" of one spouse by the other, or by members of the extended family, in some households and very little "supervision" in others. Probably no households have the formalized social control systems that hospital units do, though a few families may post charts to help them keep track of whether medications have been administered, temperatures taken, and so forth. And when an infant requires nursing care at home, the routines that incorporate nurses into the household and that coordinate the work of a team of nurses approximate the routines of a hospital unit, though some of that administrative routine is located outside the hospital in a home-health agency. But households with only a single adult member, or in which only one adult assumes responsibility for the child, may provide fewer social incentives, either positive or negative, for doing a good job of caring for a demanding and perhaps sick infant. The variance in social control is higher in homes than in NICUs, with families providing both the most careful monitoring on the widest variety of indicators, at the high end, and inadequate care with little monitoring and consequently little hope of corrective action, at the low end. NICU social control systems ensure higher floors than some families can provide but are unable to duplicate the one-on-one attentiveness that raises the ceiling in other families.

Finally, there is less variability in the congruence of interests between NICU care providers and infants than between parents and infants. NICU care providers are usually not passionately concerned with the futures of the infants, given that they care for them only briefly, and even then intermittently. Parents, in contrast, have a long-term stake in their own children and, once the babies are discharged from the hospital, are stuck with caring for them night and day until they become self-sufficient. Parents might thus be expected to be more deeply concerned with a baby's welfare. The pain experienced by the baby is in some senses their pain, and many parents gave poignant testimony about their distress at their infant's suffering. "No one can love your child the way you do," one mother explained. "When your child is in pain, you feel it. The other person can't. I mean they sympathize, they understand the child's in pain, but there's a different feeling. When your child wants or needs something, you can almost sense it because they're a part of you" (1039F, p. 33). One father explained why he cried while his child was in the NICU: "I didn't feel sorry for myself, I felt sorry for the baby. What has he done that he has to deserve, go through this, and the fact that you can't do anything for the baby" (2033M, p. 33). The mother of this same child reported that she cried every time she looked at her son, "because he was so little and so helpless" (2033F, p. 15), adding that "the baby must be suffering, they got to be" (2033F, p. 16).

Parents also are more likely to find that their interests, or those of other family members, conflict with those of the child. Any baby can stretch its parents to the limit, but some former NICU patients are especially likely to do this. If they need a lot of special care, are unusually fussy, become ill often, or cannot supply the rewards offered by other infants, former NICU patients can cost their parents more while giving less back than most babies. NICU nurses and physicians may also become exasperated with a baby, but they can leave the baby behind at the end of the day and console themselves with the reminder that a particularly burdensome infant will not be part of the unit population for very long. For the NICU employee, the opportunity costs of caring for any particular baby are lower than they are for parents. The NICU employee has to care for some baby during his or her workday, and it may just as well be this one. For the parent, the opportunity costs are higher. Time with the baby is time not available for housework, employment, sleep, caring for another child, or recreation.

In pointing out these differences between the NICU and the household to which the baby goes, we wish to suggest that once we leave the close regulation of an intensive care unit, substantial variations in parental responsibility are likely. It would be hard to exaggerate the variability among the families we studied, and we present statistical profiles of the two groups of interview families in Table 7.1. Briefly, our study included the very poorest families as well as the very richest. The mean family income was about $31,000 a year for the families we interviewed from City Hospital, and just over $48,000 a year for the families we interviewed from Suburban. Several families had no regular source of income other than welfare, several fathers were unemployed, and a few parents were unemployable because of disabilities.[1] Other families had two employed parents; one family was difficult to interview because the father's international work led them to be often abroad. Families also varied a good bit on educational measures. While some parents had completed only elementary school, others had postgraduate degrees. Parents from Suburban Hospital were much better educated overall than parents from City. As Table 7.1 shows, over 30% of parents at City Hospital had not completed high school or its equivalent, while the figure is less than 4% at Suburban. Some infants lived

1. Edin and Lein (1996) report that welfare recipients often cannot make ends meet if they rely on their welfare income alone. These women often supplement their welfare income in a number of ways, including working at side jobs, obtaining cash from friends and relatives, and relying on community groups and local charities, but hide such supplementation from caseworkers to keep their benefits (1996:254). In the 1980s and early 1990s, when we did our research, welfare payments in the metropolitan area in which City and Suburban Hospitals are located approximated the national average; nevertheless, families who received public aid had great difficulty getting by on their welfare checks. It is interesting to note that some of the women we interviewed who received welfare benefits were initially skeptical about the reasons we wanted to interview them. Despite our repeated assurances that we had no affiliation or alliance with state child-welfare agencies, some feared that talking to us would jeopardize their payments.

Table 7.1 Profiles of two NICU sample interview groups: City Hospital and Suburban Hospital, ca. 1990

	City Hospital (N = 28)	Suburban Hospital (N = 21)
Mother's education (percentage)		
No high school degree	32.1	0
High school graduate or GED	21.4	37.0
Some college/associate's	17.9	48.1
College graduate or more	25.0	14.8
Missing data	3.6	0
Father's education (percentage)[a]		
No high school degree	32.1	3.7
High school graduate or GED	17.9	3.7
Some college/associate's	25.0	33.3
College graduate or more	17.8	44.4
Missing data	7.1	14.8
Mother's unemployment (percentage)		
Not employed at birth	39.3	14.8
Not employed at interview	60.7	18.5
Father's unemployment (percentage)[a]		
Not employed at birth	10.7	0
Not employed at interview	21.4	3.7
Mean annual family income (dollars)	30,552	48,041
Marital status (percentage)		
Married	67.9	74.1
Unmarried	32.1	25.9
Infant's race/ethnicity (percentage)		
White	57.1	88.9
Black	21.4	3.7
Hispanic	14.3	0
Other	7.1	7.4

[a]In some cases, information about fathers was supplied in interviews with mothers.

in two-parent nuclear households; others lived in large extended families. Some parents were married or divorced and remarried; others had never been married. Roughly two-thirds of the parents we interviewed from City Hospital were married, while nearly three-fourths at Suburban were married. Some infants lived with their mothers and their children but with no other adults. Some children shuttled between households. Some families had only a single child, while others had many children, not always the products of the same union. Some mothers did all of the child-care themselves; in other families fathers or grandmothers helped. Still other families hired helpers, either by sending their child to a babysitter or by incorporating a nanny into their household. Households also varied a great deal in what kinds of material objects were present, and we particularly noted the presence or absence of books and toys. All of the households had televisions, but not all of them had books or telephones (which might be essential for summoning emergency medical help). Some households were scrupulously clean and very tidy. Others were disorderly and even dirty; a few were in such bad repair that they were dangerous.

Approaches to child rearing varied quite a lot as well, with different levels of planning the child's daily activities, approaches to discipline, and amounts of time spent in interaction with the parents or other adults rather than with siblings or other children. Parents varied in levels of concern about such matters as growth and weight gain, language acquisition and cognitive development, social skills and relations with peers, physical coordination, and attainment of developmental milestones. Some parents were thoroughly convinced that their child was going to have a tough time and need considerable medical attention, others were intensely concerned about early indications that something might be wrong, and still others thought that their child was doing fine even though their level of concern was not perfectly correlated with "objective" indicators or the child's medical history. Finally, parents varied in how they felt about their child's early medical problems. Nearly all experienced the hospitalization as a trauma, but some parents seemed to have recovered from the experience, and others were still deeply troubled. One mother, whose child had been transferred at birth to another hospital, continued to wonder whether she had been given someone else's child (1032F, pp. 1, 3, 4, 10, 14). Several women were reluctant to have another child either because of fears about their own health or intense anxiety about having another critically ill infant. One family (2025) was concerned that the addition of another child might make their first, who had cerebral palsy and was unable to walk, feel that he was not "normal." For them a "perfect" child now seemed much less desirable.

Our examination of the NICU in this book has been, in some senses, an examination of the social organization of responsibility in a structured situation in which personnel are selected because of their capacity to take on a particular task and rewarded for devoting themselves to that task, in which conflicts of interest between parties are minimized, and in which the social system is engineered to facilitate the kinds of supervision and coordination that are required for reliable performance. We have noted that parents do not always find it easy to fit into the NICU routine.

As we discussed in chapter 5, NICU staff members have definite notions about how parents should behave and try to make parents conform to their model of a responsible parent (see also Heimer and Staffen 1995). Over the course of an infant's hospitalization, parents begin to take over responsibility for their child, as we described in chapter 6. Sometimes this transfer of responsibility begins simply because the child is approaching discharge or because parents whose child is hospitalized for a long time gradually come to feel that they have some expertise. But sometimes the transition occurs for other reasons, for instance because some problem leads parents to feel that they must be more watchful. It can be a delicate matter for parents to carve out roles for themselves when their child is being cared for by a team of experts. While some hospital staff members may welcome parents' participation, others may have more hostile reactions to parental intervention.

Parental roles shift dramatically when the baby makes the transition from the hospital to the home. Once the baby comes home, parents are on their own turf, no longer needing to defer to the authority of flocks of doctors and nurses. But at the same time, without those care providers following their carefully planned routines, parents are likely to discover that it is hard to get all of the work done, keep track of what has to be done when, and be sure that all of the bases are covered. Households typically do not have an adequate infrastructure for caring for a child with special needs, though of course they usually would not formulate the problem that way. We turn now to an examination of the social organization of responsibility in the relatively unstructured, highly variable situation of the households we studied, beginning first with a discussion of what the responsibility tends to entail.

Taking the Baby Home

Getting the baby home is a central goal for most parents during their child's NICU stay. But once the baby is home, many parents describe themselves as feeling overwhelmed by the responsibility. Staff members recognize that the transition is traumatic and remind parents that the NICU is open twenty-four hours a day and that they can call any time of day or night if they have questions or are concerned. A few primary nurses even give their home phone numbers to parents they've grown especially close to. Many parents reported that they did in fact contact the unit, sometimes only to share news with a favorite nurse they had promised to keep informed about the baby's progress, sometimes to consult a trusted doctor about a bewildering occurrence. Many parents reported their calls with the shamefacedness that other parents display in talking about their ignorance in their days as new parents. But parents also talk about difficulties adjusting to the level of attentiveness and expertise of ordinary pediatricians after receiving deluxe medical care from experts. For some parents this contrast between the care provided by an ordinary pediatrician and the care provided by the NICU staff was the stimulus that made them aware of their own capacity to evaluate medical care, to make crude assessments about whether some medical practitioner had sufficient knowledge or experience to care for their child, given its peculiar medical history.

The transition from hospital to home also raises new questions about who will care for the baby. Though parents may have spent considerable time caring for their baby during the hospitalization, suddenly they must provide twenty-four-hour coverage. No longer can they take an evening off, take a break if they are discouraged, plan on an uninterrupted night's sleep, go to work without worrying about arranging child care, or even make a quick trip to the grocery store. Such adjustments must be faced by all new parents, but for the parents of NICU graduates, the adjustments are likely to be particularly difficult. A quick trip to the grocery store is always less convenient with a baby in tow but may be completely impractical if the baby is tethered to an oxygen tank or ventilator. An evening out is often logistically difficult for new parents but may be impossible when grandparents have not been trained to do CPR. And though new parents are famous for their conviction that no one else can provide adequate care for their newborn, such normal concerns are exaggerated among those who have very nearly lost their baby and who are intensely aware that a large team of medical specialists worked hard to sustain the baby's life.

How Well Is an NICU Graduate? How Onerous Is the Responsibility?

We should reiterate that this study focuses on the healthier part of the NICU population—we interviewed the parents of babies who survived. It is crucial to remember that in the twelve-month period for which we have data, 15% of babies admitted to the NICU of City Hospital died before being discharged, as did nearly 9% of those admitted to the unit at Subur-

Table 7.2 Disposition of infants at first discharge (percentage)

	City Hospital (N = 379)	Suburban Hospital (N = 566)
Discharged to parents	44.6	65.9
Discharged to mother	20.3	6.5
Discharged to father	0.5	0.2
Discharged to foster or adoptive home	1.1	0.9
Discharged to long-term care facility	0.8	0.2
Discharged to another hospital	17.4	16.3
Deceased	15.0	8.7
Missing data	0.3	1.4

Note: Data for this table were collected from the infants' medical records.

ban.[2] As we document in Table 7.2, another 16%–18% are discharged to another hospital (often to "feed and grow" closer to home) before being sent home or are sent to a long-term care facility. Only about 66% of babies admitted to City Hospital and around 74% of those admitted to Suburban Hospital can be sent home (or to a foster or adoptive home) at discharge, and some of those are subsequently rehospitalized for further treatment, sometimes for months at a time.

Infants can be categorized, as we did in chapter 3, according to whether they went home as "well babies," continued to have a few problems associated with their early hospitalization, or still had quite significant health or developmental problems. By that categorization scheme, roughly 59% of the babies whose parents we interviewed had suffered an initial crisis but were really "well babies" by the time of our interviews, roughly 16% continued to have relatively minor problems, and about 24% had serious problems of one sort or another. Another way to examine the question of how much special care a baby needs is to ask what special training or instructions the parents were given when they took the baby home. When a baby is discharged home or sent to a foster-care facility, a discharge summary is prepared and placed in the infant's medical record. In addition, the medical record typically includes information about the instructions parents were given. We coded the information from these documents to provide some sense of just how the situation of a newly discharged NICU patient differs from that of a healthy newborn.

2. Recall that City had on average somewhat more serious cases than Suburban.

Most of the infants whose parents we interviewed went home needing some kind of special care, assessment, or monitoring (on average 3.3 items from a list of 11 at City, and 2.4 from the same list at Suburban Hospital). The most common items mentioned in the discharge instructions were medications (other than vitamins, which were ordered for nearly all infants) (22% at City and 14% at Suburban), various kinds of mechanical monitors (13% at City and 47% at Suburban), special assessments or interventions (35% at City and 37% at Suburban), and physical or occupational therapy (17% at City and 21% at Suburban).[3] Many families also were referred to a service that would send a visiting nurse to their home to monitor the infant's progress (57% at City and 42% at Suburban) or were referred to a follow-up program (78% at City and 100% at Suburban). Other instructions—such as about how to care for an infant with a tracheostomy tube (which creates an artificial airway) or for a ventilator-dependent baby, or how to feed a baby with a gastrostomy tube (a tube inserted into the stomach)—applied to a much smaller number of infants but were very serious matters in those families.[4] These data are shown in Table 7.3.

For parents these discharge instructions mean that in addition to the usual round of diaper changes, feedings, wakeful nights walking a disconsolate baby, and visits for well-baby exams and shots, many parents must also learn to administer medications, track the schedule of medicines (including deciding whether to delay the medicine or wake a peacefully sleeping baby), learn to read and respond to monitor alarms and how to deal with false alarms from a malfunctioning monitor or detached monitor leads (both very common), perform some physical and occupational therapy routines, discuss the baby's situation with a visiting nurse or therapist and receive instruction from this person, and take the baby to specialists for therapies, assessments, or emergencies.

Caring for a normal infant is a time-consuming job and includes the time spent in child care and the extra time added to household work by

3. Although Suburban infants are considerably more likely than those from City to go home with a monitor, we believe that this reflects different discharge practices rather than differences in the health of infants at discharge. Our conjecture is that middle-class Suburban parents are more likely to insist that their children come home with monitors and that their insurers are more generous than Medicaid in paying for such equipment.

4. Although our table indicates that none of the infants were initially sent home on a ventilator, several babies went home on ventilators after subsequent hospitalizations and were still ventilator dependent at the time of our interview. So Table 7.3 may understate the seriousness of illness in some cases.

TABLE 7.3 Special care required by infants discharged home from hospital (percentage)

	City Hospital		Suburban Hospital	
	Total	Sample	Total	Sample
Proportion of cases in which discharge summary or instructions mentioned item				
Medications (other than vitamins)	21.9	17.9	14.0	40.7
Special feeding technique (e.g., reflux precautions)	8.0	4.0	0	5.0
CNG, NG, or G-tube feedings	11.0	13.0	1.0	5.0
Care of colostomy, ileostomy, ureterostomy, etc.	6.0	4.0	1.0	0
Tracheostomy tube	4.0	13.0	1.0	0
Ventilator	2.0	0	0	0
Oxygen support	3.0	9.0	2.0	11.0
Apnea/bradycardia monitor, event recorder, Holter monitor, etc.	11.0	13.0	26.0	47.0
Condition requiring knowledge of special assessment or intervention techniques	44.0	35.0	17.0	37.0
Physical or occupational therapy	19.0	17.0	6.0	21.0
Other special care	11.0	9.0	4.0	11.0
Mean no. items mentioned	3.47	3.30	1.14	2.37
Standard Deviation	1.70	1.77	1.22	1.98
Range	2-11	2-7	0-9	0-9
Proportion of cases in which a referral was made at discharge to				
Visiting nurse	47.0	57.0	18.0	42.0
Follow-up program or clinic	77.0	78.0	75.0	100.0
State child-welfare agency	3.0	4.0	1.0	0
Other	9.0	88.0	10.0	26.0
N for which discharge information available	(255)	(23)	(377)	(19)

Note: Excludes infants who expired, who were discharged to another hospital, or about whom discharge information was missing. It is crucial to keep in mind that the infants for whom discharge information is available are the ones who were well enough to be sent directly home rather than to an intermediate-level nursery. Further, some infants were rehospitalized after brief stays at home and went home with additional equipment. Although this table suggests that no ventilator-dependent families were included in our interview sample, in fact at the time of our interviews, two of the babies from City Hospital were on ventilators.

the infant (e.g., in extra laundry). An NICU graduate often adds more work than another baby just coming home from the hospital, and probably always adds more worry. How much work and worry are added is impossible to say, and the burdens are clearly quite variable.

At one extreme are families who had the help of teams of nurses who worked regular shifts in the home. That such nurses were paid for by insurers or by the welfare system suggests that even bureaucracies can see that sometimes the care of a child is more than a family can manage by itself. But neither insurers nor public aid tends to be generous in supplementing family labor. Although quite a few families had some nursing assistance when the baby first came home, only a few continued to receive nursing help for very long. Just after discharge seven families had nursing care paid for by their insurer or with public funds (1009, 1017, 1031, 1036, 2003, 2016, 2024); another family privately hired a nursing student to watch their child during the night when he first came home from the hospital (1028). For most families nursing care was quickly cut back or eliminated, though several families still had nurses working regularly in their homes at the time of our interview a year and a half or two after the child's birth (1009, 1017, 1031, and 1036), and one family had only very recently stopped receiving home nursing (2024). One couple, Marta and Ricardo (1017), described their disputes with their insurer when it cut back on nursing help, making it necessary for Marta to care for Cassandra, who was ventilator dependent, most of the weekend after working full-time all week at the job that provided the family insurance coverage.

For couples such as this one, life with their NICU graduate bore a striking resemblance to life in the NICU or the ventilator-dependent unit of the hospital. Though they no longer spent their evenings and weekends in the hospital, the hospital had colonized their home. Cassandra's room was filled with medical equipment; the day and week were organized around nursing schedules and the relay-race transitions in which responsibility for Cassandra was transferred from one care giver to another; time was further ordered by schedules for therapy, the administration of medications, and checking and maintaining such vital equipment as the ventilator. Marta was now no ordinary mother. She was also a medical worker, regularly taking her turn in the rotation of nurses, supervising the work of other nurses, and even dismissing nurses who did not perform up to standard. Though Marta has no formal medical certification, and may not have the general background of a nurse, her on-the-job training places her high in the hierarchy of those who regularly care for a ventilator-dependent child in a medical outpost. She could not at this point qualify for a job in another medical outpost, but we should nevertheless not be misled into believing that she is only the child's mother.

For Marta and Ricardo, family life was fundamentally reshaped by the presence of the NICU graduate. The workload was much too high for the parents to manage alone, so specialized workers had to be brought into the home, with all of the disruption that entails. Though in many ways a nurse caring for a baby or toddler functions much like a babysitter, there are crucial differences. The nurse will not accept responsibility for other children, so child-care arrangements still have to be made for any siblings. The labor contract is also quite different from an ordinary child-care labor contract, because workers are not formally employed by the parents but are instead hired by a separate contractor and paid with funds that come from an insurer or from the government. Nevertheless the parents retain some supervisory duties, though these often must be exercised in tandem with the formal supervisor in a home-health agency. And here we see that the problems created by the agency chain explored in the context of the NICU in chapter 6 do not cease when a child is discharged home. Parents must still act as intermediaries between their infant-principals and other agents on whom they depend for crucial goods and services.

To describe the extra hours of nursing care is to understate the responsibility, though. Cassandra's parents were concerned with much more than just keeping their daughter alive. Though Cassandra was blind and suffered from serious respiratory problems, Marta and Ricardo wanted a normal life for their daughter. They talked about hoping to wean her from the ventilator and their expectations that she would eventually learn to walk and talk, but they also talked about their hopes that Cassandra would one day attend college and would have a boyfriend and even marry. These are universal dreams. But what is different here is that Marta and Ricardo recognize that their child cannot hope to achieve these ends without help—very considerable help—from them. While parental intervention to accelerate child development is fashionable these days, we are not here talking about infant exercise programs like Baby Gymboree. Cassandra's needs are closer to those of Helen Keller than to those of the average toddler. Consequently Marta and Ricardo contemplate filling their days with learning about education for the blind, finding ways to supply a balanced diet to a finicky eater whose natural responses have been disrupted by endotracheal tubes (inserted into the mouth and down the airway for mechanical ventilation) and by nasogastric tube feedings, providing motivation for the child to progress without pampering her, and figuring out how to steer a careful course between the Scylla of excessive optimism and the Charybdis of resigned acceptance. But even this is not enough. An active six-year-old has a right to a full and happy life, too, and Marta and Ricardo scheme valiantly to save time and money for Ricky, Cassandra's brother. Marta pays Ricky's parochial school tuition in full at the start of the year so that family emergencies do not consume what she regards as his share, and Ricardo is careful to take Ricky along to the sporting events he continues to participate in. But as Marta sadly notes, "I try to give them equal. But you know, it don't always work that way because the fact is she needs more" (1017F, p. 19). In families like this, then, what siblings often get is explanations from exhausted parents about the difference between "fair" and "equal."

Though Cassandra's case is an extreme one, several other families faced similar situations or had faced them earlier. But even when families did not have (or had never had) home nursing, their homes often had some of the other features of medical outposts—medications had to be administered regularly, diaper changes were supplanted or supplemented with colostomy bag changes or catheterizations of the bladder, medical supply companies made visits to check equipment or deliver supplies, and procedures that needed to be performed regularly, such as checks of the shunt removing excess fluid from the child's head, had to be routinized and fit into a daily schedule.

For still other families, modifications to family life were smaller but nevertheless required that the parents be able to recite the litany of the child's medical history to new physicians (e.g., in emergency rooms), make extra doctor visits, increase their attention to weight gain and developmental progress, or be vigilant about colds because of lung damage sustained in early infancy. Even parents whose children now seemed quite "normal" (as gauged by developmental screenings, for instance) continued to worry about what might be discovered in the future about the correlates of extreme prematurity, the consequences of administering a particular drug to a neonate, or the effects of frequent X rays in the neonatal period. And a few parents continued to be sufficiently troubled by the trauma of the early days that they attended parent-support groups, to get the latest information about problems they were experiencing (e.g., hearing loss from antibiotics in the NICU) or might experience (e.g., high-risk pregnancy) and to discuss their experiences with others who had endured similar ordeals.[5]

Bringing a baby home from an intensive care unit is thus an experience that bears some resemblance both to ordinary parenting of a newborn and to working in an NICU. As is clear from newspaper accounts, not all parents rise to the occasion when faced with a normally demanding infant. Similarly not all parents rise to the occasion when faced with the extraordinary demands of a baby newly released from an intensive care unit. But we need to know more than this. We need to know something about the personal characteristics, resource pools, strategies, and networks of those who are able to shoulder responsibilities that others might shirk or evade. We also need to know how parents' conceptions of good-enough parenting vary, how parents decide what and how much to do for their infants, and how they explain their decisions to themselves and others. Some of the variation we observe between parents cannot be explained by paying exclusive attention to the parents' individual characteristics. We must also bear in mind that parenting often requires that parents draw on services and resources provided by others. We must also pay attention, then, to the variation between the organizations parents encounter in how easy or difficult it is for them to secure those contributions and take responsibility. We turn now to an assessment of these variations among parents and among families.

Responsibility as a Social Product

If we believe that an NICU and its staff can responsibly care for a critically ill infant, we presumably believe the outcome is a profoundly social one. No individual can produce that outcome alone. Instead, what is required is a variety of individual inputs (skilled actions, attentiveness) that are coordinated with one another by a division of labor, protocols for procedures and medications, and elaborate organizational routines for staff meetings, medical and social service rounds, intake and discharge procedures, payment processes, record keeping, and quality assurance and accreditation reviews. The division of labor in turn depends on inputs that are to some degree standardized through training programs and motivated by salary

5. Wuthnow (1994) documents the increasing popularity of support groups of all kinds across the United States and reports that up to 45% of the adult female population claims to be involved in one. Taylor (1996:3) analyzes the support group movement that has developed around postpartum depression and reports that up to 80% of women have at least some form of depression following delivery.

systems, formal review processes, and informal sanctions. Elaborate monitoring, partly arranged by overlapping obligations (e.g., nurse and physician share some tasks; physicians review their work with other physicians), increases the likelihood that errors will be caught and corrected and that people are kept on their toes. While the effort, ingenuity, observations, and commitment of individuals are important, they alone are insufficient; the NICU's capacity to care responsibly for critically ill infants is produced jointly by these contributions and by the supra-individual mechanisms that coordinate individual efforts and make them predictable and reliable.

Responsibility is similarly socially produced in families, though the mechanisms are less transparent than those of a formal organization, and mechanisms that produce responsibility in some families may be entirely absent in other families. In previous chapters we have examined the relationship between the family and the NICU, looking first at how the parents fit into and are disciplined and evaluated by the NICU and then at how families gradually take a larger role in the care of their child and even begin to evaluate, criticize, and attempt to reform hospital care providers. In examining how responsibility is produced in a family, we look simultaneously at the social processes that produce responsible behavior in individual parents and at how the contributions of individual parents are supplemented or matched by the contributions of the other parent, family members, friends, or paid care providers.

The core of our argument here is that responsibility is not simply an individual attribute but rather is bolstered by certain kinds of social arrangements and undermined by others. This is equally true in the NICU and the home. However, there are some important distinctions between the production of responsibility in an organization like the NICU and its production in the home that should not be overlooked. First, as we emphasized in the opening pages of this chapter, the homes to which children are discharged are much more variable than the NICU. It is not that the personnel and procedures of NICUs never change but rather that NICUs are more formal and predictable organizations than families.

Second, the type of responsibility that is being produced in the two settings varies quite a lot as well. As we outlined in chapter 4, both NICUs and parents have an ultimate responsibility for their patients and their children, respectively. But the responsibilities are clearly different. While the NICU has a responsibility of relatively short duration and narrow scope, the parents' is of long duration and broad scope. The mechanisms that produce responsibility in NICUs (and other formal organizations) are unlikely to translate well to families. Organizations, for instance, are interested in inducing commitment to jobs, not to particular projects, problems, or in our case, patients. In fact, overcommitment to a particular project or patient may hinder job performance. In families, in contrast, it is precisely this commitment to individuals that is crucial. Thinking about the future is also clearly different for the staff of the NICU and the parents. Medicine in general, and NICUs perhaps in particular, are roundly criticized for not taking a longer-range view of their patients' lives. While there may be formal organizational mechanisms that encourage organizational members to think and strategize about the future, it is mainly about the future of the organization rather than the future of any one patient. This is to suggest not that the people who work in NICUs are unconcerned with the eventual fates of their patients, but only that their first imperative is to get them well enough to be discharged. The future beyond discharge is largely someone else's problem. Families' responsibilities to their children, in contrast, are (to say the least) not so neatly bounded.

Finally, the production of responsibility in formal organizations like NICUs differs from that in families in a third way. We have already argued that what it means to be a responsible care provider in an NICU and a responsible parent in a home are quite distinct and that the orientations to those roles are also likely to be quite different. But what this also means is that NICU staff members and parents are likely to err in different directions. Parents develop a commitment to a particular child, but NICUs treat many infants who just happen to become their patients while they're critically ill. NICUs are, therefore, likely to view the infant as an instance of a bureaucratic category, as a patient or member of a specific diagnostic category, whereas parents are likely to refuse to see their child reduced to so many numbers in a chart and will treat the child instead as an individual with particular needs, likes, and dislikes. This difference is often at the crux of the social control efforts just detailed in chapters 5 and 6. The NICU tries valiantly to get parents to fit into the organizational routines, in part by insisting that they respect the hospital imperative to view the child as a member of bureaucratic category. Procedures and protocols must be followed for every patient; other patients must be cared for as well; idiosyncracies cannot be indulged. Parents, in turn, try valiantly to get the NICU staff to see their infant as not just another patient. Rules were made to be broken; my child needs to learn to eat from a bottle even if it takes more time; in short, my child should have the best, not just adequate, care. Responsible parenting, then, requires people to take the view of the organizations on which they depend for crucial services and at the same time to encourage those organizations to see the uniqueness of their child when that is what's needed.

The NICU plays a crucial role in teaching parents some of the skills they will need to care responsibly for their children following discharge. In addition to learning the medical skills they will need at home, parents get some important lessons about how to parent in the normative system of a large medical organization. Parents can't help being transformed by the experience of having a critically ill child. Much of their approach to parenting is emergent, as they learn new skills, work out definitions of their roles, make adjustments and adaptations to life with an especially needy child. But parents also have fairly durable cultural conceptions of parenthood that may be more resistant to change. Responsibility is socially produced in either case—emerging as the result of situational adjustments to new contingencies or enduring as the result of life-long learning about the proper role of parents.

Our task in the rest of the chapter is to examine what mix of situational adjustments and cultural conceptions of parenthood tend to shore up or undermine responsibility. Drawing on our interviews with parents, we will examine each of the dimensions of responsibility elaborated in chapter 3. As readers will recall from that earlier discussion, taking responsibility for someone (or something) entails taking account of others' interests as well as one's own, accepting a diffuse definition of one's role, thinking about the long term, using discretion and tailoring one's inputs to the situation so that contributions of time or effort or other resources are appropriate to changing circumstances, and accepting resulting variations in one's own welfare as the needs of the other person increase or decrease (see also Heimer 1996b). Responsible orientations and behavior can come about in a variety of ways. There is no single route to responsible parenting, and it is therefore imperative to search for the paths that seem most likely to lead there and to determine how different resources or experiences or ties substitute for one another as suppressors or amplifiers of responsible impulses, orientations, or actions.

Taking the Baby's Needs Seriously

We have argued that a key part of taking responsibility is treating the needs and interests of another person (or group of people or organization) seriously. Whether a member of a large-scale organization or a small family, in order to be responsible, one must take others' interests into account as well as one's own. Unlike the more universalistic and bounded responsibilities in organizations, however, parenting is a particularistic and unbounded responsibility. Parents are expected to take their baby's needs seriously and to balance their baby's needs with the needs of the rest of their family. Responsible parents are also expected to take their baby's needs at least as seriously as they take their own needs and interests, so seriously that the misery of their child makes them miserable too. A central question, then, is how this commitment to meeting the baby's needs is produced.

Among the parents we interviewed, a group who on the whole are quite committed to their children, we found some variability in expressed commitment to the child and to meeting his or her needs.[6] At one extreme were parents like Mike (1018), whom we first met in chapter 3. On the one hand, Mike said he would never abandon his son, Robert, and felt obligated to have a relationship with the child because "he's mine" (1018M, p. 39). On the other hand, he also thought it quite likely that he would lose all contact with Robert if the mother moved. Mike did not visit Robert in the hospital and at the time of our interview had not seen his son, who resided in the same town, in the previous month. According to Mike, Robert "didn't seem like he was in too much pain" (p. 10) in the NICU, and he had little to say about his relationship with Robert (though more to say about his irritation with Robert's mother Gloria).[7] At the other extreme are parents who describe indicators of how the child experienced the hospitalization ("she winced every time someone touched her foot"), worry about how this early experience will shape the child's life ("she still doesn't like anyone to touch her face" or "other kids can be so cruel; how will they talk about his scars in the locker room in junior high?"), and report how anxieties during the early days and in the present affect their own well-being ("I didn't really sleep at night until he was home").

We believe that commitment to a child and to meeting its needs ordi-

6. We believe that less committed parents would be harder to locate (given that we were locating them through medical records) and less likely to consent to an interview about the child once we did locate them.

7. Though Robert had spina bifida and was very developmentally delayed, Mike minimized his problems: "To me he seems normal, I mean, all but his legs and the shunt that's in his head. Other than that he seems normal to me" (1018m, p. 38). Further, Mike believed that the doctors had more to do with shaping Robert's future than he and Gloria did: "I mean, they're, we're not doctors so we don't know what, I mean what's going to be wrong with him. . . . All I can say is if Gloria takes him to the hospital or doctor when he's supposed to [go], then I feel that nothing will happen to him" (1018m, p. 34).

narily arises as an empathetic response. But what is important about this observation is that there are a variety of ways that such a response can be stimulated. Our conclusions here recombine the insights of other scholars and show how the processes they describe occur together in a natural setting. What factors help account for attachment to the child and empathy with it? We argue that the keys are a cognitive apparatus to help process the information that the parent gathers through observation of the child, sustained contact with the child, so that the parent can observe what the child is experiencing, and some mechanism to make the parent believe that the child belongs uniquely to him or her.[8]

The cognitive apparatus that facilitates observation and coding of the child's experience may come from a variety of sources, including feminine socialization, middle-class ideologies about children's needs, sustained discussion with a spouse or other kin about the child, or discussions with hospital staff members. LaRossa and LaRossa (1981) noted the difference between how men and women interacted with their infants. Fathers were comfortable leaving the baby in the crib for long periods while they did other things, but mothers felt more compelled to interact with the child. For fathers, they argue, the infant was an object; for mothers, the infant was already a person, capable of real interaction and entitled to many of the interactional courtesies extended to other people. Rossi and Rossi (1990) echoed some of the same points when they discussed gender differences in intergenerational contact. But they went further and showed that gender differences in providing care are largely accounted for by differences between men and women in emotional expressivity. Those men who were particularly emotionally expressive resembled women in the extent to which they had contact with and exchanged services with kin, and women who were less emotionally expressive resembled men in having less contact and providing fewer services across generational lines. This

8. Although it is beyond the scope of this book, we by no means intend to suggest that there is no biological basis for parent-child attachments. On the ways in which biological and social factors might mesh, see, e.g., the work of Alice Rossi (1977, 1985). And although we emphasize that contact with the child helps stimulate the parent's empathy and commitment, we wish to acknowledge that parent empathy and commitment can arise long before a child is born. Observation is not the only route to empathy or commitment, but observation (e.g., of fetal movements and changes in the mother's body) also occurs prenatally. Many parents thus feel strongly attached to their children before birth and grieve deeply over pregnancy losses. Grief over pregnancy losses is not always acknowledged by others, and pregnancy losses may even be blamed on the women themselves (see, e.g., Layne 1990; Letherby 1993; Reinharz 1988).

suggests that feminine socialization in emotional expressivity is one, but hardly the only, route to empathy.

The mothers we interviewed were somewhat more likely than the fathers to think of the baby as a person, capable of experiencing pain and even of interacting. Quite a few parents described interaction with the child as central to their feelings of attachment. Although parents proudly reported on physical indicators that the baby responded positively to their presence (e.g., 1017F, pp. 17–18; 1017M, pp. 7, 28; 1025F, p. 11; 1030M, p. 7; 1031F, p. 6; 1036F, pp. 76–77; 1039F, p. 13; 2034F, p. 65), eye contact and touch are central to the parents' experiences of interaction with their child. What is important to them is the experience of communication when the baby met their eyes (e.g., 1015F&M, p. 8; 1016F, p. 28; 1030F, p. 7; 1036M, p. 52; 2002F, p. 42; 2021F, p. 45; 2024M, pp. 10–11) or squeezed their fingers (2023M, p. 3; 2025F, p. 4; 2025M, p. 4).

Often the parents even went so far as to say what message they felt the baby was communicating. Describing the first time she saw her daughter, one mother noted that she "had her eyes open and like looked right at me and like 'Hi, Mommy,' you know, and the one hand was even out, you know, and it was just kind of like 'Hi, Mom, hi, Mom, I'm going to be okay.'" (2034F, p. 22). One father reported that right after delivery, "She looked, it's like 'Dad, what's going on?' She was holding my finger, holding on to it real tight . . . just looking at me, and I was looking and I was crying" (2011M, p. 2). A few parents reported both sides of the communication. One mother wouldn't let relatives visit unless she believed that they would be positive and upbeat: "She seemed to know me, and she kept . . . trying to look at me and—this is the hardest part—she would roll her eyes back and forth, like this, desperate: 'Get me out of here.' And . . . she was crying, but there was no fountain [tears][mother very choked up], you know, because she was begging me to help her" (1008F, p. 16). The mother responded with long explanations. She told the baby that she was her mother, described their home, and assured her that this wasn't what life was going to be like: "I figured that for her to survive, we had to make it clear to her that she had to fight and stay with it and not think that this is what she was created for" (1008F, p. 18).

While this is undoubtedly parents projecting positive messages onto their tiny, fragile infants, this process of projection should not be dismissed as mere delusion. Clearly, small, sick infants cannot literally communicate the messages their parents conveyed in these interviews. However, this kind of projection is an important part of constructing the humanness of their infants. And although causal direction is difficult to untangle here, some parents stated that their sense of attachment and of their child as a person arose very directly from interaction with the child: "I mean I don't remember feeling like this strong attachment. I remember feeling more duty bound because, like I said, he was paralyzed [by drugs], he was asleep, his eyes were closed. It wasn't until that first time I saw him in the hospital and he like looked at me that I was like, all of a sudden it was like, 'Oh my God,' you know, there he is because I'd never, I mean he was just, might as well have been a cardboard picture. . . . Like I said when I first saw him, he was just a cardboard frog" (1016F, p. 28). Following this experience, the mother's "maternal instincts" kicked in (p. 28). This mother also reported herself as having been especially concerned that hospital staff members use the baby's name, because she "just wanted to make sure that he was a person" (p. 20).

A second route to empathy is more directly cognitive. Conceiving of children as having developmental needs and believing that their early cries are crude methods of communication led parents to be more attentive both to cries and other reactions as signals about the baby's state. Parents who had read books about pregnancy or child rearing or who subscribed to parenting magazines were more likely to talk about developmental milestones and to remark on the extent to which the child was "behind" because of prematurity and needed additional stimulation to help him or her "catch up." They were also more likely to connect early babbling with later speech and to conceive it as their job to help children with these developmental tasks by providing appropriate toys, structuring situations to elicit repetitions of behaviors that would help children develop, and rewarding developmentally appropriate behaviors. These cognitive categorizations of infants' behavior were more likely to occur in well-educated than in poorly educated people but were also more common among women than among men. Both men and women noted that women read more about pregnancy, child development, and their child's specific situation than men did and that women were the family leaders in seeking out materials and in pointing men to the sections that even they must read.

Though middle-class understandings of child development provide people with a rudimentary understanding of developmental milestones and equip them to assess their child's progress, this basic framework can be supplied and reinforced in other ways. Spending time on an NICU leads to exposure to the talk of nurses, physicians, and therapists. Parents often reported to us what the nurses or therapists had told them. For instance, parents reported on physical indicators of stress or relaxation in their baby and how these were apparently correlated with their presence on the unit. Physical therapists, working to increase the range of an infant's movement might, for instance, also report to the parents on whether the baby was "organized" or could "console" itself.[9] With this enriched understanding of what was happening with their baby, parents would now be equipped to observe their child's responses to them.

Finally, this enriched understanding can arise from the need to report on or discuss the baby's progress with other people. This means that in addition to the moral support that a parent receives from a spouse and from the baby's grandparents, such people increase the acuity of the parent's observations. If a baby is sick enough to be in an intensive care unit, other family members will rarely be satisfied with the answer that the baby is "fine." Marriage and a strong extended kin group thus increase the likelihood that parents will be asked to describe their own observations of the baby and explain what physicians and nurses have reported. We believe that this requirement to report to the spouse (coupled with the fact that married mothers visit more often than unmarried mothers) helps explain why the descriptions of the child's hospitalization produced by married mothers contained far more details than those produced during interviews with unmarried mothers.[10]

We have hypothesized here that people need a cognitive framework that permits them to notice things about the baby and suggested that this cognitive apparatus can be supplied and elaborated in various ways. But clearly a cognitive framework is by itself insufficient if the parent has little opportunity to use it. Without observations of the child itself, a cognitive framework can only create an abstract understanding of a child's situation.

9. We were never given a formal definition of *organized* by the physical therapists who used this language, but the contrast between organized and disorganized infants was made clear to us as the therapists pointed out aspects of infants' reactions. An infant who is organized moves in a coordinated way and has a consistent, coherent reaction to stimuli and some capacity to attend to one stimulus without immediately being distracted by others. In contrast, a disorganized infant "goes ten directions at once."

10. It is hard to tell the extent to which these differences were accounted for by age and education. Unmarried mothers tended to be younger and less educated than married mothers. But among the young, poorly educated mothers, those who were married or living with the fathers of their children were more likely than those who did not live with the baby's father to give detailed accounts of the baby's hospitalization. It is far more difficult to report on differences between married and unmarried fathers. We were unable to interview many unmarried fathers. The medical record did not always contain sufficient information for us to locate them without the assistance of the mother, and when the parents were no longer a couple, mothers were often, though not always, reluctant to help us locate the father.

Contact with the child is crucial in creating the kind of emotional response that Zajonc (1980) argues really underlies our actions and that Latané and Darley (1970) seem to believe explains why (in experiments) people who have had even brief contact with a "victim" are more likely to intervene to offer help than are complete strangers (see also Mynatt and Sherman 1975; Rutkowski, Gruder, and Romer 1983).

We must note here that the variables that we believe affect the likelihood of thinking of a baby as a person rather than an object and so taking its needs and interests seriously do not operate independently of those that influence contact. Women are somewhat more likely than men to visit their hospitalized infants (according to the data we presented in chapter 2), and married parents more likely than unmarried parents.[11] We have already noted that both groups (married people and mothers) also are more likely to think of babies as people. Clearly the effects are multiplicative rather than additive here (so that, e.g., the difference between married mothers and unmarried fathers is larger than one would expect by summing the effects of gender and marital status), though we suspect that each has some independent effect. Parents who visit are more likely to see things that make them think of their baby as fully human. But, of course, those who think of their baby as a person are more likely to visit—and to tell interviewers that in addition to believing that they should be there, they believed that their presence was important to the baby's well-being.[12]

Finally, when a parent believes that he or she has a unique tie to the baby, the parent is more likely to take the baby's needs and interests seriously and feel compelled to act so as to improve the baby's lot. Again, mothers were more likely to make statements that suggested that they viewed their tie to the baby as unique and their contribution to the baby's welfare as irreplaceable. In some instances, parents (particularly mothers) talked about believing that the baby "knew" them—for example, recognizing parents' voices from hearing them during the pregnancy. More commonly, parents talked about worrying that the baby would be treated as just another patient if they didn't visit and keep track of what was happening. By virtue of their attachment to a single child in the intensive care

11. Interview reports that are harder to quantify suggest that the data from the nursing notes understate gender differences here. Mothers more often than fathers reported spending most of the day at the baby's bedside, but fathers were more likely to visit more briefly before or after work.

12. Of those with whom we discussed the matter, 81% of mothers and 58% of fathers believed that their visits mattered to the baby's well-being. (When the mother and father were interviewed together, we have attributed the view to both parents unless one disagreed.)

nursery, parents thus saw themselves as having a role as vigilant overseers of the health-care team, as we described in chapter 6.

We believe that it is this feeling of unique attachment that helps explain an otherwise anomalous finding, that while increases in the burden associated with caring for a child might be expected to predict that a needier child would get less adequate care, in our sample needier infants on average got more care.[13] Although the standard economic prediction might be that the amount of care would not vary much with a child's needs (on the grounds that a parent had implicitly agreed to spend only a certain amount to "purchase" this "good"), we observe a direct relationship between amount of care needed and amount supplied. Infants who are unusually needy get better care than those who need less. We believe that this occurs partly because the plight of the child requires parents to pay unusual attention even if they have no well-developed conceptual scheme for thinking about child development. In addition, though, sicker infants are more likely to elicit parental commitment because parents are fully convinced that no one else will rise to the occasion to care for so needy a child. Few arguments are so compelling as a belief that one must care for a child because no one else will.

People are more likely to see another's needs and interests as being as important as their own and are more likely to feel that their own well-being depends on helping to meet the other person's needs, we have argued, when they believe that others are as worthy as themselves (for infants, this means that others consider them to be fully human), when they have conceptual systems that permit them to observe and understand the other person's experience (a process that requires varying degrees of translation, depending on the differences between the people), when they are brought into sufficient contact with one another that they are familiar with the other person's experience, and when some mechanism forces people to see another's welfare as a problem that belongs uniquely to them. Whether a parent poignantly describes the plight of a premature baby or discusses with more detachment how babies will not remember the pain of their early days should help predict how much responsibility the parent takes for the baby who is finally home.

13. It would be foolish to make too much of this point. Clearly, sicker children are also more likely to be institutionalized and so to take less of their parents' time and attention. Further, our data are surely subject to a selection bias—parents who are less devoted to their children were probably less willing to be interviewed and are surely underrepresented in our study.

Though much of our discussion here stresses the ideologies, observations, emotional responses, or cognitions of individual parents, we wish to highlight their social aspects. Though we cannot point to anything as concrete as prescribed organizational routines that exist in all cases or are mandated by some accreditation society, we can nevertheless point to routinized practices of families or of larger groups. When a husband and wife report that the wife reads the parenting books, discusses them with the husband, and highlights the sections he must read, they are reporting on a household routine that ultimately, we believe, increases the likelihood that parents will take responsibility for their child. This routine helps parents to refine their conceptual categories and thus may increase the acuity of their observations about their child.[14] Other routines that similarly bring the parents into contact with the child ("I went to visit every evening after I got off work") or that entail collection of information about the child ("I called every day just before I went to bed and when I woke up in the morning") and discussion of that information with others ("Whichever one of us talked to the nurse on the phone gave the information to the other one") support attentiveness to the child's experience. And though many of these routines for acquiring information about child development, for reporting and assessing observations about the child, and for "creating" the child's personhood are routines that are especially likely to occur in couples, they may occur elsewhere as well. In principle, a particularly supportive grandmother, aunt, brother, or friend could do the same things and presumably often either supplement or substitute for a spouse in reinforcing the parent's sense that the child is a real and worthy person.

In essence we are arguing that the construction of the child as a person undergirds parental commitment to meeting the child's needs and that the constructive process does not automatically occur. Philippe Ariès (1962) argues that childhood is a relatively recent invention and that before the invention of childhood as a separate phase of the life cycle, infants often were treated as less than human until they had passed a certain age. Until that point, parents remained somewhat detached from infants, not even giving them names. Whatever one may think of the historical accuracy of this argument, it nevertheless is a salutary reminder that the humanness of any person is at least partly a social product. Other scholars have also

14. We do not mean to ignore the possibility that refined conceptual schemes may also lead to misperception, as parents attempt to fit their observations into the conceptual categories they have now adopted. But even a misdiagnosis may increase responsibility by increasing the closeness of observation.

documented the historical shift in our views of children (see, e.g., Boli-Bennett and Meyer 1978; Pollock 1983; Zelizer 1985). Contemporary and historical debates about when life begins and historical discussions of differences between the sexes and races offer similar evidence of the social construction of humanness. Not everyone thinks of a very premature or sick baby as a person, but our argument is that those who do are more likely than those who don't to worry about what such protohumans need and what they as parents can do to protect and nurture their offspring both during the hospital stay and after the baby comes home.[15]

The humanness of the NICU patient and the baby who goes home with its parents from the NICU is thus produced by uncertain and imperfect social technologies, precariously routinized, and adopted and supported by only some of the parents and their families and friends. We have tried to show here what characteristics of people themselves and what features of the ways they conduct their lives increase the likelihood that this particular social product—the humanness of a fragile child—will be produced.

Thinking about the Future

Jaques's (1972) analysis of responsibility in industry is one of the few to link responsibility to planning for the future. But when Jaques analyzes the relationship between responsibility at work and the time period over which an employee is expected to plan, he does not emphasize enough that such planning is on behalf of a group. People rarely plan asocial futures. Thinking about the future tends to occur in solidary units. There usually has to be a "we"—whether a work group, a firm, an educational institution, or a family—to make such planning worthwhile. This observation about how planning is organized around collectivities is crucial in explaining differences among the parents of NICU patients, because only some of the parents conceive themselves to be part of a solidary unit with a joint future.

What group constitutes the "we" that typically plans for children's futures has varied from one historical period to another and from one society to another. In societies in which children are considered to belong to the father's kinship group, it is these groups that are responsible for the children, particularly when the nuclear family does not reside in a separate

15. See Heimer and Stevens (1997) for a discussion of how NICUs help construct the humanness of these tiny, fragile infants. Parents are encouraged to name their children, to bring in pictures of themselves and other family members, to dress their infant in clothes brought from home, to decorate their baby's crib or isolette, and the like. Even the rituals surrounding death reconfirm the humanness of the infants.

dwelling unit. In contemporary American society, the locus of responsibility for a child varies with the marital status of the parents and the composition of the household in which the child resides. Legal capacity to give consent for medical treatment, for instance, resides with the mother when the parents are unmarried, though either parent can give consent if the parents are married. When the parents live together, whether they are married or not, they are assumed to bear joint responsibility for the children. But when the parents are not together, the mother usually has primary responsibility, and the extent of the father's obligations varies a good deal with whether the parents were ever really a couple and what legal arrangements have been made if married parents divorced (Arendell 1986, 1995; Gerson 1985, 1993). The assumption that children "belong" to their mother if a marriage dissolves is a recent invention in America, as Friedman (1995) shows, and indeed the convention that a divorced mother will have custody of and responsibility for her children is being challenged by some divorced fathers.

Conventions about who has primary responsibility for children and who has a joint future influence people's sense that they are appropriately situated to make plans for their child. Such conventions also affect the stability of plans. In contemporary American culture, a mother and her children typically are not a stable and well-institutionalized "we" partly because the boundaries of the planning unit may at any point expand (or be expected by others to expand) to include a man or shrink to a smaller unit when a liaison doesn't work out. If a mother and her children are a somewhat precarious planning unit, unmarried, noncustodial fathers are even less likely to constitute a planning unit with their children.

Adults plan futures together. Some consumer durables, such as houses, are purchased primarily by units that consider themselves families (Heimer and Stinchcombe 1980). Similarly, joint planning for the future of children is more likely to occur between adults who believe enough in their joint future—whether they are married or not—to dream, hope, and plan together. These plans often include children, who may sometimes be participants in the discussion. But the elaborateness of plans varies substantially with whether more than one adult shares in the planning and whether those adults believe that they have a future together. Insofar as planning occurs in discussions with other adults with whom one might construct that future, simply having other adults around may not solve the problem if they are not the ones that one envisages spending the future with. A young mother living with her mother might not be a unit that planned a future.[16] Both might anticipate that the young mother would in the long run form her own household. The elder's attempts to participate in planning might then seem like idle interference.

In suggesting that single mothers (or, for that matter, single fathers) are less likely to make detailed plans for the future of their children, we raise some questions about social policies that would concentrate resources on the caregiver-child (or other dependent, perhaps) dyad as the fundamental familial unit. Fineman (1995), for instance, argues forcefully for such a policy, urging the replacement of sexual unions by caretaking ties in social policy. But such a substitution fails to acknowledge how parental caretaking, particularly paternal caretaking, depends on the sexual tie between parents. If, as Rossi and Rossi (1990) argue, it is emotional expressivity that makes people feel sufficiently attached to others to attend to their welfare, then we must ask how emotional expressivity is elicited. As Rossi and Rossi acknowledge, women are somewhat more inclined to be emotionally expressive than men. If it is also true, as many allege, that men are more emotionally expressive with those with whom they have a sexual tie, then the attachment and caring that are correlated with emotional expressivity will, for men, be concentrated in relationships that are sexual themselves or are mediated through sexual ties. We thus ignore the importance of sexual unions at our peril—that is how men become attached to children. While, for women, gossip over coffee, telephone calls to friends and relatives, and the rituals of cards and gifts (DiLeonardo 1987) all are occasions for talking about children, developing and renewing their commitment to them, and fantasizing about their futures, for men pillow talk may serve the same function, though it is important to note that the circle included in pillow talk is considerably more restricted.

Our argument that men's ties to their children are mediated is consistent with medical record data on parental visiting patterns in the NICU. As we first described in chapter 2, fathers in general are slightly less likely to visit than mothers, but unmarried fathers visit considerably less frequently than married fathers. Further, both unmarried and married fathers are more likely to visit with the mothers of their infants rather than alone. In our interviews with parents, mothers often reported visiting for long periods during the day, whereas fathers often visited at night after returning home from work.

16. Analyzing the effects of unwed teenage childbearing on mother-daughter relations, Kaplan (1996) argues that teenage motherhood can produce long-term family conflict and is not simply condoned by the adult mothers of the black teenage mothers she interviewed.

Our point here is not that single parents make no plans whatsoever. Rather, we argue that if they are not engaged in joint parenting with another adult, single parents' plans for children's futures are likely to be less fully elaborated. Padgett and Ansell (1993) argue that goals—and therefore, plans for the future—are properties of roles, not of persons. Further, they note, there is no particular reason to assume that the goals of these various roles are consistent. By this argument, the plans an adult makes as the parent of a young child may not be fully consistent with the goals and plans that are formulated by the same adult in other roles, such as lover or spouse, employee, or student. Consistency may be more likely, though, if as an occupant of a variety of roles a person interacts repeatedly with the same cast of characters. That is, a parent's plans or fantasies about children's futures may be less likely to conflict with plans for his or her relationship with a romantic partner if that partner is also planning the future for those same children.

Plans for the future may also be absent or undeveloped for three other reasons, all related to our argument about how stability facilitates planning for the future. First, some of our observations about marital status and capacity to plan are undoubtedly explained by social class. Single mothers are more likely than married mothers to be poor, and poorer people experience more overall uncertainty. If one's energy is consumed by getting through tomorrow and next week, then how can one think sensibly about next year? While the cultural and intellectual resources of middle-class people no doubt enhance planning, middle-class people are also more likely than poorer people to inhabit a world where planning pays off.

Further, when social ties are especially fragile, a person may, as a simple defense mechanism, retreat from planning. If a father expects the mother to exclude him from the family circle or to block his access to his children, his failure to plan may simply reflect despair about his future with the children. If fathers' ties to children typically are mediated by mothers, then discord between parents can easily divide father and children. Recall that the tension between Gloria and Mike (1018) made it much more difficult for him to maintain a tie with Robert (despite his ex-wife's urging). We ordinarily consider it foolish or even delusional for people to construct plans for relationships that do not exist. Though fathers usually have some capacity to maintain ties with their children despite the mothers' opposition, the motivation to do so may nevertheless disappear if the costs are deemed too high.

Finally, planning may seem grandly beside the point when a child's health is precarious or when there is substantial uncertainty about the child's capacities. Obstetricians and midwives breathe a sigh of relief when a pregnant woman passes such milestones as the period when most miscarriages occur (the first trimester), the point of viability (around twenty-five weeks during our research), and the point at which most premature infants will survive intact (around thirty-two weeks). The fetus is a "keeper," and they now can advise prospective parents to announce the pregnancy, choose names, and buy baby clothes. This sense of security ends abruptly with the birth of a premature or critically ill infant, and parents sometimes experience a "tentative parenthood" mirroring the "tentative pregnancy" that Rothman (1986) describes.

Parents typically talked about "taking things one day at a time" during the early crisis, and some who described themselves as having been "planners" now felt unable to plan. Capturing the futility of making plans when one's child is critically ill, one mother (whose child had spina bifida and hydrocephalus and was severely developmentally delayed) explained why she and her husband had given up planning: "You can plan for the future, and what do you do if it doesn't go that way?" (2011F, p. 36; a similar sentiment is expressed on p. 31). In telling us how she had to give up plans to return to school or work after Kenny's birth, Janet commented: "When I was pregnant, I made plans. Before my pregnancy I was a planner. After he was born, I no longer planned for anything. . . . I think of day to day. Mostly when I think of him, I think of where he's been and where he's at now. I don't think too much on the future" (1036F, pp. 108, 111). Contrasting the period just after her daughter's discharge with the present, one mother gave a carefully nuanced explanation of how she still can't make day-to-day plans but can now at least think about the future: "[Just after the child was discharged,] we didn't have any plans. We still don't make plans. We don't plan more than a couple of days ahead. And then we always leave the clause 'if everything's okay, if everything works all right'" (1039F, p. 28). "We think about the future a lot more [now]. Still, because of financial or other problems, we kind of go day by day" (p. 39).

The perceived end of the crisis occurred at different points for different people. Many parents indicated a radical change in their feelings about their children after discharge; only then did their children come to feel like "theirs." One mother confessed that she had worried her child "would end up calling somebody there [in the NICU] mommy instead of me" (2001F, p. 30). Though many parents expressed the feeling that the baby wasn't quite theirs during the hospitalization (e.g., 1026F, 2001F, 2017F, 2025M,

2031M, 2037F), it was articulated especially clearly by one father who used the language of bonding to explain the shift in his feelings after he brought his twin daughters home: "Not until you really got them home . . . you have any what they would call bonding, you know. . . . Yeah, I think that's it, until you take complete control of them yourself and you have complete responsibility for them yourself, there's a little bit of detachment perhaps. Because you go there and everything is done for you" (2037M, p. 11). Such a statement acknowledges a shift in custody and "ownership," but it also signals that parents could start to plan because the future was now in their hands, insofar as it was in anyone's. But even after infants came home, large uncertainties remained for many families. Parents talked about their decreasing anxiety as the child began to meet developmental milestones—to roll over, sit up, walk, and talk. For those parents whose children had yet to pass such milestones, even though their infants had reached eighteen months or more, planning for the future tended either to focus on other children or other areas of life or to take the form of fantasies in which the child was essentially "normal."

To care for a child well requires that a parent make choices that take account of the child's future. A baby needs more than food and warmth—it also needs the kind of attention and stimulation given by someone who recognizes its developmental possibilities and responds to a random movement of its mouth as if it were a smile. When parents think of babbles as communication, precursors of the conversations they will later share, they are more likely to treat the child as a full human being and to adjust their own actions to improve developmental outcomes.

Here we have asked about the conditions under which parents think about and plan for their children's futures. We have argued that such projections into the future are especially likely to occur when a parent is able to share planning with a co-parent, typically a spouse or lover. But we must recognize that planning can be elicited by other social arrangements. In particular, if the baby's grandparent or aunt or uncle feels responsible for the parent, helping the parent plan for the child may be simply an extension of helping a daughter or sister finish growing up. Similarly, teachers or social service workers may take it as their charge to help a parent plan for her (or, less commonly, his) child's future. But because parenthood often marks a transition to adulthood, only those who are willing to be heavy-handed and intrusive or who have exceptionally close relationships can engage in the sort of joint planning that typically occurs in the intimacy of marriage or marriage-like relations. We have stressed here that thoughts of the future occur in a social context rather than only in the isolation of individual minds and hearts. In addition, thinking about the future is often done in an organizational context and so must be sensitive to organization-specific time horizons. For instance, the NICU urges parents to think about the future, but only the near future, because otherwise plans may be unrealistic given the degree of uncertainty about the child's health and well-being. Responsible thinking about the future is not then just an individual trait.

Broad versus Narrow Conceptions of Parenting and the Adjustment of Means to Ends

Describing the social origins of planning for the future or of conceptions of the child as a person does not fully answer our question about variations in the acceptance of responsibility for a child. We also need to consider how parents come to conceive of themselves as managers of their children's lives, responsible for figuring out what is best for the child and capable of arranging for what would best serve the child's interests. In this section, we discuss these two related dimensions of taking responsibility: how parents come to define their obligations diffusely and what encourages parents to use their discretion flexibly to adjust means to ends.

As we noted earlier in this chapter, not all parents "do parenthood" the same way. Some parents, like Gloria (1018), whom we first met in chapter 3, see their job as parents quite narrowly. Children need to be fed and clothed, taken to the doctor, and kept out of trouble. Other than that, a parent shares the household with the children and watches them grow up. Not too much intervention is called for, and when something unusual is needed, a specialist such as a doctor or teacher is the appropriate person to provide it. Robert needed more than most of the children in our study, because he was quite seriously developmentally delayed. But Gloria had done little to adapt to his special needs. It was the employer of Robert's father who had arranged Robert's first visit to the hospital where he was being treated at the time of our interview. Gloria wasn't really sure what the doctors were going to do for him—except that the concern was his inability to walk. If there was anything to be done, the physicians were the ones who could do it, not she. Her job was to take Robert to the doctor episodically but apparently not to track what they were doing or to assess their competence. Gloria had made few adaptations to Robert's disability except to treat him as she would a considerably younger child. At eighteen months, he was cared for more or less as if he were only a few months old, with little thought about how that might affect his development.

In sharp contrast, Maureen (1008) felt that what her job entailed depended on what Caitlin needed. That meant that she needed a basic understanding of child development to give her some idea of what to expect and some way to assess whether Caitlin was "on track," but it also meant that she expected to learn new skills as she went along. What parenting entailed would depend on Caitlin's age and the nature of her needs at each stage in her life. Maureen expected that parenting an infant would be different from parenting an adolescent, and that parenting a child with special needs would be different from parenting a "normal" child. But at each of these stages, Maureen would very likely believe that her daughter needed a great deal of attentive parenting—more than other parents would believe was needed by their children in comparable circumstances. We argued earlier that how much attention parents believe infants need depends on whether they think of babies as people or as objects. Maureen, whose "communication" with Caitlin was reported at some length earlier in this chapter, was extreme in attributing personhood to her child. Knowing that she would adjust—perhaps even overadjust—to a child's needs and that she would define those needs expansively, Maureen told us that she would never adopt a disabled child because she would be overwhelmed by the need to maintain her own high standards about childcare.

Gloria and Maureen are extreme cases, though each thought of herself as a good mother. Gloria had a narrow conception of what a mother is supposed to do, but Maureen defined her job very diffusely. Gloria made little adaptation to Robert's situation, but Maureen watched carefully and put a lot of thought into how to adjust her inputs to produce the outcomes she wanted. Most parents fall between these two extremes, and our job in this section is to show how parents come to resemble Gloria or Maureen or to adopt a model of parenting that falls somewhere between these two poles.

Once again, cultural frameworks are crucial. Just as people have different notions of what a child is, so they also have varying conceptions of what it means to be a parent. Although all of our respondents would agree that parents should provide such basics as shelter, clothing, and food, they would be less likely to agree about what else a parent should do. They would disagree, for instance, about what exactly is within the capacities of parents, where parental obligations end and the those of various professionals such as pediatricians and teachers begin, how the work of parenting should be divided between mother and father, and how parental obligations shift as a child matures.

When confronted with the obligation to care for the NICU graduate, parents have quite varying reactions—partly because they have radically different notions of what is possible. Some treat the baby's medical difficulties as akin to a developmental stage and expect that the child will grow out of most of the problems. The paralysis of the lower limbs associated with spina bifida may thus be seen as similar to an extended babyhood. Such a view does not require that the parent do anything special for the child—the child will simply learn to walk when he or she is "ready." Others seem to assume that the condition is permanent and that the baby and family must simply accept the baby as it is. If the baby's lower extremities were paralyzed, then, the parents might expect that they would always be paralyzed, and mobility aids such as wheelchairs might be used, but physical therapy to increase the use of the lower limbs would not be considered. Finally a third group of parents believes that thoughtful intervention might well improve the child's condition. A baby with paralysis of the lower extremities might in the long run learn to walk, but only with a finely tuned program of physical therapy. Parents who believe in the efficacy of intervention still vary in their conviction that substantial improvements are possible, some believing that with intervention improvements might occur, others convinced that improvements will occur.

These different orientations are associated with differences in what the parents do, or feel it is appropriate for them to do, in caring for their baby. Parents who think that their child is irrevocably disabled react differently from those who think that the child's situation might improve if they intervened in just the right way. Parents come to the task with different orientations to parenthood (which, as Cindy's [1001] rapid maturation following Jason's birth shows, may be radically altered by the experience of having a critically ill baby) and vary a good deal in their intellectual preparation for caring for a disabled child. Different orientations and differences in intellectual preparation limit how parents conceive responsibility, what they think is possible, and what they think they can enlist others to help them do. Such constraints must be recognized and analyzed. We may firmly believe that a child will be better off walking than relying on a wheelchair. We might therefore argue that parents who do what they can to increase the mobility and independence of the child are doing a better job—behaving more responsibly—than those who, for whatever reason, do not try to improve their child's chances of walking. At the same time, though, parents' reasons for not intervening are important. While some parents define the parental role narrowly because they are selfish, many others adopt a limited conception of parenthood because they believe that parenthood is about meeting basic needs and giving plenty of love, or because they lack resources, have other obligations, believe that the baby's problems are immutable, or have been taught that "time heals all."

Conceptions of what parenting entails are, once again, social constructions (Hays 1996). Such conceptions are partly shaped by situational adjustments and partly shaped by broader cultural notions of parenthood. This cultural component may be thought of as scripts that are enacted in particular circumstances, scripts that vary by gender, class, race, and ethnicity. But scripts don't tell the whole story. They are sometimes modified when they don't fit the situation or when others involved in the same drama seem to be following a different script. Mothers are, for instance, more likely to find their script acceptable if they are paired with a father who is willing to accept a role as breadwinner. Despite the legitimate criticisms that the traditional division of labor has received, the sort of devoted parenting that some former NICU patients need is more likely to be supplied if a parent willing to stay home is paired with a person willing to supply financial resources. Gloria (1018) might have done more for Robert had she not needed to devote so much time to worrying about where to get money for the next box of diapers rather than focus on his developmental problems. But, as we've described, she struggled to support herself and Robert's two siblings on public aid and his disability payments, while Robert's absentee father only occasionally provided financial assistance. We are, of course, not advocating a traditional division of household labor, where mothers do all of the unpaid domestic labor. We are, however, noting that it is easier to meet the demands of domesticity if there is a partner who shares at least some responsibility for providing what the children need.[17] Finally, hospital staff members, physical and occupational therapists, visiting nurses, and teachers in zero-to-three programs may also play an important part in shifting parents' conceptions of what parenthood is all about. When parents discover that the role they must play is different from the one they had imagined playing, professionals provide valuable information about exactly what this alternative form of parenthood entails.

17. We also would not align ourselves with those, like Popenoe (1996), who believe mothers cannot make good homes for their children without fathers.

Parents vary a great deal in how easily they learn their new role, and not all of them are able to convince others to go along with the modifications. One couple (2025) described their family's rejection of their disabled son, a bright engaging child whose cerebral palsy made it impossible for him to walk. Some mothers sadly told us that their husbands didn't help with the physical therapy, had never mastered colostomy changes, or couldn't "see" the baby's problems. Maternal roles had shifted more than paternal ones, perhaps because in most families maternal roles are defined more diffusely than paternal roles, perhaps because the new chores seemed to be closer to what mothers ordinarily do than to traditional breadwinning, perhaps because mothers were more likely than fathers to experience sustained exposure to the cognitive frameworks of health-care and child-development professionals. Undoubtedly, mothers received more pressure from the NICU staff and from family to expand their role than fathers ever did, as we argued in chapter 5. Whatever the cause, mothers were more likely than fathers to adopt new conceptions of what parenthood entailed and therefore to be able to provide what their child needed.

Cultural frameworks are important for a second reason. If one is to adjust means to ends, one must have some conception of what the goal is, how to tell when one has achieved it, and most important, what intermediate indicators show that actions early in a sequence are producing the desired results. Parents varied widely in their understanding of child development and in their willingness to attribute importance to early indicators. At one extreme, though Kenny was very developmentally delayed, Janet and Ken nevertheless expected him to overcome his early problems and end up attending an Ivy League college (1036). Was this brave optimism, an expression of love, the parents' attempt to demonstrate to university interviewers that they too subscribed to middle-class educational goals, ignorance about child development, or denial of reality? It is hard to tell, particularly when such optimistic statements were coupled with discussions of evidence of Kenny's responsiveness, perhaps indicating that Janet and Ken were basing their predictions on information that they thought undermined the validity of more standard assessments of developmental potential. But Janet and Ken seemed not to have a clear conception of cause and effect in muscular and skeletal development either, for instance seeming unaware that placing Kenny in an infant seat for hours on end was exacerbating his curvature of the spine. It is also difficult to tell whether the parents might have been focusing on some other goal. They might, for instance, have noted that Kenny could interact more with his parents and sister when he was in the chair rather than the crib, that he could see more of what was going on, or only that he seemed more content. Janet and Ken might thus have been choosing social development over physical development. Or they might have understood instinctively that their child's time was limited (Kenny later died) and that whatever happiness and short-term comfort were possible should not be sacrificed to pipe dreams of normal development.

If parents varied in their capacity to judge whether their child was developing normally or whether some sort of intervention was needed, they differed also in their capacity to tailor their activities to produce desirable results. Raising children is an inexact science under the best of circumstances and probably becomes less exact as new goals are introduced. If we have little idea of how we "teach" our children to talk or walk, we have even less idea of how to help them learn these fundamental skills when they have had trouble with such rudimentary ones as sucking and swallowing or turning over.

Nevertheless, parents who had clearer conceptions of developmental milestones and of the relationship between such milestones were more likely than others to adjust their behavior in an attempt to assist their child in mastering key skills. Discussions of physical therapy provided the clearest evidence here. Some parents described themselves as going through prescribed routines—"Yes, we do his exercises with him"—without commenting much on what the routines were supposed to accomplish or whether they seemed to be producing desired results. Other parents talked about the goals of the therapy, the nature of the exercises, discussions with the therapist about the child's progress, modifications of the routine over time, and their own estimations of the success of the therapy. Marta (1017), for instance, described a variety of activities she had worked out with a therapist to provide sensory experiences for Cassandra, who was blind. Maureen (1008), attempting to help her daughter, Caitlin, overcome a tendency to tilt her head to one side, exhibited considerable ingenuity in overcoming Caitlin's resistance to the exercises. Exploiting Caitlin's natural curiosity, Maureen placed the baby on her belly in the stroller with her head facing the direction they were walking. To see the sights, Caitlin had to hold her head up. Her neck muscles quickly became strong and the problem was soon corrected.

Maureen's adaptation of Caitlin's physical therapy shows parental discretion at its best. Maureen understood the problem, had mastered enough of the rudiments of physical therapy to understand cause and effect, had a good relationship with a physical therapist who here functioned as a consultant, and had an excellent understanding of her daughter's physical problems and of how to motivate her. But this case is unusual. While it is not unusual for parents to have a thorough understanding of their child, and particularly of how to motivate the child, parents vary more in their mastery of the technical aspects of the child's problems. It is not uncommon for parents to be better than the average medical care provider at providing some of the care their child needs. For instance, Sue (1009) did a better job with Tiffany's tracheostomy than most of the nurses and was also good at detecting when Tiffany was getting sick. Grace and Roger (2016) both were more skilled than the hospital staff at catheterizing Tammy and in fact would not take her to just any emergency room when she got into trouble. But we talked to many other parents who were less skilled and had a weaker grasp of their child's problems.

It is in the fine-tuning of therapeutic interventions, the modification of routines to increase the odds of success, that NICUs and homes differ most. NICUs are wonderful institutions for encouraging innovation in the care of sick, fragile, or congenitally disabled newborns. Such innovations are so plentiful that they are obvious even to casual visitors. A surgical mask might double as a diaper for a really tiny baby and parents (like 2017) were urged to bring in Cabbage Patch doll clothes for especially tiny premies. More subtle, and no doubt more important, are the innovations in feeding regimes, in the development and adaptation of pharmacological fixes for neonates, and in the refinement of surgical techniques for babies weighing less than a kilo. Such innovation and adaptation arise through the research that is carried out in tandem with patient care, of course, but are also facilitated by the division of labor that allows a person to specialize in one set of tasks or one part of physiology so that he or she encounters the same problems repeatedly and can see what works and what doesn't. And though personnel may feel overworked, NICUs are required to have adequate numbers of staff. Staff members therefore almost always work as part of a team, have sufficient time to reflect on and learn from their experience, and have interested and informed colleagues with whom to discuss possible innovations. Adaptations of routines—within the limits of protocols—are thus extremely likely.

The NICU's concentration of expertise obviously is not duplicated in the household. A household is in some ways ill suited for innovation, but it has one strength that the NICU lacks. While the NICU's expertise is extensive (its staff includes experts in respiratory problems, nutrition, neonatal surgery, genetics, and the like), the expertise of the home is intensive (the parents are experts about a particular child). The sort of innovations made by Maureen are then more likely to occur in a home than in the NICU because they build on a mother's deep understanding of her own child rather than on a therapist's understanding of physical processes or of what seems to motivate children in general.

We argued earlier in this chapter that NICUs were less variable than households and that variability among households means that they are not equally able to adapt sensitively to the needs of particular children. Some parents instead supply inexpert enactments of the routines taught to them by hospital staff members, neither rising to the minimum level of competence of hospital staff members nor supplying the sharp perceptions that arise from knowing the patient well. But what accounts for this variability among households? To make the sharp observations about a child characteristic of the most responsible parents requires, first, an understanding of the medical problems. One mother, who participated regularly in a parent-support group (observed as part of the preparation for this project), was regarded as so expert on her daughter's endocrine imbalances that the physicians routinely consulted her when making decisions about what further to do. Her opinion was taken more seriously than the opinions of other endocrinologists not familiar with the case. Most parents have not achieved that level of mastery, but a substantial proportion are at least regarded as competent and as having a sufficiently general understanding of the problem that they can be relied on to interpret signs of trouble correctly.

Without exception, though, the parents with a flexible understanding of their child's troubles had gone beyond the information supplied to them by the NICU staff. Some parents went to the hospital library and pored over medical journals. Others joined support groups and sought contacts with parents whose children had similar troubles. Still other parents consulted people in their personal network (friends, family members) who had some medical expertise. A few parents kept extensive notes on their baby's progress, regularly read the medical record during the baby's hospital stay, obtained a copy of the record after discharge, and assiduously questioned doctors and nurses about anything they did not understand and bravely pointed out discrepancies or suggested modifications of therapies.

Acquiring a deep understanding of one's child's medical situation is not like going to medical school, however. There is no set curriculum, and there are no established prerequisites for beginning the course of study. Parents who became expert in their child's medical condition were not all well educated—high school dropouts and parents with postgraduate degrees both were represented in this group. But what educational strategy parents employed varied a good deal with what skills and contacts they brought to the situation. One parent whose job required him to process a lot of information simply transferred his well-honed note-taking skills to the new situation (1005). And recall that Cindy (1001) was a high school dropout who received a great deal of help from her sister, Diana. Diana and her husband both worked in medicine and were able to act as tutors in the mother's independent study, guiding her in her early explorations of the medical library. But understanding the medical phenomena is not in itself sufficient. Anspach (1993) argues that nurses and physicians draw on different kinds of information in making their prognoses about NICU patients. While nurses rely on information from their observations of and interactions with infants, physicians are more likely to employ information from tests and monitors. That parents more closely resemble nurses in how they use information is important because parents, like nurses, are only able to make assessments when they have direct contact with the child.

Understanding the child's medical condition in the abstract is unlikely to lead to adjustments of routine or innovations in therapy unless the parent also has enough contact with the child to collect information about early indicators to note what is and what is not working. Parents busy with other children, preoccupied with marital difficulties, or employed outside the home have less chance to observe their child. They are therefore less likely to be able to state confidently that the child is behaving oddly and so perhaps has a blocked shunt (which would ordinarily drain fluid accumulating around the brain), to assert to a therapist that the child seems to be in pain during a prescribed exercise routine, or to suggest that a feeding regime needs to be modified because the child is willing to eat under one circumstance but not another. Armed with a detailed understanding of her child, Sue (1009) was able to stand up to physicians' suggestions that Tiffany would be gaining weight if only her mother were more adept at feeding her and to suggest that the problem lay elsewhere. In another case, the mother's attentiveness focused less on adapting routines than on ensuring that the hospital did not give up on her child. Charlotte and Bruce (2024), whom we first met in chapter 6, became extremely wary after physicians seemed ready to "write off" their daughter Ellie, who they believed could survive and do well. To give Ellie every chance, Charlotte negotiated access to a room in a hospital-affiliated building, moved in, and was watchfully present nearly around the clock. Charlotte's continuous presence allowed her to offer evidence about Ellie's condition that the staff might otherwise have missed. Although this particular example occurred before Ellie went home for the first time, for parents whose children have continuing medical problems (e.g., Roger and Grace [2016], Marta and Ricardo [1017], or Cindy and John [1001]), "moving into the hospital" is not an uncommon event. Indeed, such parents seemed to feel that the special knowledge that comes from being an attentive parent gets its most important use during a medical crisis.

Responsible care giving in an NICU does not require that staff members adopt diffuse definitions of their roles. Though we must be careful not to overstate our point here, a relatively narrow definition of the job is compatible with responsible care giving in a hospital, because one staff member's efforts are supplemented by the contributions of others. But once the baby goes home, responsible care giving cannot be produced in the same way. When the care of a child falls exclusively or almost exclusively on the shoulders of the parents, the consequences of parents' adopting a narrow definition of their role are much more serious. In the NICU, then, the bases are covered by an elaborate division of labor. In the household, in contrast, the bases are covered only when parents embrace a broad definition of parenting.

But how do parents come to define parenting diffusely? We have described several different routes to such diffuse conceptions. We have suggested that for most parents motherhood tends to be defined more broadly than fatherhood and that it is therefore somewhat "easier" for mothers than for fathers to accept new tasks as appropriately falling into their domain (although we would never suggest that this is naturally so). We have also pointed out that there seems to be some tie between how parents think about children (e.g., as needing help with developmental tasks) and how they think about their jobs as parents. In addition, we believe that there is a connection between how parents think about illness or disability (as an immutable condition or one in which intervention might be efficacious) and how they conceive their jobs. In some cases, parents come to define their job more broadly when a health-care provider points out to them that child development sometimes requires parental prodding or that a physical impairment will be less disabling in the long run if the parent faithfully exercises the child. Hospital interventions have only limited effects in changing parents' notions of what parenting is about, though, as we noted in chapter 5. The NICU has only limited resources to expend on resocializing parents. Social class variations are important here—middle-class parents are more likely to arrive in the NICU already knowing a great deal about child development, but other parents will only be brought up to a middle-class standard if they are eager learners who master material quickly once the core ideas have been introduced. Parents who arrive with less cultural capital, are less facile, or are less motivated are likely to retain their initial narrower conceptions of parental roles.

Finally, we have pointed out that the source of innovation is different in the home than in the NICU. NICU innovation is grounded in specialization in a particular procedure or aspect of physiology, but household innovation is instead based on specialization in a particular child. In both cases, though, innovation requires careful observation and thought. Just as some nurses are more innovative than others, so some parents are more likely than others to adapt general procedures to fit the needs of their particular child. Such parental creativity requires both a general understanding of the child's condition—usually an idiosyncratic medical education—and intensive contact with the child.

The Community of Fate

Families are groups of individuals whose fates are tied together. Though families differ in the extent to which internal variation in circumstances is tolerated, with some gender and age variation in circumstances being quite common, nevertheless members of families are usually a community of fate (Heimer 1985), affected by the same shifts in fortune, facing the fat and the lean years together. But the differences among families in their toleration of internal inequality tells us, once again, that the familial community of fate is a social creation that need not exist and indeed does not always arise. The birth and hospitalization of an infant may typically lead family members to pledge their loyalty and resources to the new addition but may sometimes instead lead people to sever family ties and refuse to accept the sacrifices in welfare entailed in sharing scarce resources with such a needy member.

Among the families we studied, we were surprised to find that relatively few seemed to feel that incorporating the new and needy child entailed sacrifice. We had expected to find soul searching about how to reorganize lives given the need to abandon or defer dreams in order to care adequately for the baby. Given the demands on parental time and on family financial resources, parents might need to cut back on work time or give up paid work entirely, postpone a return to school, temporarily give up cherished leisure activities, make painful choices about which child's needs would be met when, and cut back on personal consumption. We had expected to find more parents echoing this father's statement about the effect of the unreimbursed $3,500 of medical bills on the budget of his large family: "Oh, yeah, I think that it's hard on the whole family. I mean, uh [laughs], uh, you can't do much now, because there just ain't nothing to go around. I mean, we got our house right now and this furniture's gonna be here a long time because there ain't going to be no new furniture. [Laughs] It takes a toll, you know. Like I said, my cars are going to run until the tires fall off now because there ain't [going to] be no new tires, no nothing no more" (1011M, p. 41). But most parents described the sacrifices as less substantial than we had expected. Incorporating the new baby into the family pinched less than we had anticipated. Our investigation shifted its focus somewhat as we began to ask why meeting the new baby's needs seemed to entail so little sacrifice.

To be sure, some families did feel the pinch. Among the parents we talked to, probably Grace and Roger (2016) felt it the most. Further, because Tammy's health remained precarious and she still faced a lengthy program of surgeries, they talked about the difficulty of their family circumstances with a poignancy missing in the accounts of those for whom the sacrifice was largely in the past. The family had recently moved from one house to another in order to cut expenses. Roger worried about keeping his job and their health insurance. The parents seemed somewhat less aware of the toll that Tammy's needs were taking on the rest of the family. Tammy's brother, a cherubic eight-year-old, was already forging checks and slashing other children's bicycle tires. His parents recounted these stories with worried fatigue but seemed not to register the message that he needed some of their attention. But with Tammy in and out of the hospital, it wasn't clear that there was any time or attention to spare.

Other families clearly felt considerable pressure—Janet and Ken (1036) eventually divorced; Marta and Ricardo (1017) both seemed tense and unhappy (though she was more open about her unhappiness than he); Cindy and John (1001) discussed the difficulty of making ends meet and paying for the speech therapy that their older child needed when their younger son's needs were so pressing; and Donna and Kurt (2017) nearly divorced and were anxiously awaiting the birth of a second child, hoping to avoid a second very premature birth. Many were still deciding whether to have more children, all too aware now of what could—and sometimes did—go wrong. But many other families seemed to be under less pressure than we had expected. They took their troubles in stride, adjusted to the demands of the new baby, and lived more homebound lives than they had previously. We noted in the early parts of this chapter that the families we interviewed were hardly uniform in financial circumstances or educational backgrounds. These differences in material circumstances, educational backgrounds, and occupational situations were correlated with different adaptations to the demands of a needy infant.

For some families, meeting the demands of the infant was less costly than we had expected simply because the opportunity costs of time spent on child care were rather low. Despite the reputation of Americans for active participation in civic life and voluntary associations, very few of the parents we interviewed claimed to have any regular involvements outside the house except paid work. With few exceptions, our respondents were not regular churchgoers and were not involved in musical groups, bowling leagues, the PTA, amateur sports, or political campaigns. For many parents, staying home with the baby meant mainly giving up "partying" with friends, and most of them conceded that they had been ready for a more settled life anyway. Some commented that the group of drinking buddies had in any case disbanded as other members acquired familial obligations. But a few spoke nostalgically of their friends and arranged to go out to bars occasionally.

By and large fathers' employment was not disrupted by the birth of the critically ill baby. Fathers did not quit their jobs, though some lost jobs in the normal course of events. Fathers who were only marginally employed typically did not enter training programs or seek additional work because of the need to support the child. Not surprisingly, mothers' work lives were much more affected by the baby's birth, though mothers varied a good bit in their responses to these disruptions. Some mothers continued to work (in a few instances, after a brief maternity leave), sometimes because the family depended on their income, or because the family insurance was provided by the mother's employer, and sometimes because the mother was committed to working. In a few cases mothers felt strongly pressured by their husbands to return to paid employment even when they did not wish to or to stay home and devote themselves to child care even when they wanted to take jobs. In many cases, though, mothers stayed home to care for their children, either giving up jobs or delaying plans to seek employment. Few of the mothers spoke with much regret about giving up these jobs—whatever their expectations when they first entered the work force, work had not ended up being all that attractive. This is not to say that they intended to stay home permanently, only that the costs of staying home temporarily were not all that high given that these mothers had jobs rather than careers and would have had to pay for child care out of their meager salaries.[18]

What this says so far is that the costs to families were somewhat lower than we expected. Because people's lives were somewhat more impoverished before the birth of the child than we had anticipated, we did not encounter stories of sacrifice as often as we expected. Yes, some mothers reported feeling very constrained, particularly if they were young and facing child rearing alone. But even they reported that what they lost was not all that valuable and that the gains more than compensated for the losses. As a caveat, we note that in some instances the costs were lower because of the way the parents carried out their child's care. Accepting a child's limitations rather than striving to improve the child's lot often costs less, at least in the short run. The narrower conception of parenting that we described in the previous section then tends to be "cheaper" for parents—to require less investment of time, energy, and even money. Costs were often lower because parents chose the low-investment route.[19]

Here the experiences of the various families diverge somewhat. All of the parents spoke of their children with considerable affection (though in a few cases with little detail). The affection they felt for their children and that they believed the children fully returned was an important compensation for whatever sacrifices the parents had to make. But for some parents there was more to the story. For a substantial number of parents—and especially for those whose children continued to experience serious medical problems—the illness of the child was a turning point in their lives. Consciously accepting responsibility for the child was an impetus for reorganizing and rethinking their lives. Sue and Will (1009) decided to train as nurses. Through her confrontations with incompetent hospital staff members, medical suppliers, and home nurses, Sue came to see herself as an intelligent and powerful advocate for her child. Cindy and John (1001) both reported a transformation in their relationship: a joint commitment

18. This finding is consistent with Gerson's (1985) conclusion that often the world of paid employment provides few opportunities and even fewer rewards for women, for whom staying home to raise their children may then become the more attractive alternative.

19. *Chose* is not quite the correct word here. People don't really "choose" their understanding of what parenthood entails, though they may sometimes brush aside suggestions or hints that there are other ways to parent.

to raising the children (only one of whom was John's biological child), careful plans about how to manage future crises, investment in training to improve their earning capacities, and a new sense of the importance of financial planning. By Cindy's account, all of this started when she realized that she, and not someone else, had the obligation to make her child's life work: "When I had my first child, I still acted emotionally out as a child instead of as a mature adult. And then when I had Jason, it really sunk in that I am a mother, I have a five-year-old child, and I have a baby that's got all of these problems, and I'm just going to have to straighten my shit up and that's it, you know" (1001F, p. 47). Continuing her commentary during John's interview sometime later, Cindy explained that she finally realized that it was time for her to assume responsibility, to stop relying so much on her older sister. As she put it, "Nobody can do this for me except me" (1001M, p. 37).

Such testimonials were echoed in the accounts of other parents. They were proud of their capacity to master complex medical information, their newfound confidence in interacting with medical professionals, their endurance and personal strength in the period of crisis, and their ingenuity in working out solutions to an astonishing array of problems that ranged from interpersonal difficulties to malfunctioning machines to diagnosing what was wrong with the baby. In its psychological effects, caring for the NICU graduate (at least for the first year or two) sometimes resembled project work. The effect of devotion to the collective enterprise is to minimize the experience of costs and magnify the experience of benefits, much as Goffman describes as occurring in those sites that seem to their participants to be "where the action is" (Goffman 1967; Heimer 1986).

What we discovered is that the creation of a community of fate in which parents agreed to hitch their fates to those of their child was quite a different matter than we had imagined. Opportunity costs tended to be lower than we had anticipated, and parents reported that other costs were lower than we had believed. Further, parents reported the benefits to be much larger than we had imagined, largely because they gave the child credit for the personal growth and redirection of their lives that followed the birth of the baby and its stay in the NICU. Though they did find that some resources, such as time and money, were sometimes in short supply, parents found that new ones had been added, so that their overall experience was as much one of surprise over what they had gained as of dismay over what they had lost. When caring for an NICU graduate becomes a "project" for the parents, the problem of social control recedes in importance.

When they care deeply about the project outcome, people need little policing, except perhaps to ensure that they do not commit too many resources to the project, robbing other worthy enterprises. The problem of how to balance multiple responsibilities is always a challenge.

NICUs are not communities of fate in the same way that families are. Because the commitment of the staff to any one infant is more limited, working in an NICU tends not to involve the psychological investment or personal sacrifice that parenting entails. But because they have come to their tasks well prepared, NICU workers also are less likely to experience the deep satisfaction of having to stretch, learn, and grow to meet a truly unexpected challenge.

Social Control and Responsibility at Home

We have argued in this chapter that the social structure that supports responsible parenting once children go home from the intensive care unit is rather different from the social structure that provides reliable care inside the NICU. In both cases responsibility is a social product, and in both cases the oversight and participation of other parties are crucial. But the social processes by which responsible behavior is produced and sustained are quite different in the two settings. In the NICU, responsible behavior is produced through an elaborate division of labor, careful recruitment of personnel, and orchestration of the efforts of individuals through job descriptions, review processes, job ladders, rotations and work schedules, protocols, written records, and the like. In the home, responsibility arises instead through empathetic identification with the child, joint planning for a collective future, radically individualized instruction programs, intensive observation of a single child, and the experience of the personal growth that results from learning to care for a needy child. But each of these in turn is socially produced and maintained. Intense observation of a child, for instance, is more likely to occur when mothers and fathers discuss the child's condition or when other family members repeatedly ask a parent for reports on the child's condition. An interested and supportive social network thus produces a more observant parent.

Because the raw materials—the labor force and the resource base—from which a responsible household must be constructed are so variable, no single protocol or blueprint will work in every case. But that only means that responsible parenting is a more complex social product than responsible care in an NICU.

EIGHT

Responsible Individuals in an Organizational World

ALL PARENTS LOVE THEIR OWN CHILDREN. The nearly universal love of parents for their children means that we cannot look here for an explanation of why some parents take responsibility and others do not. Popular culture to the contrary, love is not all you need. As social scientists, we have at least two choices if we want to understand why some parents take more responsibility than others. One option would be to develop more refined ways of measuring the affection that people feel for their children in the hope that improved measurement would reveal a relationship between responsibility and love that could not be detected with crude measures. In theory we would then be able to compare the levels of affection that various parents feel for their children (or that an individual parent feels for different children or that two different parents feel for the same child), and this improved measurement might give us some purchase on the question of why some parents are more responsible, others less so. Not only do we find this project unpalatable, but we also believe that it leads us to look for causes inside individuals rather than in social systems. We prefer the second option: looking first for variations in people's social circumstances and then exploring the ways in which individual variations in acceptance of responsibility, capacity to act responsibly, or even feelings of responsibility arise from or are suppressed by particular social arrangements.

Inequalities between rich and poor, male and female, white and black, old and young, employed and unemployed, married and unmarried, and better educated and those with fewer years of schooling all affect both a person's capacity to take responsibility and the pressure put on them by others to take responsibility. In many cases, though, organizations play important mediating roles in translating inequalities into differential pressures, for instance by assigning responsibilities to some categories of people but not to others or by accepting excuses from some people that would not be accepted from others. Organizations and people's relations to them color assessments of what the responsible course of action is, who should take a particular responsibility, how parental behavior should be evaluated, what kinds of pressures should be applied, and what kind of support should be given.

Further, inequalities between people affect their capacity to function effectively in organizational settings. Younger people may have to convince others that they are mature. People less accustomed to bureaucratic settings may find it hard to know which details about forms, payments, or appointment times are important and which are not. People whose speech suggests that they have had little education or are from foreign countries may be patronized or demeaned by busy and insensitive workers. People who know their rights, and who have the social skills to insist tactfully that those rights be honored, may be treated better than others. Preexisting inequalities thus shape people's experiences in organizations, but organizational processes also create new inequalities and modify the effects of old ones.

Much of the work of caring for a baby who is or has been critically ill either takes place inside formal organizations or depends on forays across organizational borders. Organizational influences shape the capacity and inclination of parents to take responsibility and also who experiences what pressures, who applies the pressures, and what kind of pressure is brought to bear. Because so much of the action is either inside formal organizations or at organizational borders, negotiations between parents and other actors (such as hospital personnel, equipment suppliers, home health nurses, employees of insurance companies, or government employees who administer benefits programs such as social security) are strongly stamped by bureaucratic categories and organizational routines. We argue, then, that we cannot fully understand the process by which responsibility is assigned and embraced or shrugged off unless we look closely at organizational influences and at the interfaces between organizations. We therefore revisit key points, now focusing attention on the organizational thread that runs through the book.

In judging parents appropriate or inappropriate, the NICU staff faced crucial organizational constraints. The shortage of social control resources shaped staff members' routines for assessing parents and making decisions about when to exert pressure on them. Staff applied varying standards to mothers, expecting less of younger than older, unmarried than married, poorer than richer, and African-American than white mothers. Because bringing everyone up to the same standard would entail considerable work, NICU staff members economized by adopting standards that varied with their understanding of the modal behavior for different groups of parents. Because teenage mothers were expected to visit less frequently than older ones, they tended to be held to a lower standard of behavior than other mothers. One could argue that varying standards show tolerance for diversity in parenting styles and respect for parents' rights to raise children as they see fit, and NICU staff members do air such arguments. But, we suggest, no one believes that visiting a baby infrequently is really acceptable, and the policy of accepting divergent parenting styles arises more from resignation than from tolerance. The practice of placing most of the responsibility on mothers similarly arises partly from an attempt to conserve organizational resources. When the NICU staff has to bet on someone, they bet on the mother. Here gender stereotypes (to some degree grounded in true statistical variations, of course) combine with scarcity of resources to form working routines that put different amounts of pressure on mothers than on fathers.

But organizational influences did not stop there. In addition to being evaluated as parents, mothers and fathers were also evaluated as organizational participants. Did the mother make it easy for the nurse to complete her work, or was she disruptive? Were parents able to contain their emotional displays while on the unit? Did parents respect the claims of other infants on the staff's time, or did they insist that their child receive a disproportionate share of the attention? In some cases, annoyed staff members lost perspective, claiming that disruptive parents would be bad parents, when evidence suggested only that they might have difficulty interacting smoothly with organizational representatives.

If organizational influences shaped staff members' understanding of responsible parenting and their expectations of the members of different groups, they also shaped parents' expectations about staff members. Here, the most important influences derive from the effects of organizational boundaries which define some people as members and others as outsiders. Members of an organization are much more likely to be sufficiently acquainted with organizational routines to know how to exert influence, and by virtue of being assigned a position in the organization they acquire allies, co-workers, bosses, and subordinates with whom to strategize and share information. Parents as outsiders face an unfamiliar organization and face it alone. No one shares with them the inside dope on whether a particular therapist or physician is skilled or reliable. Parents thus have less capacity to judge whether their troubles are idiosyncratic or whether intervention is warranted. And they lack infrastructural support for transforming isolated observations into the materials for social control. While they can always praise staff members, it is much harder to marshal evidence to support an accusation.

This problem of being outsiders who must nevertheless do some of their work inside organizations continues to plague parents after their child's discharge. Important variations arise among parents and in the experiences of individual parents. Just as a parent whose child remains hospitalized for a long time becomes in some respects an insider to the NICU, so parents become acquainted with the routines of other organizations throughout their child's infancy and childhood. Parents come to prefer one hospital over another partly because they feel they can function effectively in that organizational context. When parents told us that they would avoid the local emergency room or the local community hospital at all costs, they were talking as much about their own capacity to interact with staff members as about the skill levels of the physicians. If parents were adept at catheterizing their child or changing the tracheostomy tube and the emergency room staff was not, then parents found it more difficult to communicate across the organizational divide and to translate their observations and actions into something that made sense in this medical environment. Oddly enough, the local emergency room was more "foreign" than the NICU, and parents were better able to function effectively in the higher tech environment. Although more skilled medical workers would know the language of medicine and medical routines sufficiently well to be able to work in a variety of environments, parents are not so versatile. Because they are at the bottom of the medical hierarchy in both skill and status, they can function well only in a medical environment whose routines are familiar and where their role as parents of an NICU graduate is well understood. In short, as ancillary medical workers, they are likely to have difficulty in any organization except the one in which they were trained.[1]

But, of course, variations among parents remain important. We might expect, for instance, that better-educated parents would have sufficient knowledge of medical phenomena or organizational practices to translate across organizational boundaries when less-educated parents could not. We might also expect that lower-status parents would find the transition from one hospital to another difficult because hospital staff were unwilling to give them the benefit of the doubt and would make them earn the re-

1. By this argument, parents whose child did not spend its first days in an NICU—"normal" parents, in short—would be more likely to have difficulty in an NICU than in a community hospital.

spect automatically accorded higher-status parents. Similar arguments can be made about other organizational interfaces.

Coleman (1974, 1982) pointed out some time ago that the balance between two categories of actors, organizations and natural persons, has shifted. A world once populated largely by natural persons has given way to a world in which considerable wealth and power lie in the hands of corporate actors. For our purposes the problem is less that substantial resources are now controlled by corporate actors than that people now must flexibly shift modes, functioning sometimes as individuals and sometimes as members of organizations. Arguing that families, governments, and complex organizations are simply different types of organizations, Ahrne (1994) suggests that an organization is essentially defined by a repetitive schedule and a menu of activities carried out in a dedicated location. Because people are members of many organizations, a key part of managing an organization is managing its relations with other organizations (Aldrich 1979).

By this argument, family life is as much about managing the interface between the family and other organizations as about the relations among family members, and parenting is about managing the child's relations with the outside world as well as about affectional and nurturing ties between adults and children. In this concluding chapter, we argue that one of the chief differences between loving a child and taking responsibility for a child is that while love is often thought of as primarily a dyadic relationship, responsibility looks well beyond the relationship between parent and child (or between husband and wife, or close friends, for that matter). A key part of taking responsibility is moving between the dyad and the external world, retaining a particularistic relationship with the child while translating the particular needs of the child into universalistic claims on the child's behalf. The capacity to imagine the child as a member of several bureaucratic categories, as a cog in the machinery of several organizations, is then as important to responsible parenting as is the capacity to imagine the child as a unique and irreplaceable member of the family.

Personal Responsibility in Impersonal Settings

A responsible parent cannot simply assume responsibility for his or her child within the four walls of the home. But if mothers and fathers must do their parenting in the border regions between organizations or even within the boundaries of other organizations, then they must take account of the rules, routines, and cultural practices of these other organizations.

We return to our discussion of distinctions between more and less responsible parents, showing how the need to function simultaneously in the private world of the family and the more public world of formal organizations requires modification of parochial notions of parenthood.

Particularism and *Universalism*

While this is not the place to wax eloquent about parental love for children or to attempt a thoroughgoing definition of love, we nevertheless need to examine the dilemma of parents who must believe that their child is unique and incalculably valuable while recognizing that others do not think of the child in quite those terms. We noted in chapter 7 that people are more likely to take on responsibilities when they believe that there is some compelling reason why they, rather than someone else, should assume a responsibility. Love is about the tie between one person and another in which a person constructs the other as unique and inherently incomparable with others. One father captured this point well in describing his tie with his children and contrasting his feelings about their irreplaceability with his feelings about his wife: "I love my wife. My wife can be replaced. You know—no offense intended, but there's enough women out there to please any man. They can be replaced. Kids can't" (1036M, p. 39).

The notion that one's children are unique, intrinsically valuable, and incommensurable with other people or objects is a defining aspect of parenthood.[2] Children are "constitutive incommensurables," according to Joseph Raz (1986:345–57), because their incommensurability is crucial in defining how people should relate to them. Drawing on the work of classical Greek thinkers, Nussbaum (1986) argues that incommensurability is crucial to commitment to other people: the more we regard one person as interchangeable with another, the less we invest in developing and preserving our relationships with those we love. Children are not in all ways incommensurable, of course, but their incommensurability is sufficiently important as a defining property so that infringements of this general principle are disconcerting. Zelizer's (1985) account of the cultural transformation of children from economically useful to emotionally priceless illustrates how incommensurables can sometimes be "priced" (as children are in insurance). But she also shows how emotionally charged such practices (and particularly changes in them) can be.

2. See Espeland (1992, esp. 37–44) for a careful and wide-ranging discussion of commensurability.

"Knowing when to treat a child as unique is an important aspect of parenting, and one that stems from our understanding of children as incommensurate," Espeland (1992:40) explains. Such knowledge does not come easily for many parents, though, partly because it often develops in the context of pressure from others to understand children as members of a category. When such agreements to treat one's child as a member of a general category arise under pressure from others who may have less interest than the parents in the child's welfare, parents are justifiably concerned that they may have compromised too much. Although they may have to make claims on universalistic grounds, and so acknowledge what their child shares with others, responsibility also requires particularistic attention to the unique needs of their child (Heimer 1992a).

Many of the parents we interviewed told us, in one way or another, that their children were unique. They told us of their agony during the child's hospitalization, of their whispered promises to the child that life was not just one painful episode after another, of their bargains with God, and of their memories of the first time the child's eyes met theirs. They also told us that they had been transformed by these experiences, had committed themselves to providing, to the best of their ability, what the child needed.[3] Recognizing the uniqueness of a child and committing oneself to providing what that child needs does not, however, necessarily equip a parent to meet that promise. The difficulty here is that the language of love and commitment is a language of relations among individuals, but taking responsibility for a child is about carrying the commitment of particularized relationships into an organizational setting.

Chambliss (1996) argues that we have misunderstood the ethical problems of nurses by constructing ethical dilemmas as individual decision problems. But that is not the form that moral dilemmas take for workers who must simultaneously care for patients and follow their superiors' orders. Similarly, the individualized lens through which we look at parental love doesn't quite capture what parental responsibility is about. Parents must simultaneously love their children as individuals, attending to their unique needs and retaining a commitment to them as unique beings while working on their behalf in settings in which they are not unique individuals but members of categories. Parenthood, then, is about double vision.

3. One father, struggling to express the depth of his commitment to his family, told us this: "I think—I don't know, it ain't got this deep yet—but I think if really push came to shove, I would get it [money to support the family] one way or another. If I had to walk into somebody's house with a pistol in my hand to support mine, I would get it" (1025M, p. 18).

Parents must retain an image of their child's unique features while simultaneously seeing their child as an instance of bureaucratic categories. Both parts of the vision are essential, for without a sense of the child as an instance of a bureaucratic category the parent cannot claim resources, and without a sense of the child's uniqueness the parent cannot tell whether the child is properly categorized.[4] To return to the comparison with Chambliss, parents face both the moral problems of nursing (they are low-level participants in organizations) and the moral dilemmas of doctoring (they bear ultimate responsibility and are at some points the ones who must call the shots).

We argue, then, that some of the variability in the acceptance of responsibility arises from a mismatch between our folk understanding of what loving and caring for a child are about, on the one hand, and the task of child rearing as it is in fact presented to parents in contemporary societies, on the other. That gap presents itself sooner to parents of critically ill infants than to parents of normal newborns, and looms larger for them—as it would for anyone in circumstances that force him or her into frequent contact with the world outside the home. Our models of parenthood are models that stress affectional ties and dyadic (or at most familial) relations. But just as nursing is not really about facing moral dilemmas in the form in which ethicists describe them, so the challenge of responsible parenting does not really take the form that the popular press, parenting guides, or ethicists suggest.[5] Instead, responsible parenting requires that parents sus-

4. Ribbens (1994) discusses some of these same points. She writes of New and David's (1985) "image of the mother as looking two ways at once—towards her child, and towards others, with the woman herself placed between the child and these others, mediating the demands and requirements of each as she understands them" (Ribbens 1994:199). Ribbens recognizes variability among women in their willingness and capacity to take on the intermediary role of broker, advocate, or agent; in whether they define the boundary between private and public as permeable or impermeable; and in how assertive they are in public settings. She also notes that as intermediaries, mothers can identify themselves more clearly as advocates for their children, seeking sympathy and understanding for children's viewpoints, or as representatives of the wider society, attempting to bring children into conformity with outsiders' expectations. This last point would apply much more to mothers of older children than to those of infants.

5. Popular parenting guides, such as Brazelton (1983); Eisenberg, Murkoff, and Hathaway (1989); Leach (1983); and Spock (1976) have extensive discussions of the relations of the parents with their child. Although all of these books now stress the importance of paternal involvement, they also all continue to write as if the expected audience is female. Although these authors discuss "bonding," and endorse hospital policies that permit parents to spend time with their newborns immediately after birth, they also often express considerable skepticism that parent-child relations are deeply shaped by what happens in the first few hours of life. They are similarly skeptical about the importance of the tie between biological mother

tain their double vision, focusing both on the child as an individual and as a member of a category, and that, Janus faced, they gaze at once into their household and out into the world. But all of the rhetoric about parenthood, and perhaps especially about motherhood, is about the portion of parenting that goes on in the domestic sphere. Not that working out a relationship with a child is easy or that everyone has the maturity and self-control required. Still, the point is that the true task is actually harder because it requires something more than and different from what the baby books imagine. Parenting is now less about family self-sufficiency and more about mobilizing resources and orchestrating the efforts of other people and organizations (Campion 1995).

Exactly what portion of this package of tasks people have difficulty with probably varies from one person to another. If, as has been argued at least since Freud, fathers are the representatives of the moral system of the outer world, then they may have less difficulty with the perspective that sees the child universalistically as a member of a category and so subject to the rules of the various bureaucracies the child will encounter. And mothers may, correspondingly, have less difficulty with the part that sees the child as unique, irreplaceable, not interchangeable with anyone else.

Time Horizons—Long, Short, and In Between

Although we have argued that responsibility entails thinking about the long term as well as the present, parents are sometimes pressured to take a very short-term view. During the early days of their baby's hospitalization, many parents are urged by hospital staff members not to think too much about the future and the uncertainties it holds but instead to take

and child, stressing instead the importance of continuity in care providing in the early years, and even suggesting that it is healthy for both mother and child if other adults (whether fathers, grandparents, or paid caretakers) supplement the mother's labor. But what is largely missing from these pages is a discussion of how parents must interact with others outside their homes on their children's behalf. The main exception here is Eisenberg, Murkoff, and Hathaway, who carefully discuss how to choose a pediatrician, how to negotiate a relationship with this medical expert, and how to tell when one should switch pediatricians. Spock also comments on day care and schooling in discussions of children aged three to six and older. Guides for parents of premature or hospitalized infants (e.g., Harrison 1983; Lieberman and Sheagren 1984; or material in the packets handed out by NICUs and parent-support organizations) contain somewhat more information about the organizations and professionals that parents will encounter. But parenting clearly is still conceived as mainly a set of tasks organized around a dyadic relation and carried out primarily inside the home. For a close textual analysis of some of these same popular books on parenting, see Hays's work on the ideology of intensive mothering (1996).

things one day at a time. While NICU staff may urge a temporary suspension of long-term planning during the baby's early crisis, the rules and routines of other organizations may disrupt planning beyond this point. The rules of Medicaid, for instance, undermine financial planning for the future by denying coverage to families with savings. Further, Medicaid "spend down" rules may encourage inappropriate expenditure patterns, partly because they force people to think only month to month.[6]

The work lives of hospital staff are carefully geared to a complex series of schedules. Nursing shifts, the taking of vital signs and the administration of medications, nurses' report at shift change, morning and evening rounds for physicians, weekly interdisciplinary rounds, rotations of physicians and residents on- and off-service, "grand rounds," mortality and morbidity meetings, continuing education classes, certifications and recertifications, periodic salary reviews, site visits by the Joint Commission on Accreditation of Health Care Organizations and other accreditation bodies, and professional conferences all occur on predictable, but different, schedules. Many of these periodic events are irrelevant to NICU patients and their parents, but because organizations are so rigidly governed by schedules, parents must learn about these schedules and fit into them whenever they need medical services. They must learn what hours the doctor's office is open and how far in advance they must schedule an appointment, as well as track the occasions that call for a doctor's appointment or phone call (e.g., regular well-baby visits, a follow-up visit after an illness, the expiration of a crucial prescription). In addition to tracking the time line of services, parents also must track the time line of payments for services. Doctor bills may be due at one point and preschool payments at a different time.

Although the inflexible periodicity of organizational schedules poses problems for most parents, the constraints imposed by organizations are harder on families with fewer resources. Families with fewer resources cannot look for interaction partners with more compatible schedules, for instance changing pediatricians if they are dissatisfied with the way a pediatrician's office staff manages the scheduling of appointments or handles calls about a sick child. They also cannot as easily comply with the financial

6. See Abraham (1993) for a very accessible discussion of Medicaid rules. Briefly, because Medicaid is only available to poor families, those who would not otherwise qualify for benefits (their monthly incomes are above the limit, or they have savings account balances that are above allowable levels) can sometimes become eligible by "spending down" their resources until they are below the limits.

demands of organizations and so may be constrained by budgetary considerations to seek services only when they can afford them. When we add together the constraints of organizational schedules and of scarce resources, it is easy to see how planning for the future might be undermined. Keeping track of what needs to be done today or next week may be the most people can manage when they have a sick child, lack resources, and are required to operate on the schedule of a half-dozen organizations.

Parenting Outside the Home

An expansive sense of what parenting is about looks different when parenting occurs within the confines of the home than when it invades the territory of other workers. Hospital staff members might endorse the notion that babies need exposure to a variety of sensory experiences but nevertheless balk at a parent's request to put cotton balls soaked with bacon grease or lemon juice into an isolette to increase the variety of olfactory stimuli. (Such a request was in fact made by a couple we encountered in a support group.) Similarly, although some medical procedures such as circumcisions are considered to be at a parent's discretion, surgical residents are nevertheless outraged when parents take the initiative to schedule such procedures. For instance, when one family inquired about whether their son could be circumcised before leaving the NICU, the chief surgery resident was irate. "What do they think this is—a gas station? They can just tell us what they want done and we'll do it?" she asked (see Heimer 1992b:166–68 for a fuller discussion of this event).

In chapter 5, we pointed out how parents are labeled "inappropriate" for lapses as both parents and organizational participants. The boundaries between parenthood and other roles are ill defined, particularly when a child is hospitalized or when its condition requires frequent contact with professionals. Parents are responsible for ensuring that their child is well served in his or her contacts with these other professionals, so they cannot be too respectful of professional jurisdictions. But even putting aside the social control of professionals by parents, the boundaries must be fluid for another reason. Because professionals cannot do their work without information from parents and without the cooperation of parents who carry the practice of medicine into the home, rigid separation of the work of doctor, nurse, therapist, or teacher from the work of parent simply is not feasible.

We must recognize, though, that parents face two quite different pressures in carrying parental roles outside the home. On the one hand, they must enlarge their notion of parenthood to include the supervision of professional workers and the performance of the work ordered by those professionals once the child comes home again. On the other hand, parents often face professional hostility to both parts of this enlarged parental role. Professionals may not welcome the critical gaze of parents as they oversee the services their child receives, and they may also not welcome the (limited) competition from parents who become confident that they can do some of what they once felt compelled to seek from professionals.

Parents must then work out their understanding of what exactly parental roles entail in negotiation with other people. While there might be consensus that parental roles should be diffusely defined, they are not unboundedly diffuse. When parents encroach on the jurisdictions of others, they learn that diffuse definitions of parenthood are supported only insofar as they do not interfere with someone else's capacity to manage and control his or her own work. Parental rights and obligations are thus worked out in negotiation. Parental roles may be very clearly defined in certain times and contexts, but because the job of parent is often defined in counterpoint to other roles, what exactly parenthood entails varies with the organizational context and the jurisdiction of the interaction partner.

Parents are not alone in having their roles defined in counterpoint to others'. The work of a secretary similarly varies with context. Legal secretaries, secretaries who work as members of a pool in a corporation, personal secretaries of executives, and secretaries in academic departments of universities all have quite different roles. Some of the tasks are the same (typing, answering the phone, filing), but the mix of tasks and the rules for how to treat people and objects (e.g., how to preserve the confidentiality of legal documents and letters of recommendation, and which groups are permitted to see confidential documents and which are not) vary. But when people are inducted into an organization, they usually receive both formal and informal instruction in how to do their job. Because parents do not become members of many of the organizations in which they must enact their roles as parents—they are clients rather than employees, for instance—they are less likely to receive guidance about their tasks, rights, or obligations in those settings. It would be presumptuous for organizational members to give too much instruction to interaction partners at their borders, and indeed those interaction partners might well resist or reject instruction. But our point remains: interactions at the boundaries between organizations are unusually ill defined. Because parents, and particularly the parents of children who are or have been critically ill, so often find themselves in these border regions, we must reassess our claim that responsible parenting requires a diffuse definition of the job. That is true enough, but we should clarify the point now by noting that parental roles take more definite shape. But what shape they take varies with the particular context and may be the outcome of substantial negotiation. A key part of defining parenthood diffusely, then, is seeing the need to work out the content of the role in cooperation with other participants in a setting. Parents who start off defining their roles narrowly may be less likely to engage in these negotiations and so may do less parenting when they are outside the home.

Claiming the Right to Use Discretion

People often are reluctant to modify someone else's routine. When people visit in others' homes or take a new job, they inquire about the details of how even common things are done in that setting. This is partly a matter of simple deference but is also an acknowledgment that routines are adapted to local conditions in ways that may not be obvious to visitors or newcomers. In their own homes, parents formulate their own routines and adapt received routines to their own needs. An infant's medication schedule might, for instance, need to be adapted to the child's patterns of eating or sleeping. How difficult it is to use discretion, then, varies from one situation to another. In situations in which no "canned" routines are provided, people have little choice but to use their discretion. Parenthood is, of course, a role for which many scripts are available, from people's own parents, child-care books or magazines, pediatricians and other professionals, support groups, religious groups, and child-care classes. So many alternatives may in fact decrease the authoritativeness of any one script, making it easier for parents to modify or invent their own routines.

But parents' confidence in using their discretion probably varies with their respect for the authority promulgating any particular routine, their sense of competence in the area to which a particular script applies, the way in which they receive a script (they might be commanded to follow a routine exactly, or a routine might be offered as a suggestion about how to solve a problem), where the script is enacted (in the home or in some other setting), and who else is present when the routine is implemented. Some scripts or routines are offered to parents for their use—parents are expected to implement them and even to adapt them. Other scripts are enacted by others, with parents as bystanders. The more that parents are treated as bystanders or novices, the more difficult it will be for them to use their discretion in adapting routines later or in interrupting the routines of others if they believe something is amiss. That so much of the work of parenting takes place outside the home, often in the work space of others, means that using discretion requires claiming the right to use discretion, not simply adjusting or reworking inappropriate scripts.

Family Fates in an Individual World

While it may be relatively common for family members to think of themselves as having a common fate and drawing on a common pool of resources, we believe that such tendencies can be undermined. When parents do not live together (because of divorce or because they never shared a residence), for instance, a noncustodial father may be reluctant to pay child support if he believes that his money goes into a pot that helps support the mother as well as the child (see, e.g., Arendell 1986, 1995; Gerson 1993). In some cases, the policies of organizations also may militate against family solidarity. Financial support often is provided to individuals, not to families, and the effect of a disabled child on the family welfare is not considered relevant in determining the magnitude or the conditions of the support.[7] Thus if a child requires more than his or her share of the mother's attention, or consumes a disproportionate share of the family budget, this is not the concern of social service agencies, which regard themselves as at most obligated to provide meager support for the target individual. When transporting a sick child to an emergency room means that there is no money to pay the family rent, a welfare system focused only on whether the child qualifies for Medicaid will not be concerned with how its stinginess affects the rest of the family. We pointed out earlier how such policies can encourage parents themselves to adopt a narrow and uncharitable view. Recall that Robert's father (1018) expressed outrage that Robert's social security might help pay for the roof over the head of the rest of the family. He seemed less aware that this same roof could be jeopardized in those months when Robert's needs were especially great.

Some families, recognizing the tendency of social service organizations to concern themselves only with a target individual, devised ways of pro-

7. Seligman and Darling (1989) criticize the practice of treating only the disabled member of a family rather than looking at how that child fits into the family. Their point is that outcomes for all family members are interdependent. The illness of a child has an impact on the family, but the family similarly plays a role in the health and well-being of the disabled child.

tecting the interests of other family members so that resources were shared more evenly. One family (1017) paid their son's parochial school tuition in a lump sum at the beginning of the school year as a way of ensuring that his interests were not always sacrificed to his sister's. Another family (1001) had at various points done things to protect crucial resources for both of their children. As we mentioned before, during a particularly lean period, the mother had stockpiled food for the child who had been hospitalized, arguing that he could not eat just anything. At another point, she scrimped to pay for the speech therapy Medicaid would not cover for her older son.

Our point here is that when families must seek resources from a variety of organizations, some of which may not recognize the family as a single consumption unit, they can respond by either allowing inequalities between family members to increase or developing their own compensatory policies to readjust the welfare of family members so that inequalities remain within a tolerable range. We must also recognize, though, that not all organizations focus so exclusively on the family member who has been designated as their chief concern. The staff at City's NICU urged parents to consider their own well-being as well as that of their child, suggesting to parents that they could do little for their child if they allowed themselves to "burn out."[8] To encourage parents to spend an occasional evening away from the unit, the NICU provided meal tickets for dinners at local restaurants. These occasional corrective impulses are just that, though—occasional. For the most part, organizations myopically focus on the person who falls into their domain—as is their mandate, of course—leaving families to figure out for themselves what is fair when some family members are targeted for extra resources or have unusual needs. Parents may be willing to accept sacrifices in welfare for the sake of an especially needy child, but they may nevertheless be reluctant to accept an organization's unthinking assumption that the needy child should have first claim on familial resources and should always have priority over other children in the family. From the parents' point of view, you can't have it both ways—it isn't fair to treat the family as a consumption pool when an organization wants family resources to be available for the baby during its hospitalization or after discharge but not to treat the family as a unit when resources are flowing the other direction.

8. According to Gilligan (1982), an important step in moral development is learning to include oneself among those who need to be cared for.

Organizational Effects as Explanations of Variations in the Acceptance of Responsibility

We have argued in this chapter that responsibilities often cannot be met by individuals operating in isolation. Because we live in an organizational world, responsibilities often cannot be met without crossing organizational boundaries. But what does that tell us about who will or will not take on responsibilities? That is, does the embedding of responsibility in organizations help explain any of the things we have learned in this investigation?

To answer these questions, we turn to three distinct ways that organizational effects appear in this study. People are different, they have different relationships to organizations, and organizations are different. And these differences provide the raw materials for three kinds of effects of organizations on people's capacities to take responsibility. We turn first to traits of individuals. Organizations do not treat all people equally. Personal characteristics, made salient by cultural definitions, shape the ways that people are treated by organizations. Organizations do not treat rich and poor, young and old, or male and female alike. Here we show how some of the differences between mothers and fathers either originate in or are reinforced by the ways that organizations treat men and women. People also have quite different roles in organizations, and we have argued that one of the most basic distinctions is between people who are considered regular members of an organization and those who are considered outsiders. Members of organizations have very different participation rights than outsiders, though of course important differences remain in the participation rights of different categories of insiders. Here we ask what difference organizational membership makes for a person's capacity to take on responsibility, noting that when people must draw on resources and skills which they do not themselves have, crossing organizational boundaries becomes necessary. Finally, we look at differences among organizations themselves, asking how these variations affect people's capacity to meet their obligations. Here we are not so much concerned with the content of these differences as with the simple fact that there are differences. Clearly some organizations have many written rules of procedure and others have few, some are more open to change and others are more resistant, some are more comfortable for participants and others more hostile, some are more egalitarian and others more hierarchical, and some of these variations will have important effects on whether members or clients find it easy or difficult to take responsibility. But for people who must function in a variety of organizational settings, simple variability among organizations by itself poses an impediment to meeting obligations.

Differences among People: Gender and Organizational Boundaries

On the average, the mothers we interviewed for this study take more responsibility for their children than the fathers do. Further, differences between mothers and fathers are exaggerated when parents are not married and do not live together. Marriage and cohabitation are not perfectly correlated, and the ties created by formal marriage and by sharing a residence are not identical. Nevertheless, among our respondents, all of the parents who lived together regarded themselves as having a long-term tie whether or not they were married, planned to marry in the future, or anticipated that they would never formalize their union. For now we wish to examine the boundaries around the family unit and how these vary with the nature of the parents' relationship and with the gender of the parent. The location of boundaries is important because those who are located inside boundaries are subject to different pressures than those outside.

As we pointed out in chapter 5, when parents are not married, the hospital staff is legally obliged to get the mother's consent for medical treatment. When parents are married, parents are legally interchangeable and the consent of either parent is sufficient, although many staff members believe it wise to verify that the parents are in agreement. This legal rule is fully consistent with general social practice. Socially, the tie between mother and child is not equivalent to that between father and child. Those who are not well acquainted with a particular family will conserve their resources by betting with the stereotypes. As we argued in chapter 5, unless hospital staff members have information to the contrary, they will invest their scarce instructional and social control resources in preparing the mother to take the baby home.

Hospital staff members are not unique in this regard. Teachers (ranging from preschool to high school) ask for the mother when they call a child's home, whether they are calling to discuss the child's school performance, report on an accident, request a contribution of labor or goods, or talk about the child's antisocial behavior. Nannies usually negotiate with the mother (Hertz 1986). Emergency calls are routed to the father only after the mother cannot be located. Questions about birthday parties and birthday gifts are directed to the mother whether they are from relatives or the child's friends. Fathers often hear the news from the outside only through the mother's mouth. Fathers' ties with their children's myriad care providers—whether they be physicians or swim coaches—are thus mediated ties. In contrast, mothers have direct ties both to children and to children's other care providers; their identities as mothers may thus be reinforced rather than diminished when mothering occurs both inside and outside the home. Fathers' ties are diminished when children have outside ties, while mothers' ties are augmented because their identities and tasks as mothers exist both inside the family sphere and outside it.[9]

But what exactly does this have to do with responsibility? Ties between teachers and parents, between health-care providers and parents, or between grandparents and parents can transmit practical advice about child rearing or information about schedules. But they also transmit expectations about what parents should be doing and praise or criticism of their performance as parents. When fathers mostly have mediated ties, any pressure they might experience and any praise they might receive is filtered through, and perhaps diluted or amplified by, a third party. Because mothers are so often the intermediaries, fathers may dismiss criticism by suggesting that it really comes from the mother, not from some outsider. Often fathers simply receive less pressure and less praise than mothers do because both praise and criticism are aimed at mothers. When child rearing is thought to lie largely in the province of women, it is women to whom sanctions will be directed and women who will be prepared to receive and interpret the snide comments, whispered asides, catty remarks, and innuendos.

If praise and criticism, as well as more neutral exchanges of information, are disproportionately aimed at mothers even when parents are married or cohabit, such gender differences are even more exaggerated when fathers do not reside with their children. Teachers or relatives who might somewhat reluctantly agree to speak to a father if a mother was unavailable to discuss the child will surely not go out of their way to contact a father. Fathers who do not live with their children share with residential fathers

9. The stereotype about men is that they mediate the family's ties to the outside world. Earlier we seem to be agreeing with that stereotype when we argued that fathers might be more comfortable than mothers in seeing their child through the universalistic lens of the outside world. But here we have argued that mothers have the larger role in forging their child's connections with the world beyond the home. Are these statements inconsistent? We believe not. Although fathers may be more comfortable with the universalistic orientation of the public sphere and so less likely to bristle when others treat their child as a member of a category, and in many families they still bring in the majority of the financial resources, mothers are nevertheless the ones who do most of the work of building the child's ties to the rest of the world. To oversimplify, fathers bring the world in, while mothers take the child out.

the experience of not being specifically sought out for discussions about the child or about child care. But they are further disadvantaged as parents in not experiencing the chance encounters that residential fathers experience when the costs of contacting the mother are sufficiently high that talking with the father becomes the preferred alternative.

No doubt causes and effects are deeply entangled here. Fathers marry mothers and live with mothers and children partly because they wish to take responsibility for children. But in addition, marrying the child's mother and living with her and the child make it more likely that a father will be assigned responsibilities, receive the information he needs to contribute to child rearing, and receive the rewards and punishments that support responsible parenting. People certainly make some choices about how to configure their lives, but once those social arrangements are created, they have independent effects.

The gender differences we observed should not be swept under the rug by suggesting that this is "just the way men and women are." Differences in "personality" often are situationally produced, as Becker (1960, 1964) argued was the case for commitment. He suggested that instead of concluding that some people are just more "committed" than others, we should look for the situational pressures that might produce behavioral consistency, for instance making some people appear more stable than others. Becker points to the "side-bets" that people make in pensions, friendships with colleagues, the acquisition of knowledge about local merchants, ties to children's schoolteachers and classmates, and so on as factors that make inconsistency so expensive that it ceases to be a realistic alternative.

But, as Becker astutely noted, insofar as the possibilities to make commitments are afforded by social structures, we should expect that people would end up with different perspectives. If, for instance, commitment is the result of a series of situational adjustments, structural changes that require different situational adjustments then would produce different levels of the behavioral consistency that looks like commitment. And, as we have argued above, if women must make different situational adjustments than men, and men who live with their children (and the children's mothers) must make different ones than men who do not live with their children, then responsible behavior can be produced by a series of relatively small and partially independent situational adjustments rather than by some deeply embedded difference in orientation to children. Our argument, then, is that in treating women differently than men, organizations require women to make a long series of side-bets that constrain their behavior and shape their perspectives so that they are more likely than men to take responsibility (and to take more responsibility) for children. A similar argument can be made for the differences between married (or coresiding) fathers and unmarried fathers.

Such an argument of course implies that changes in situations will produce changes in situational adjustments and changes in perspective. As Becker argues, if a perspective is produced by participation in a situation, then we should not expect people's outlooks to be substantially more stable than the situations that produce them. Should there be structural changes that made it expensive for men to behave irresponsibly (because of the side-bets they had made) or that decreased the cost for women of behaving irresponsibly (by altering the kinds of side-bets they make), we would expect some decrease in the gender difference in taking responsibility for children who were or had been critically ill. To take a very simple example, if men developed fuller relationships with NICU staff, then each failure to visit would require a payment in the form of an explanatory phone call. Relationships with staff members are one of the side-bets that help sustain women's patterns of frequent visits. Changes in employment patterns, in hospital routines about consulting and training parents, and in residential patterns of parents all could produce different situational adjustments and so differences in the likelihood that men or women would take responsibility for their children.

The thrust of this book is clearly that taking responsibility is good and shirking is bad. And, given the empirical focus of the research, we are clearly saying that it is good for children to have someone take responsibility for them. When children are or have been critically ill, "good-enough" parenting is not sufficient; responsible parenting is what is needed. But it is just as important to be clear about what we are not saying. Responsible parenting is costly. We have frankly acknowledged that caring for a sick baby consumes the time, thought, emotional energy, and financial reserves of its family. But of course, providing responsible care for such children typically drains mothers more than fathers. In saying that it is good for children to get such attentive care and in describing the supports and pressures that predispose some people to accept responsibility and others to shirk it, we are not saying that we think it is a good thing that such pressures to take responsibility for children fall more heavily on women than on men. Rather, in pointing to the ways in which such gender differences arise, are made to seem natural, and are sustained, we hope to point the way for change. But the change we advocate is not less care for needy children, but a fairer distribution of the burden between the sexes.

Differences in Relations with Organizations: To Whom Does the Responsibility Belong?

One of the chief difficulties that parents encounter in assuming responsibility for their hospitalized children is that there is substantial ambiguity about whose responsibility it is to care for the child. If parents too assertively claim that the child is theirs and therefore their obligation, others may accuse the parents of poor judgment and of claiming expertise they do not have. But if parents are too deferential to authorities or experts, or if they too quickly relinquish a child to the care of hospital (or later, school) personnel, they are accused of being uncommitted or uninvested in their child's welfare. Ambiguities about the ownership of a responsibility change character once the baby leaves the NICU. While the child is hospitalized, parents often feel that the baby's welfare is largely in the hands of the hospital staff. As the balance between parents and staff members shifts, parents wonder less who owns the baby and more what it means to be a parent on someone else's turf. If parents once believed that they left their parental rights at the doorstep of the hospital, many of them now believe that they continue to have rights and obligations but remain uncertain about exactly how to enact their roles as parents outside the home. In settings such as NICUs, follow-up clinics, and schools, parents are something more than bystanders and something less than participants. "Real" participants have defined roles that bear somewhat clearer relations to one another. In a hospital setting, relations between roles are defined both by task domains and by hierarchy. But parents have no clearly defined tasks and no position in the hierarchy. What they are supposed to do remains unclear. To understand how people come to define a responsibility as theirs, then, we must look at how organizations and their boundaries shape people's sense of where they belong and what they can do.

The ambiguity that parents experience as outsiders has some benefits, though. Ombudsmen and troubleshooters have no clearly defined tasks and no clear place in a hierarchy; the boundaries of case management and primary nursing are loosely defined. In these occupations tasks are not clearly specified because the object is to assign global responsibility for a problem or person. That, of course, is what parenthood is about too. But occupants of such roles will face substantial uncertainty about exactly what falls within their purview and will be unusually likely to encounter resistance from others whose task domains are more clearly defined.

Ombudsmen, case managers, and primary nurses share a trait that parents lack, though. They are legitimate members of the organization, with all of the basic rights that membership confers. They have identity cards, directories listing phone numbers and room assignments of other members of the organization, maps of relevant buildings, calendars of important events, and easy access to appeals channels. Cialdini (1984) points to the deference elicited by titles, uniforms, and other insignia of authority, and this is surely one explanation of why parents find it so difficult to find their way on others' turf. The uniforms of parenthood do not elicit deferential behavior (even from children) the way that doctors' coats do. Without these markers of legitimacy, parents must continually reassert their right to be there before they can even begin to claim a right to intervene. As parents become acquainted with a particular setting such as a school or an NICU, they learn how to "pass." When they can bustle down the hall because they know exactly where they are going, ask for the person they need to see by the correct title, and perform such medical rituals as scrubbing and gowning with sufficient expertise that they do not invite correction, then parents begin to feel that they have earned the right to participate. They are clearly not insiders, but they are no longer intensely and continually aware of their status as outsiders.

Parents who are less adept organizational actors will have more difficulty making claims about their rights and obligations as parents, however deep their feelings of attachment to their child. This is as much a matter of gut reactions as of carefully worked out responses to organizational rules and routines. The same NICU may be experienced quite differently by different parents. To one parent the NICU may seem like an efficient, well-organized place that can be trusted to oversee the baby twenty-four hours a day. It may seem like a clean, comfortable, safe place to visit the baby while someone else provides the care it desperately needs. To another, equally concerned parent, the NICU may seem like a bewildering and uncomfortable place—foreign territory where one has to leave one's baby for its own good. But it might not seem like a place to *parent,* and so parenting might be deferred until the baby is "returned" to the parents. Just as parents protect their children by sending them out of a war zone to live with strangers, so one might temporarily relinquish one's child to a hospital team.

Ambiguity about who "owns" a responsibility affects the likelihood that anyone will act responsibly. Experimental research on the diffusion of responsibility, looking at the conditions under which bystanders will offer help, shows that anything that makes a bystander feel that he or she has some unique obligation increases the likelihood that help will be offered (Latané and Darley 1970; Mynatt and Sherman 1975). That is, bystanders who "own" the obligation behave more responsibly.[10] Similarly, Clarke (1989) shows that some of the delay in getting organizations to clean up or contain a toxic accident occurs because of negotiations about who owns the obligation. People who feel like outsiders are less likely to feel that they can or must claim ownership.

But ownership of obligations is not the only question. We also know that people would not all agree on what course of action is the responsible one. To some degree views on what responsibility entails depend on where one stands in relation to the key institutions that share the obligation to care for a child. Here, again, it matters who is inside and who is outside the organization, but roles inside the organization matter as well. Hospital staff members have a different understanding than parents, for instance, because each group is rendered myopic by the lens of its own role. Hospital staff members may forget how strange and intimidating the NICU is to new parents, and parents may not realize that the doctors and nurses have to ask intrusive questions in order to fulfill their obligation to discharge the baby to a safe home with caring and competent parents. Variations in acceptance of responsibility thus depend on people's understandings of what their obligations are, and such understandings arise partly in response to signals from others about what one is or is not supposed to do. Chambliss (1996), for instance, points out that nurses are deeply concerned about the welfare of their patients, but they also feel constrained to follow doctors' orders. Their sense of what it is responsible to do is fundamentally shaped by their position as subordinates in the medical hierarchy. If staff members explicitly or implicitly tell parents to confine themselves to nonmedical matters, are parents less likely to pay attention to the medical details they will have to track after discharge? Are they less able to assume full responsibility for the child when it comes home?

If many parents initially feel that they are outsiders with only limited capacity to intervene productively, we need to ask how they subsequently

10. Rutkowski, Gruder, and Romer (1983) show that although the presence of many bystanders usually decreases the likelihood that anyone will offer help, this is not the case when the bystanders know one another. This may be because such bystanders are able to negotiate about how help should be provided and by whom.

come to feel that they are the ones responsible for their child. How, then, do parents come to feel that they have rights to intrude on the turf of medical care givers? Although parents play little role in the medical decision making that gets their child admitted to an NICU, by the time of discharge, parents must be ready to take over responsibility for their child, even when that includes making decisions about when to consult medical professionals. Parents' responsibility thus grows over the baby's hospitalization, although for many parents this is not a gradual evolution, but a punctuated one. Mistakes (or perceived mistakes) are one of the ways that parents are jolted into feeling that they cannot comfortably leave medical matters only in medical hands. Variations among medical protocols also suggest to parents who have experienced more than a single medical regime that there is less-than-perfect consensus about "technical" matters and that they may therefore be capable of intervening.

But increased feelings of responsibility also arise from a growing relationship with the baby. Although for most parents those feelings grow over the baby's hospital stay, parents do not respond uniformly to hospital experiences. They are differently equipped by virtue of both social class location and idiosyncratic biographical experiences to respond to the events in the baby's medical course. Some parents may be looking for mistakes; others may not see even the most blatant errors. Some parents may keep their own records so they can evaluate progress; others do not notice interhospital differences in treatment regimes. Parents who are not present in the unit, who have not "boned up" on the baby's medical condition, or who have no familial allies to support them may not respond with an increased commitment or willingness to intervene when other parents would confront staff members or aggressively claim a right to transfer the baby. In their struggle over what it means to parent within the confines of the NICU, parents take different routes. Some gradually come to think of themselves as insiders as their own expertise increases; some come to think of the professionals as possessing less expertise than they had originally believed; some develop ideologies of parenting as a distinctive role; and some bide their time waiting for the day when the baby is really "theirs."

Whatever has gone before, parents again experience a kind of parity when they take their babies home and responsibility for the child is unambiguously theirs. A few may be called on by visiting nurses or child-welfare workers. But like all new parents, those taking a baby home from the NICU suddenly confront the weighty reality that this child depends on them. To some degree the equality among parents at this point is an illusion. Though nearly all experience a sense of inadequacy, nevertheless there are important differences among parents in the kinds of resources they bring to parenting. Although key resources such as money, education, time, and a supportive relationship with a spouse surely make the assumption of parental responsibility easier, the absence of such resources does not spell disaster. While even they cannot squeeze blood from a turnip, parents who are determined to take responsibility for their children are surprisingly resourceful. Further, parents' sense that the child is really "theirs" is to some degree temporary as well. While their status in the NICU no longer matters, parents quickly discover that there are many other organizational borders to negotiate and that parental rights and roles are ill defined in those organizational settings as well.

Differences among Organizations: Normative Systems and Organizational Boundaries

We have argued that infants and those who care for them live in an organizational world. One consequence of this is that they also live in a variety of normative worlds (as well as having to deal with other important variations among organizations). The normative order of the NICU is not the same as that of the home, which in turn is not the same as that of the school, the zero-to-three program, the insurance company, the parent's employer, the hospital emergency room, the pediatric intensive care unit (where NICU graduates are likely to go if they return to the hospital for critical care), the visiting nurse association, the social security administration, or the state child-welfare department. One important respect in which parenting in contemporary America is different from parenting in previous generations is that parents must negotiate more organizational boundaries and adjudicate the contradictions between normative orders at the boundaries of these various systems. What is responsible depends partly on one's worldview and on whose interests and needs have to be taken into account (other family members', other clients'). Others may be unwilling to recognize and respect such ambiguity, and families with unconventional beliefs (e.g., about alternative health care) or unusual affiliations (e.g., with religious sects or political movements) are especially likely to have their notions of responsible behavior challenged by others (Frohock 1992).

Schools, an institution all parents will encounter in some form or other, illustrate this problem well. Schools and parents are both prone to ask the other to enforce *their* rules in the other setting. Schools want parents to support school homework policies and policies about how to interact with peers, for instance. While this may sound innocuous enough, parents may be chary in an era when sexual harassment policies have begun to penetrate elementary classrooms and substance-abuse policies are occasionally extended to cover caffeine and mild analgesics (see, e.g., *Economist* 1996:31; Page 1996:15). Schools may endorse the principle of respecting cultural and familial differences but are in fact reluctant to take on the conflicts that result when distinct dietary regimes mean that some children are excluded from participation in holiday celebrations, or when the dispute-resolution strategies of different parents mean that some children wish to settle disagreements by themselves, while others believe in calling in the authorities.

In the first few years after parents take their child home from an NICU, the most important organizational boundaries are those between the household and medical care providers, and between the household and social service agencies. And here we find important differences among parents. Having a sicker baby means having to manage interfaces with more organizations. A baby sick enough to require home nursing is one whose parents will be in constant negotiation with medical suppliers, home nursing organizations, private insurers, Medicaid, a follow-up clinic, a pediatrician's office, and a host of medical specialists who plan and carry out additional interventions.

Each of these boundaries is likely to be contested. Can the mother really "fire" a nurse who sets the alarm on her watch and sleeps most of the night rather than stays awake to watch the baby (1036)? What should the mother do when the medical equipment supplier delivers the wrong supplies so that equipment repeatedly malfunctions (1009)? How can parents get physicians to respect their knowledge of their child even in situations that are usually in the medical purview (2016)? And, from the other side, how can a visiting nurse get parents to follow feeding regimes that are safer for the child (1025)? What can a physician do to get mothers to follow an appropriate schedule in getting inoculations for the child (1018, 1024)? And to what degree should health-care providers try to reshape the behavior of parents when that behavior harms the health of a child? Can a health-care provider insist that the parent of a ventilator-dependent child enroll in a class to help him or her give up smoking, for instance?

Parents often feel vulnerable when confronted with the authoritative statements of organizational representatives. Organizations are likely to have written policies spelling out the conditions for their engagement with parents. Parents must apply for public aid if they do not have insurance, some hospitals insist. One child's discharge was delayed for six months while her mother's insurer battled with Medicaid over who exactly was going to pay the bills (1017). Parents are weak players in these games. They do not arrive on the scene with their own rules for engagement, but it would matter little even if they did. As we pointed out in chapter 6, although the parents are the baby's main representatives, contrary to what some agency theorists imagine, they nevertheless are not the ones who write the contracts for how others will behave or the conditions under which various goods and services will be bought.

Parents may not be quite as weak as they imagine, though, and one of the points of difference among parents lies exactly here. Some parents, frustrated at having to learn the schedules and rules of so many organizations, simply retreat. Gloria (1018), for instance, did not receive services to which she was entitled because she was unable to track her interactions with the various organizations. Robert's spina bifida might have been detected prenatally had Gloria followed up when an expected notice about an appointment failed to arrive. Her vagueness about when Robert was supposed to be seen at the Shriner hospital, and her inability to keep the children up to date on their shots, suggested that her failure to have scheduled prenatal tests was not an isolated incident. Although it is hard to know how to allocate the blame, almost certainly a host of people and organizations should share the blame with Gloria for the poor care Robert was receiving. Stingy welfare resources meant that she could not afford a phone. An irresponsible father meant that she was obliged to track the baby's medical care alone. A disengaged team of health-care providers had failed to convince her of the importance of getting care and had not designed a system of reminders that compensated for Gloria's inadequacies.

In contrast to Gloria, some parents learned that they did have some room to maneuver despite rigid organizational policies. Janet (1036) was told by the discharge planner that her son would have to stay in the hospital because no home nurses were available in her area. She advertised at a local nursing school and managed to put together an adequate team. Roger and Grace (2016) figured out how to pick and choose among health-care providers and used the services of only those they considered both highly skilled and appropriately respectful of the parents' contributions. Tammy relied on her parents to keep her alive; if physicians could not accept that Tammy's parents knew a lot about her medical condition, Roger and Grace reasoned, Tammy would not be safe. But no hospital protocol provides for such detailed consultation with parents, and Grace and Roger learned how to work the system by bitter experience and by paying a high cost in alienating some health-care providers and in a decline in their family's financial circumstances.

Thus far we have focused primarily on the difficulty that parents must operate simultaneously within the normative systems of organizations such as hospitals and day-care centers and those of their own households. It often is not easy to reconcile the demands of two or more organizations, particularly when one is disadvantaged by being the weaker party, as most parents are when interacting with representatives of formal organizations, and when one is not armed with written policies. In comparison with claims that "this is what our family believes," the written policies of the hospital are powerful bargaining tools. Schelling (1960) pointed out that negotiators who can claim that they can make no further concessions are much more able to dig in their heels stubbornly than are those who have no way to make or back up such a claim. Parents cannot make their demands stick because they usually cannot claim that their hands are tied. Jehovah's Witnesses are an exception here, and the presence of church leaders helps reinforce parents' claims that they are obliged by church law to refuse blood products for their child. It is probably no accident that the legal mechanisms that allow medical staff to resist parent demands are exceptionally well developed here, and that the level of inequality between parents and staff members remains roughly constant. Parents are then weak participants because they arrive at the negotiating table (figuratively speaking, usually) not knowing their own minds, without clear and authoritative statements if they do know their minds, and without any of the supports that will make it possible to insist that they cannot be the ones to back down.

Parents may be further disadvantaged by the effects of institutional memory and records. In hospitals it is not just medical conditions and interventions that have sequelae. Parents may find that their reputations follow them—from one nurse to the next, from one hospital unit to the next, and even from one institution to the next. Once they are classified in the organization as irresponsible, as difficult, or "inappropriate," such reputations are likely to follow them. Medical records, with commentary on parents as well as on their offspring, necessarily follow the child from one site to another, and workers at one site may telephone workers at another for clarification. Such communications link cognate workers in different institutions—physicians telephone physicians, and social workers consult with other social workers. While such communications are not routine (health-care workers, like workers in other settings, may not read every page they receive), they also are not unusual. But just as people often are surprised to learn that "old" problems have not disappeared from their credit ratings, that errors made by tax authorities continue to appear years later as unpaid taxes, for instance, so parents often are unaware that their child's medical records contain hints that mothers may have used drugs during pregnancy, comments on the reliability and competence of parents, evaluations of the parents' interactions with the child, or discussions of conflicts between the parents and the staff. Oblivious of the existence of these "data," parents cannot defend themselves against the "charges" or provide definitive evidence that things have changed. They may be baffled by health-care workers' suspicious reactions to them or wonder why they are always treated as if they couldn't manage their own affairs.

Parents of course make similar evaluations of hospitals and of individual staff members. But such evaluations are less consequential for staff members—in no case is a staff member facing a sanction as important as being denied custody of a child—because parents control fewer rewards and punishments. They may be able to bring suits, although few do; they may be able to make a staff member's work life unpleasant for a few days, but staff can ask others to take their place; and they may transfer their child to another institution, but one child is usually only a small proportion of the patient load in any given institution. Parents may commit their thoughts to paper, and may even keep systematic notes complete with dates, times, names and titles, actions, and consequences, but because they are not "professionals," their records will carry less weight. Parental evaluations also tend to remain isolated. Parents could share evaluations in support groups, but few parents attend these groups. As we pointed out in chapter 6, social control by parents is a radically individualized enterprise. Parent evaluations simply do not travel between institutions or pass from one parent to another the way that the evaluations of parents by staff members do.

Normative systems are hardly static—indeed the thrust of contemporary sociology and anthropology is to emphasize that normative systems are the product of negotiations among participants and so should be expected to be somewhat fluid. But we wish to stress that not all participants have an equal say in shaping the norms that govern any setting or in the interactions that occur in it. Although parents are not powerless when they enter the NICU, a school, or their pediatrician's office, they also cannot completely rework the rules of engagement. For instance, parents are largely powerless to write the contract that governs the relationship between their family and the professionals who are hired to act as the child's agents in supplying medical care or instruction. The contract, supplied by the hospital or school, is shaped much more by organizational rules and procedures than by parental wishes. Such constraints are difficult for parents to untangle or even understand. Surely this is one meaning of hegemony. When the "contracts" between parents and the professionals who care for their child are so deeply embedded in the organization's routines and so entwined with other contracts between one organization and another, the constraints become invisible. The parents may feel trapped in these invisible webs of rules, these concealed constraints, and may feel powerless even when they care deeply about the outcome. NICU staff members are intensely aware that parents do have some power. An occasional parent does throw a temper tantrum that would do a two-year-old proud. But just as adolescents' rebellions do little to reshape the system, so parents' rebellions are weak moves in negotiations about the normative orders of complex organizations.

Social Control and the Production of Responsibility: Generalizing to Other Settings

In this book, we have been concerned with how to get people to take responsibility. We have developed our arguments in a thorough examination of the case of families who have had critically ill infants; now it is time to move beyond this case. We have stressed the role of the law in setting minimum standards but pointed out that the law must be articulated with other, suppler normative systems to achieve higher-than-minimum compliance. We have examined responsibility in the hospital itself, where the objective of legal and normative systems is to get physicians and the other members of a health-care team to juggle a variety of obligations to patients, the hospital, and other team members while providing the best possible care. And for parents, the dual objective of the law is to ensure that parents' rights to raise their children as they see fit are protected at the same time that parental obligations to provide minimally adequate care are enforced. But for both the parents and the medical team, the real goal is to increase the likelihood that parents will bring home a healthy child who will thrive and be able to live a full and happy life. Neither group would be satisfied merely to keep the child alive or to decrease marginally the child's impairment. To achieve such a goal requires much more than just following the rules about medical care or parenting; instead both parents and medical staff must keep their eyes steadfastly on the goal, asking continually what more must be done and when protocols must be abandoned because they are inappropriate to the situation. These questions about when to follow rules and when to break them and how to motivate thoughtful attempts to achieve the goals of a legal or other normative system are universal. We have looked at them in neonatal intensive care only because it is a setting in which the costs of unthinking adherence to rules are particularly apparent.

But how do social control systems induce people to take responsibility? How are incentive systems shaped, standards established and modified? How are people made to feel that particular responsibilities belong uniquely to them and that it would be shameful to neglect those obligations? This section draws on the previous empirical investigation to address more general questions about the production of responsibility.

Responsibility, we have argued, is about following a problem across organizational boundaries. But the fainthearted, those less savvy about making their way in organizations and those whose participation rights are restricted in one way or another, are less likely to cross organizational boundaries when core participants fail to welcome them or actively discourage them for one reason or another. Less sophisticated actors may not notice subtle shifts in their relations to organizations. Parents may, for instance, generalize inappropriately, assuming that the experiences they had while their infants were hospitalized are "normal" hospital experiences. Of course these experiences are normal in some respects, because they are instances of a relatively common class of interactions, namely those between lay people and professionals. But even within that general class of relations, variations are important. Parents of hospitalized infants are at the mercy of the NICU, depending on staff to care for the medical and everyday needs of their child. But once the baby goes home, a subtle but substantial shift takes place. Yes, the parents are still laypeople who must draw on the expertise of hospital staff. But now, rather than medical care being provided automatically without further parental intervention, parents must request the assistance of the hospital staff. When the baby moves across an organizational border as physical custody shifts from the hospital staff to the parents, a different party bears the responsibility for ensuring that appropriate medical care is provided, and the relation between parents and medical care providers shifts correspondingly.

Responsibility, then, requires people to be sensitive to the context of their actions and make necessary adjustments. What is responsible in one setting may not be responsible in another. And, furthermore, what is required to claim the right to take responsibility, on the one hand, or to compel others to make necessary contributions, on the other, will also be quite likely to vary. The more organizational boundaries an actor must cross, the more flexibility will be required. And here is where agency is so important. Responsibility cannot be enacted from a single script. At the very least, actors must strategically choose from among available scripts and, in cases such as ours, often must construct scripts for situations where no available script seems adequate. Further, they must work out compromises that take into account the sometimes divergent perspectives of all those whose activities must be coordinated to produce a responsible outcome. Some of this divergence arises because most people have multiple responsibilities—to their employers and co-workers as well as to their families, to a classroom full of students or a nursery full of infants, rather than just a single individual.

Two features of normative systems are important to our general understanding of how responsibility is produced. The first is flexibility. We have pointed out that it is easier to make rules about floors, thresholds below which performance cannot be allowed to slip, than to make rules that encourage flexible adjustment to continuously changing situations. We have argued that such supple normative systems are more likely to occur when there are mechanisms to incorporate new developments or characteristics of individual situations into the standards. Such mechanisms are more likely to exist when several enforcement bodies draw on the expertise of other practitioners to assess performance. A shifting or evolving consensus among practitioners does not exist in all fields, of course, and where it doesn't, it is more difficult to insist on high quality performance. Without such a consensus, there is little for a court of law to draw on in enforcing standards and little for a certification body to draw on in granting a license. And, of course, there are some fields—and parenting is clearly one of those—in which no one has to have a license to practice. Thus parents can only be "fired" if their practice is so far below the standard that they are judged neglectful or abusive.

A second factor, though, concerns the permeability of boundaries. Normative systems vary in how supple they are, but in addition, actors vary in their susceptibility to influence. Occupants of roles are to varying degrees exposed to or shielded from social pressure. Those higher in social hierarchies are probably more shielded from direct social pressure than those lower down. But at the same time, the fact that higher positions carry more responsibility, are reviewed less often, are oriented to longer run values, and control the use of more substantial resources means that they may be more responsive to the influence of more general social values. Standards can be imposed in some settings, such as workplaces, much more easily than in others, such as homes. We argued in chapter 7 that households are much more variable than NICUs in the qualifications of those who work there. When NICUs try to teach parents how to care for their babies after discharge, they are to some degree attempting to export information about medical care and child development. But the NICU's capacity to impose standards on the household is quite limited. NICUs may attempt to export, but what really matters is whether households choose to import these standards, and households vary a good deal in that.

Some of the variations we have described are variations among normative systems, others among roles, and still others among incumbents in the characteristics they bring to similar roles. This book has scrutinized parenthood but has made a series of systematic comparisons to highlight the features that moderate or amplify tendencies toward acceptance or shirking of responsibility. We have thus looked at how the tasks of parenting vary depending on whether the child is at home versus in a hospital unit. This comparison has allowed us to talk about the extent to which parenting is an isolated activity versus one that must be articulated with other roles.

We have also compared the obligations of parents with those of others caring for the child, such as medical care providers. Responsibilities for one's children are of an unusually long duration and broad scope. Parental responsibilities are also (in contemporary American society) for the most part ultimately shouldered by individuals or couples rather than larger groups. These characteristics distinguish parental responsibilities from other kinds of responsibilities we might be interested in examining. Such a comparison allows us to see what difference it makes, for example, when work is formally organized, when workers are trained and screened, when workers are held to performance standards and can be fired if they do their work badly, and when their work is scrutinized by others whose work begins where theirs leaves off. Thus the responsibility of physicians, nurses, and social workers in NICUs is produced in a fundamentally different way from that of parents for the same medical procedures after the babies go home.

Finally, we have compared parents with each other. We have compared female parents with male parents, richer parents with poorer, parents with more years of schooling with those with less, married parents with unmarried, younger parents with older, parents of only one child with those of several children, and parents with many supportive kin with relatively isolated ones. These comparisons have permitted us to see which characteristics are important predictors of acceptance of responsibility, which ones make it easier to accept responsibility but do not play a determinative role, and which ones make individual parents subject to more or less pressure from other people.

One of the main findings of this book is that willingness to accept responsibility does not vary much with the magnitude of the burden. We would expect this finding to translate to other settings as well, where some undoubtedly shirk with light loads while others toil under heavy burdens. We also would expect the dimensions of responsibility discussed throughout the book to apply equally well whether the subject is responsibility in a family or in some other organization. We must recognize, however, that parenting is in some important respects a unique kind of responsibility and is motivated by something other than expected material or career gains. In addition, parents have a long-term obligation to their children that is theoretically quite broad in scope, requiring them to follow problems across organizational boundaries. In short, there is a great deal of ambiguity both about what the responsibility entails and, at various times, who owns the responsibility. We can, nevertheless, make some generalizations about variations in the acceptance of responsibility that extend beyond parenting.

Fundamentally, whether one accepts a responsibility depends less on its magnitude than on whether one has ownership of the responsibility, incentives to exceed minimum standards, the resources to secure the contributions of others, and the authority to follow the responsibility across organizational borders. Taking responsibility requires that all of these pieces come together. Nevertheless, how they come together is still quite variable, and there is no single route to responsibility. Ownership may be more or less ambiguous and may be elected or assigned. Incentives may be supplied by such different entities as kin, employers, or the state. Resources may be plentiful or scarce. And authority may be found in the law, spelled out in contracts, or arranged in hierarchies. Some may have the incentive to assume a responsibility but lack ownership, others may have ownership but lack the resources and incentives, and still others must be coaxed or coerced into taking ownership in the first place.

Taking responsibility, as we have argued throughout this book, requires that people strategize and choose among various courses of action. The question we have tried to answer is how to get people to choose the responsible course of action over another course of action. Perhaps one of the most surprising, and reassuring, findings of this book is that parents so often choose responsibility over shirking. Of course, we must keep in mind that our sample probably underrepresents the most neglectful or abusive parents, and, by design, it excludes those who quickly relinquished their parental rights. However, what we have learned here is about how agency is motivated. People are more likely to assume responsibilities, we have argued, when they believe that they in particular are needed to do the job. While the unique tie that binds parent and child is not duplicated in other settings where we may wish to understand more about responsibility, the more people feel an outcome depends on their unique contribution, the more likely they will be to take responsibility. The question then becomes how to get people to feel that their contributions are crucial. Assigning responsibilities is not enough. People must also have the resources to secure the contributions that are necessary to produce good outcomes. Telling workers they are responsible for the bottom line, for instance, matters little if they are not also given the tools to improve productivity. The practice in some organizations of referring to projects as "babies" is perhaps quite revealing, a sign that people have come to see their work as something for which they have a unique responsibility. And it is also significant that parents sometimes refer to their infants and children as their "project." Such a comment, we believe, is an acknowledgment that an unusual amount of effort and attentiveness is required and that raising the child in question is more than just living with him or her while the child grows up. Not surprisingly, this comment is often heard in the homes of NICU graduates.

While we have stressed the variation between individual parents in their acceptance of responsibility in this book, we also hope that we have shown how taking responsibility is more than an individual triumph and shirking more than an individual defeat. Responsibility requires individuals to make strategic choices but is still fundamentally social. While we have drawn on the lives and stories of individual parents in this book, we have used these tales to demonstrate how normative systems encourage or undermine the taking of responsibility. This is at once, then, the story of variations in individual grit and determination and the story of how different mixes of incentives and resources produce different results. Below, we revisit just one such individual tale, that of Sue and Will, and recount it in the light of all we have learned about the social conditions of taking responsibility.

Responsible Adaptations to the Organizational World: One Family's Story

How would we tell the story of Sue and Will differently now? Sue and Will illustrate well some of the core points of this book. They had become convinced that responsible parents follow problems across organizational borders. Because parents have the ultimate responsibility for their child's well-being, they cannot be too respectful of organizational or occupational boundaries. Parents are not absolved of their responsibility just because some task is part of another person's job. For Sue and Will, the boundary between family and medical organizations had been breached many times. Crossing the boundary had been uncomfortable. Sue was equally unhappy about having to intrude in NICU business and about having nursing care at home. She ventured into the "superintendent's" office only because she had to and invited nurses into her home only reluctantly. But this was now, to them, part and parcel of being a parent. "Who says that a baby is gonna come out 110% okay," Sue asked (1009F, p. 38). Listing all of the extra tasks entailed in caring for Tiffany, Will insisted that he and Sue had to define these things as normal: "We've got to do these things. No big deal. We got extra things to do. Let's just face it, and that's it, you know" (1009M, p. 42).

By the time she was thirteen months old, Tiffany had logged about six months (the first four-and-a-half months in a single stretch) in six different hospitals. Sue had also spent a day or two in labor at still another hospital before being transferred to the hospital where Tiffany was born. While the hospitals were the most consequential organizations in the family's life, Sue and Will also were, or had been, involved with two employers (his and hers), his insurer, the public aid department, the Katie Beckett program (a federal program providing financial resources to enable families to care for chronically ill or disabled children at home rather than put them in institutions), the WIC program (Women, Infants, and Children, a federal nutritional program), the home health organization that trained and supplied Tiffany's nurses, a medical supplier, the organization that sent the occupational therapist and physical therapist to their home, and the school where they had just begun nursing classes. Sue and Will had an unusually large number of organizational borders to cross, and in this sense, their case is not representative of normal parenting or even of parenting a child who has been in an NICU. However, most parents have to negotiate at least some of these kinds of borders at some point in their child's life. And because Sue and Will had to negotiate so many, they became unusually adept at that and are therefore especially good informants about the difficulties of living in an organizational world.

Few of these contacts with organizations were uncomplicated. Although Will and Sue were generally very optimistic and were pleased with how they had negotiated their relations with physicians and other hospital personnel, they clearly felt that their activist approach was crucial to their daughter's well-being. As Will put it, "You can't just take their word for gold because . . . this is their profession. . .you still have to look at all four corners" (p. 40). Sue and Will pressed physicians hard to consider other options: "We had to dig and like, you know, 'Is there anything else, is there anything else?'" (1009M, p. 28). When they learned that physicians at City Hospital might be able to perform a less-invasive procedure, they pressed to have Tiffany transferred for this treatment. They could not call City physicians themselves but instead had to work through Tiffany's doctors. Although they found this frustrating, Will remembers that they got some coaching and support from a nurse and several social workers.[11] Working out the details took weeks, and Sue and Will had to press Tiffany's doctor repeatedly to make contact with the physicians at City. At one point the annoyed doctor conceded that it was time to call again, commenting, "I'm gonna call him to get you people off my back" (1009M, p. 30). But Sue and Will thought their intervention paid off handsomely—while physicians at the first NICU had planned to perform three surgical procedures, physicians at City concluded that only two were necessary. Sue and Will thus saved their tiny baby one surgery.

In the opening pages of the book we described the other major conflict that Sue and Will had with one of the hospitals. That conflict took Sue all the way to the top of the organization and led to Tiffany's transfer to another hospital. Both Will and Sue were pleased that they had not tolerated shoddy care for their daughter and felt that they had behaved in an exemplary fashion in confronting staff members with the problems and insisting on the transfer. When a physician, examining Tiffany in his office, concluded that she needed to be hospitalized, he browbeat Sue with sugges-

11. Will also reported learning from other parents who were staying in charity hostels for families of sick children near several of the hospitals where Tiffany received care. In addition to inexpensive housing, this chain of charity hostels may be providing one of the few institutional mechanisms supporting transmission of information among parents.

tions that her daughter would die unless she was taken to the hospital where she had originally been treated—even though Sue and Will had concluded that the care of trach patients was dangerously sloppy at this facility. Sue levelheadedly pointed out that records could be transferred and phone calls made so that doctors at the new hospital would know Tiffany's medical history. Explaining why she felt so strongly about the choice of a hospital, Sue reviewed her discussion with Will on this subject. "I have enough pressure the way it is," she recalled telling her husband, "and I don't need a shitty hospital on top of it or, or vendors, you know. You have to be picky and choosy because, um, you know there are a lot of pressures the way it is, and that's all you need is somebody to give you a harder time" (p. 57).

Generally, Will felt that they had had to scramble to get the information they needed. When it turned out that Will's insurance covered only a small fraction of Tiffany's expenses (although the policy provided generous coverage for most conditions, it was very stingy about covering the expenses of an infant who was sick at birth), Will and Sue applied for public aid to cover their medical expenses. Ultimately they did not qualify for the program—Will's laborer salary was too high, and they would have had to "spend down" each month before they received any state contribution. At a time when they had moved in with his parents because they were paying so much for the motels, dorms, and restaurant or cafeteria meals that allowed them to spend time with Tiffany, Will found this policy ludicrous. Fortunately, they eventually learned about the Katie Beckett program, which paid many of Tiffany's medical expenses without subjecting the family to a monthly spend down. But Will seemed to feel that it was almost a fluke that they learned of the program: "We had to dig for our information to find out about the Katie Beckett Program. They didn't just come to us and say, 'Oh, we have the Katie Beckett Program.' We had to go through social service and even the lady who helped us through the social service, for the like the medical assistance, she didn't even know about the Katie Beckett Program. She had to—someone else found out about it and got ahold of us. . . . Those kinds of things should be more at hand to you, you know" (1009M, p. 67).

Sue and Will found the invasion of home health nurses sufficiently distressing that they immediately cut back on the nurses' hours. When Tiffany first came home, she was eligible for sixteen hours of nursing a day. "Sue hated to have people in our house, and so did I. But not as bad as she did," Will commented in explaining why they had immediately cut back to ten hours of nursing. At the time of our interview, they had nurses for eight hours, largely so they could go to school and run errands. Sue gave a fuller account of her reasons for wanting to cut back on nursing. Privacy was only the tip of the iceberg by her account. "Sometimes it's almost twice the job," Sue concluded as she told us about her work supervising the nurses (p. 60).[12] She estimated that they had had thirty different nurses since Tiffany had come home and that they regularly had six nurses coming to their home during any given week. Sometimes when new nurses were being trained, Tiffany's room would be crowded with a nurse, two trainees, and the equipment supplier, as well as several others. "You wake up in the morning, and that's all you want to see is the whole population," Sue complained (p. 54). Although Will and Sue could not select nurses, they did occasionally inform the agency that a nurse was not working out: "There was this one nurse I really did not like. Tiffany threw up, and I thought she [the nurse] was gonna have a heart attack, she was just so nervous around her. Just throwing up, you know—normal babies throw up—but she [mother demonstrates big gasp], you know, and she was actually shaking, and I just, 'Whoa, that is enough.' So I called up the nursing care the next day, and I said I didn't want her back in here, she was too afraid. I said, 'And if she's afraid 'cause Tiffany throws up, what's she gonna do when she has to do CPR? Or Tiffany coughs out her trach? I can't handle that, you know.' I says, 'I can't even leave the house in peace.' So, um, that way we have a way of choosing" (1009F, p. 53).

Some of the glitches were worked out over time. After she noticed that the head nurses were skipping over things they themselves didn't understand when they trained new nurses, Sue spent some time instructing the head nurses about Tiffany's equipment and clarifying her expectations about household rules. Sue still expected to spend several hours training each new nurse, although she continued to resent it when nurses asked her questions when they could have found answers in the written instructions. More frightening, though, were the mistakes nurses had made. Occasion-

12. Sue is somewhat unusual here. She defined supervising the nurses as an important part of her job as a parent. Other parents who had home nursing did sometimes discuss supervision of nursing—Marta [1017] and Janet [1036], especially, commented on supervision and training of nurses. But often parents' comments stressed their own competence as much as the nurses' incompetence. And none of the other parents seemed to spend as much time on supervision and training as Sue did. Other parents also commented on privacy issues (esp. Ken [1036]), though of course parents living in cramped apartments or sharing a house with in-laws would be more troubled by invasions of privacy than would families with more room.

ally nurses had inadvertently turned off Tiffany's oxygen supply or forgotten to give her medicines even though schedules were posted.

Sue had made valiant efforts to rationalize her interactions with the nursing staff in order to minimize the disruption to her household. We have already noted her investment in training the head nurses. "You don't know who's gonna come in next," Sue observed, explaining how she had pressed the nursing agency (in vain) to give her a weekly schedule. "We just leave the door open and they come in" (p.55), she added, explaining how they had negotiated entrances and exits with the nursing staff. She probably did not see the full symbolic importance of this capitulation. With this last concession, she ceded her right to exclude outsiders from her home.

Although she followed protocols carefully (and insisted that others do so as well), Sue also resisted therapists' gentle attempts to medicalize her relationship with her daughter. Although the therapists wrote her notes about what she and Tiffany should be doing, Sue continued "playing with her like normal people" (p. 26). Tiffany's development confirmed her view that her policy was acceptable: "I wasn't really, 'Well I gotta do this because the occupational therapists said,' you know. Not everybody has an occupational therapist when they have a baby, you know. So, somehow they learn, and I must be doing okay" (1009F, p. 26).

Sue had been particularly upset over her difficulties with an equipment supplier whose incompetent maintenance man would not accept her word about which nozzles were required, couldn't make a monitor function (Sue later discovered that this was because he had failed to remove a piece of tape), and who couldn't calibrate the machine so that it functioned for the child (to Sue's amusement, he tested it on himself, just as she had, and then was surprised when it didn't work for Tiffany). "You know I could have done his job," she exclaimed in exasperation (p. 51). At one point she telephoned him in outrage: "'This is your job,' I said. 'And if you don't know how to do it, you should have somebody else that knows how'" (p. 51). But Sue was especially outraged that the repairman could just walk away whether or not he had successfully completed his work. Once, when Sue had to leave the room briefly, he called to her, "Well gotta go, Sue, see you later." After he had slipped out, Sue returned to her daughter's room and discovered that the repairman had turned the monitor off: "He turned the monitor off, left it off her because it wouldn't work, and he left. And I said, 'That is enough.'" (p. 51). Sue and Will changed to another equipment vendor after this last incident, but they then had to go through a period of adjusting to yet another organization and its personnel.

Will and Sue's troubles were legion, but both parents specifically point to the dilemmas that they faced as outsiders trying to influence the activities of organizational members, the frustration they felt when someone charged with a responsibility was either incompetent or unwilling to do the job, and the ambiguities associated with being the parent of the child but not the employer or formal supervisor of key workers. Complaining about not being respected because of their age, Sue repeatedly identified herself as a competent person who had received training. "You know I could have done his job," she said about the equipment repairman (p. 51). Sue also clearly identified herself as both a supervisor (noting that supervision sometimes seemed to be twice as much work as just doing it herself) and trainer of the nursing staff ("They're not always taught that well because a lot of times we end up taking the time that we pay them to be here to do their job [to train them ourselves] because they don't know how to do it" [p. 53]). Will several times remarked on how he and Sue had become "semi-pros" (p. 22, 29) and eventually "pros" (p. 47) in caring for their daughter. What is interesting, though, is that he adopted this language in describing his and Sue's increased confidence in challenging nurses and physicians when they believed that Tiffany was not being cared for appropriately. To challenge professional health-care providers, parents apparently have to begin to think of themselves almost as professional parents. But concerns about the respect accorded older parents compared with very young ones or professional workers compared with parents were not matters that would have troubled Sue and Will had caring for their daughter not forced them to work in so many different organizational environments.

Like all new parents, Will and Sue had to learn how to diaper and bathe a newborn. But for them, the more important lessons were about parental obligations to care for their children even when that meant crossing organizational borders, learning new skills, and intruding on others' work. Because they had to, Sue and Will located another maintenance service when one repairman left without doing the work, trained nurses when supervisors didn't teach all the necessary material, investigated federal funding programs when hospital staff couldn't provide adequate information, and nagged physicians to make the calls to colleagues that parents cannot make for themselves. These tasks, which usually lie on the periphery of parenting, were only reluctantly taken up by Sue and Will, who would have preferred spending their time cuddling Tiffany and watching her grow. Describing her desire to be an "ordinary family," Sue yearned for privacy, for a reassertion of the boundaries of the family and the sanctity of the home, for a time when, "We can move on to another house, and just [have] *us*. I'm gonna lock the doors, shut the windows, you know, shut the drapes and it's just gonna be us for a while" (1009F, p. 60). While Sue and Will may long for a world in which they could meet all of Tiffany's needs themselves, should they be unable to provide what she needed, we can be sure that they, like other responsible parents, would fling open the door once again. And given Tiffany's situation and the organization of parenting in the modern world, that is probably what they will have to do.

Resolving the Paradoxes of Responsibility: Contributions of a Sociology of Responsibility

The social organization of responsibility is stunningly complex and revolves around a series of paradoxes—about agency and structure, essentialism and social construction, fate and opportunity, particularism and universalism, enrichment and impoverishment, and motivation and inspiration. These paradoxes juxtapose existential and philosophical matters with the concrete realities of human life. It is these paradoxes that a sociology of responsibility is uniquely equipped to explore, and our contribution, we believe, is to show how the elements of such paradoxes can comfortably coexist in social life.

On the one hand, to take responsibility means to exercise agency, to make decisions independently, to mobilize resources, to make commitments, and to make sacrifices. This is the stuff of moral theory and has been eloquently addressed by Kant, McKeon, Rawls, Nussbaum, and others. To take responsibility in this sense is part and parcel of what it means to be human, to be *social* creatures. On the other hand, we would be naive not to recognize the limitations on people's capacity to act independently, to resist others' definitions of themselves and their obligations, to work their way through bureaucratic routines, to overcome the limitations on resources and rights associated with particular social locations. The paradox may be partly resolved by Kant's observation: "The light dove, cleaving the air in her free flight, and feeling its resistance, might imagine that its flight would be still easier in free space" (1965a:47). Just as the modest resistance of the air is necessary for flight, so the resistance of the social world may be essential to the experience of agency. That is, it is precisely in shaking off the shackles of their social world that people feel the exhilaration of having made choices and influenced outcomes, but they also, ironically, feel most social in pledging themselves to others.

But how do people come to struggle, to oppose, to resist, to reshape, to choose, and to commit themselves? We have found that sustained close contact with another person (here, the critically ill infant) is a key part of the construction of the empathy that motivates action, but that other people (such as hospital staff members and spouses) often must help a person interpret the situation and construct an understanding that suggests which scripts should be adopted and which ones are inappropriate. How do they find the resources for action, and which resources end up being important? How much social pressure provides just enough resistance to make agency, individual choice on behalf of others and of our better selves, possible? And how much is too much, demoralizing rather than invigorating?

It is the humanity of other people that inspires responsibility, yet that humanity has to be constructed. This is especially clear where infants on the edge of viability lack many of the characteristics that mark creatures as people, as potential partners in a social relationship. Yet while the process by which people are constructed as people is particularly transparent here, it is hardly unique to this setting. Social life is full of instances in which we identify and cherish the particularity of those with whom we share our lives and probably equally filled with examples of our diminishment of others' humanity. If the social construction of people's humanness is essential to our feeling responsible for others, the social destruction of others' humanity is an equally important social process.

The irony here is that while others clearly provide us with the raw materials for constructing their identities and so our social relationships with them—eye contact, facial expressions, speech and other sounds, reactions to stimuli introduced in social interaction—there is nevertheless work to be done in attributing meaning to these materials. With the help of others and with the cultural materials at hand, we then construct the social beings that justify our feelings of attachment and responsibility. Social settings vary in the extent to which they provide materials for constructing the humanity of others and support the activities by which individual identities are formed and social relationships created. Social settings therefore vary in the extent to which they encourage or discourage taking responsibility. While the humanity of infants may be a social construction, the experience of the authenticity of a baby's human essence is central to responsibility.

People's reactions to fate are also paradoxical. We have argued in this book that responsibilities vary in the extent to which they are experienced as fates about which people have little choice or as opportunities which people can more freely choose to accept or reject. But, of course, hardly anything is by nature a fate (one's own death probably comes closer than anything else to being a truly inescapable fate). While responsibilities may feel like an inescapable fate, we have taken pains to show how people are made to feel that obligations are inescapable and to show that some people nevertheless do escape. Psychological research on the diffusion of responsibility suggests that responsibilities are more likely to be shirked when they are not uniquely assigned. If an obligation can be construed as belonging to several others, then in effect it belongs to no one.

Ironically, though, being the one fated to take on a responsibility is not always so onerous. An assignment of responsibility is also a right to act, to intervene, to be effective. And even when they feel obliged to take on a responsibility, people continue to feel that they make choices about how to face up to these fates. The sting of fate is thus lessened because people feel themselves to be choosing to embrace their responsibilities, to commit themselves to doing a good job of the tasks that life has handed them. But here we would guess that the social psychological experience varies with which choice a person makes. Although our research does not much speak to this issue, we would guess that a decision not to take on a fateful responsibility does not carry the social and psychological payoffs that come with a decision to embrace a responsibility. Although both are *decisions* about how to respond to social pressures, the decision to take responsibility is considerably more likely to garner support from others and to lead to the social satisfactions of being an honored and respected member of a community. Responsibilities that at first blush appear to be unadulterated opportunities may in fact require difficult moral choices. Opportunities can be exploited in responsible and irresponsible ways and so may in fact bring with them fateful responsibilities to social groups. Fates may thus turn out to be opportunities and opportunities may in fact be fates. People come to be moral beings by acting responsibly in response to their bad luck, but they also become more human by responsibly embracing their opportunities.

Appeals to take responsibility are built on claims about the universal needs of people as members of a class (here, the claim that all children need attention, food, warmth, and the like), but, ironically, it is only in recognizing the particularity of an individual that we really take responsibility. In this book we have explored a case in which the need for radically individualized treatment is easily understood. Medical people, working as a team and drawing on the contributions of ancillary professions and of parents, combine carefully worked-out protocols with more experimental procedures, as well as hit-and-miss attempts, to find what works. On the forefront of medicine it is easy to see that adjustment to the details of the particular situation matter—persistence and attentive fine-tuning could spell the difference between life and death or between a relatively normal life and a life with diminished capacities. But it is equally obvious that one cannot legitimately neglect obligations to some people on the grounds that this is the only way to meet obligations to others. Fine-tuning and adjustment are essential to responsibility in other settings as well, and they are built on a universalistic commitment to particularism. Because universalism and particularism are often considered to be opposing values and because it is much easier to institutionalize universalism than particularism, some normative systems and some ways of formulating rules and laws work better as ways to enshrine these values than do others. Here we have explored the variety of ways that particularism and continuous adjustment to changing circumstances are built into routines and made compatible with the universalism that is required for responsible balancing of the needs of multiple parties. Universalism makes it clear that all have a right to draw on the resources of the community and that we have responsibilities to many people, but particularistic values remind us that we cannot really meet anyone's needs if we try to meet them all the same way.

Responsibilities often are a drain on the resources of those who accept them. To take on a responsibility typically means agreeing to devote a disproportionate share of resources to meeting that obligation, and acceptance of responsibility often does not bring with it any additional resources. This is less true for responsibilities that arise in formal organizations than for those that are part of private life, but in either case accepting a responsibility requires some willingness to shift resources from one pot to another and especially to sacrifice one's own welfare to meet the obligation. Why then do people often describe themselves as enriched rather than drained by the experience? We would argue that above a subsistence level, what is experienced as a reward and what seems like a cost are to a large degree socially defined. While no one would suggest that a family was not impoverished by having to move to a smaller house and having less to spend on entertainment, clothing, or new furniture, we would not necessarily expect that they would be less happy just because they had fewer or lower-quality material goods. Perhaps more important, though, it matters how such decreases in material welfare come about. All things being equal, poorer people may be less happy than richer people. But if decreases in material welfare come about because people have decided to devote those resources to something they care about, in fact they may be better off. Praise for doing the right thing, the satisfaction of seeing that one's investments are paying off, and the rewards of being part of a team or project may more than compensate for decreases in material welfare if people focus their attention on social, rather than material, rewards. Taking responsibility then may lead to material impoverishment but social, psychological, and spiritual enrichment.

Finally, we have argued that responsibilities can only rarely be met within the confines of interpersonal relationships; in contemporary life, to meet responsibilities often requires intervening in organizational routines. But when people are outsiders, and especially lower-status outsiders, and when they must cross organizational boundaries to meet their obligations, they may not have the right kinds of resources to induce others to act on their behalf and may lack the information to monitor others' actions. What happens when our dependence on others' efforts is not matched with the resources and memberships that would allow us to induce them to help us meet our responsibilities?

Ironically, we have found that sometimes when people cannot offer the standard incentives (such as career advancement or money), they may get others committed to their cause in another way. As others have found in studies of projects, social movements, and some total institutions, rewards and punishments work differently in social locations that are considered to be "where the action is." When people find a project or activity inspiring, they are willing to accept fewer of the rewards that are usually expected. The inspiration effect thus acts as a multiplier of other rewards. Who can be enlisted as a participant no doubt depends on people's other commitments and on what role they are being asked to play in the project. In the case we examined here, parents would be unable to convince hospital staff members to give up other patients and to devote themselves exclusively to a single baby. But parents' enthusiasm may well motivate greater attentiveness even though parents have few other rewards to offer.

In examining these paradoxes, we have shown how moral commitments are created. Social organizations add rigidity in the form of routines that have to be followed, they add layers of hierarchy that have to be penetrated, and they mark borders which have to be crossed. We cannot understand these paradoxes of responsibility without looking at the social world in which they are resolved. By depicting these paradoxes, philosophers and social theorists have clarified why it is so difficult to design a social world in which people routinely overcomply with social obligations. But empirical investigations are imperative if we are to see how the paradoxes are resolved. When we look closely, we see that in fact constraint is the precondition for some kinds of freedom, that fates are transformed into opportunities, that the humanity and individual identity that seem so essential are at least partly the generous accomplishment of a social group, that universal claims can only be fully honored when we recognize the particularity of claimants, that individuals are enriched when they accept a different sort of impoverishment, and that the incapacity to motivate others with rewards and punishment may not matter so much when it is possible to inspire them instead.

Our central argument, then, is that when we study the taking of responsibility, the use of human rationality and generosity to live up to obligations to others, many traditional problems of moral theory become clearer. When we ask about the conditions under which people are likely to take responsibility, we are not simply revisiting philosophical debates about when people should be held accountable for their actions or what principles lead to a responsible balancing of the needs of the members of a society. Morality is not simply about compliance, and we therefore argue that the key question is not when people should be held accountable but rather what social arrangements encourage them to hold *themselves* accountable. Similarly, we argue that we must shift our focus from questions about the principles that justify various distributions of welfare to ones about how people come to care about the welfare of others and to commit themselves to doing the best they can to achieve moral outcomes in the world in which they live.

APPENDIX ON METHODS

"Discussing methodology is like playing the slide trombone. It has to be done extraordinarily well if it is not to be more interesting to the person who does it than to others who listen to it," the economist Frank Knight once observed (cited in Merton, Sills, and Stigler 1984:331). Because we cannot claim to be methodological virtuosos, we will restrict our comments here to the few topics where our experience may prove most useful to others.

The research reported in this book was, as we have noted earlier, carried out in two kinds of settings. Some of the work was conducted in hospitals, and the rest in people's homes (or in a few instances in restaurants or workplaces). The research was organized around two NICUs, where we conducted fieldwork, collected evidence from medical records (by the time we examined the records, they had been moved to the medical records departments of the hospitals), and interviewed staff members. From the medical records we collected information about each NICU's patient population and used each set of records to draw a sample for interviewing. The children of the parents we interviewed had all been discharged from the hospital; the babies had been admitted to the hospital during the year or so before we were doing our fieldwork.

Interviewing and Fieldwork as Complementary Activities

This research project actually began with work not directly reported in this book. During the very early stages of the project, Heimer attended parent-support group meetings in several hospitals with Level 2 and 3 nurseries. The object of this work was to learn what issues were important to parents of NICU graduates and how they talked about them. After several months of observing meetings, it was time to start the main research. At that point, the idea was to spend a bit of time seeing how an NICU worked and afterward to move on to the parent interviews, then conceived as the focus of the research project.

But things do not always go quite the way researchers intend. During the time when we (really just Heimer at that point) were doing fieldwork, we were also doing some trial interviews with parents from a parent-support group. By chance, two of the parents referred to a physician who was visiting the NICU where we were doing fieldwork. To our astonishment, both of these parents referred to this kindly physician as "Dr.

Death."[1] Our astonishment led us to see that we were considerably less prepared to do the interviews than we had thought, and we then modified the research plan and spent much more time in the NICU. That decision ended up being very important. Without those extra months in the NICUs themselves, we would not have been able to write chapters 5 and 6. The fieldwork provided a crucial context for the parent interviews but also let us see for ourselves how and why parent and staff perspectives are so different.

Our early discomfort in the NICU gave us a hint about how other newcomers to this strange high-tech environment must feel. At the same time, fieldwork alone would not have been enough. As other researchers have noted, it is hard to see things from the patient or family perspective when one is doing research in a hospital. Chastising himself for being too uncritical of staff accounts, Bosk (1992) pays insufficient heed to the reasons why it is so difficult to learn about patient and family views. When researchers enter the field with the sponsorship of those who are the repeat players in the system, they can ally themselves with the "one shotters" only by systematically severing their ties with their sponsors. Both Chambliss (1996) and Wieder (1983) point out that participants easily pick up clues (and not always the right clues) about who is allied with whom. Only by leaving the organizational turf is it possible to get adequate information about those who pass through as clients rather than remain as workers. Because it is not feasible to do sustained fieldwork in people's homes, interviews are a reasonable way to redress the otherwise very serious imbalance in information.

We hasten to add, though, that one can do some fieldwork in people's homes (and

1. Much later, we believed we understood why these parents had been so offended. This couple had encountered "Dr. Death" as the attending physician responsible for the care of their very premature twins. He was cautious about the prospects of these infants and informed the parents that they might not survive and that, if they did survive, they were likely to have significant continuing problems, including developmental delays and physical handicaps (such as difficulties with vision, mobility, and cerebral palsy). The parents found his "gloom and doom" stance disconcerting—they were aware of the risks the physician described but remained very optimistic. As we spoke with them (they had agreed to allow us to pretest our interview guide on them), both parents also gave poignant accounts of the birth of a stillborn daughter a couple of years before the arrival of the twins. What we finally concluded was that the physician and the parents were using different comparison points. For the parents, comparing their premies with the stillborn daughter, the twins were full of life. For the physician, the natural comparison point would surely have been other newborns or other infants in the NICU, and the twins did not fare nearly so well in that comparison.

As prospect theorists have shown, how people reason about risks depends on whether they classify a choice as leading to a potential loss or a potential gain (see Tversky and Kahneman [1974] for an early presentation of this argument; see Heimer [1988] for a discussion of how the arguments apply to decisions in natural settings). Choices that are formally identical (e.g., that have the same expected value) may be framed in a variety of ways. The location of the "anchor point"—the status quo with which possible outcomes are compared—is crucial in determining whether decision makers see themselves as attempting to avoid losses or as seeking gains. Given his grim view of the current situation, "Dr. Death" probably saw the choices as primarily decisions about potential gains. The parents, who defined themselves as the parents of living twins (rather than of a stillborn daughter), probably framed the choices primarily as decisions about how to avoid losses.

Hochschild [1989] managed to do quite a lot). Generations of survey research interviewers have been instructed to make notes about the homes of their respondents and the demeanor of the subjects during the interviews. But it is possible to do much more than that. Here, we believe that we made a virtue of necessity. Because all of the parents we interviewed had small children, we had to devise some way to conduct lengthy interviews in the face of the very substantial capacity of toddlers to disrupt any adult social interaction. Our transcribers could testify that we were only partially successful. Our interviews are full of discussions of toys, comments to and about children who wanted food, demanded comfort after hurting themselves, or required some intervention to keep them from damaging household goods or their siblings. Such interruptions are interruptions, of course, but they are also opportunities to observe. We thus have not only what parents said about their relations with their children but also some evidence about how they interacted with their children.

Admittedly these observations were not made under "usual" circumstances. Household activities were being disrupted by the intrusion of one, or more often two, strangers. Often we were clearly marked as strangers rather than friends or acquaintances by our white skin, middle-class appearance and speech patterns, and the like. We did sometimes get clear indications that we were a disruption. In one African-American household, several adult men came in during the interview, and one of them asked sarcastically, "What is this? Instant integration?" In another household, the interview was terminated abruptly when the mother said she was feeling too ill to continue. More mundanely, children became tired, meals needed to be prepared, and diapers had to be changed. Even when one household member had decided to be on good behavior for the strangers, others had not necessarily agreed to go along. To capitalize on these opportunities for observation, as often as we could we arranged for two people to go to each interview. The second person also could be mobilized to do an interview with the other parent if both parents were there and consented to be interviewed, or the second researcher could care for the children, making it more likely that the interview could be completed. We also routinely wrote or dictated field observations to accompany the taped interviews. Sometimes these took the form of a discussion between the two of us as we drove back from the interview.

There is no substitute for the kind of careful observation that informs this book. Though fieldwork is time consuming and often difficult, this would be a very different book without the benefit of our extensive observations. And, by the same token, we could not have written this book without the scores of informants and respondents who shared their work and lives with us. We wish here not simply to sing the praises of these methods of data collection but also to underscore the importance of a flexible research design. Methods, after all, are the tools of the sociologist's trade, and different jobs require different tools.

Negotiating Access to the NICU

Getting official approval from the hospitals to carry out our research was an important hurdle, but really only the first step in negotiating access. We spent most of our time in the NICU "hanging around" the patients' bedsides, watching as doctors and nurses carried out their daily activities in the NICU and as parents visited their infants, participated in their child's care, learned new techniques, and talked with doctors and nurses. Though, on the one hand, this is an easy place to do fieldwork—there are very few closed doors, and so many people pass through the NICU that a researcher's presence is not in any way disruptive—on the other hand, this is also a high-tech medical environment that takes some getting used to. Our initial shock, and in some cases horror, gradually subsided, but we are left with vivid memories of babies who died what looked like agonizing deaths, of distraught parents, and of extremely premature or disfigured infants. We both had some nightmares during our time in the NICUs we studied. And indeed, it seems hard to imagine how anyone could visit these places and be unmoved.

But in addition to the emotional challenges of conducting research in an NICU, there were other more practical challenges, as well. The NICU is a very busy, crowded place, and a person who is not doing something in the NICU is often, quite literally, in the way. While the hustle and bustle of the NICU helped shield our observations to some extent, still people are often uncomfortable when they know they are being observed. We wanted to be able to move freely throughout the unit so we could observe whatever seemed interesting while we were there, but some staff members were more suspicious about our intentions than others.

Though no one was openly hostile, we were asked several times by various staff members, "Who are *you*?" The higher the status of the inquirer, the more likely the query was to be posed as a challenge. Since the NICU has very few walls and even less privacy, barriers were constructed in other ways. Such queries may be roughly translated to: "Do you have a right to be here? And if so, do I want you to be here?" Official permission to carry out research and conduct observations is, alas, no substitute for the willingness of the subjects to be observed. There is no easy answer to the problem of gaining access to a field setting. Introductions from social workers helped, but our success ultimately depended on our persistence and our ability to ingratiate ourselves with the staff. Demonstrating an interest in what they were doing had to be balanced against the possibility of arousing anxiety, sometimes verbalized, that we were evaluating them. When a therapist asked one of us, "What're you doing here anyway? Looking for what we do wrong?" a nurse who was also at the bedside quipped, "She doesn't *know* enough to know if we're doing anything wrong!" In this case, hiding a bit of expertise and redirecting interactions toward small talk helped immeasurably in gaining the confidence of the staff at the bedside.

We believe that having two researchers was also a real bonus to helping us gain access and secure the confidence of the staff members in the NICU. Although this project began as a solo effort, for most of its life it has been a team effort. Among the many intellectual, motivational, and personal benefits of working with a co-author, it was in the NICU itself, where we spent sufficient time to become identified more closely with one group of people than another, that it was really essential to have two of us. With two field-workers, we were able to divide our labor, with one of us spending most of her time with the physicians and the other with the nurses. This division of labor (while not carved in stone) extended to which meetings we attended regularly, what we observed and whom we talked to when we were on the unit, and whom we interviewed more formally. The cautionary statement that other researchers have made about avoiding being identified too strongly with one group lest it affect one's ties with another group can thus be managed either by scrupulously avoiding being identified with anyone or by having some team members identified with some groups, others with other groups. An obvious limitation here is that teams cannot expand indefinitely. Because of the intimate connection between observing and writing, we chose not to use the labor of people other than ourselves for either interviewing or fieldwork.

We eventually did become comfortable in the NICUs we studied. Initial awkwardness was replaced gradually by a sense of belonging. We came to know the routines of the units, and they came to know ours. We developed relationships with reliable informants and were no longer shocked by much that we saw. We attended meetings as well, but gaining meaningful access to the meetings was much simpler than gaining access to the rest of the round of activities in the NICU. Once we had secured permission to attend a given meeting, our presence came to be taken for granted, and our observations and note taking no cause for concern. There was no awkwardness about where to stand, no sense of intrusion, no straining to overhear, no question about the nature of our role as observers, and no hushed voices when we were present.

Although the NICU staff members usually were quite willing to let us observe their activities and to share their experiences in formal and informal interviews, helping us with our research was a low priority compared with caring for sick babies, tending to anxious parents, and even completing administrative work. Interviews were postponed or just delayed for several hours, people forgot to inform us when meetings with parents were scheduled or rescheduled, and more than once we arrived for a regularly occurring meeting only to learn that everyone else knew that it wouldn't occur on a holiday. While these delays and cancellations served as a salutary reminder of where social science research fits into the round of hospital life, they also gave us another view of how parents, also outsiders, experience the hospital. While staff members complain a good deal about delays and cancellations caused by parents, they seem less aware of just how often parents wait anxiously for a chance to talk with their infant's doctor or how frequently parents arrive expecting test results only to be told that they are not yet available. Parents are not privy to the details of hospital schedules (e.g., which holidays will be observed and what kinds of meetings will be canceled for a holiday) and are unlikely to be part of the network of people who are kept posted on last-minute changes in the schedules of key personnel. Waiting for meetings and interviews thus not only gave us additional time to do fieldwork as we cooled our heels but also reminded us that parents would experience similar periods of waiting and wondering.

But what happens in meetings and on the floor of the unit is, of course, only part of the story. For the rest of the story, we had to be patient and persistent in order to gain the confidence of those we hoped would let us into their worlds.

Winning the Confidence of Potential Respondents and Reassuring Institutional Review Boards

We preceded our phone calls to the parents we hoped to interview with letters of introduction that explained the main purpose of the research project and informed them that we would be contacting them by telephone in order to arrange an interview. Such letters were a mixed blessing, it turns out, but one about which we had little choice—both the university and hospital human subjects committees required them and placed some constraints on their content. Although some groups of people found the letters a reasonable introduction, other respondents had clearly been put off by them. Despite the university letterhead, they were convinced we were in some way or other out to deprive them of welfare checks, Medicaid cards, disability payments, or even of their child. Official letters are not always reassuring. As field-workers have long known, official endorsements do not always help and often harm a research project, and we were often required to do repair work when contact was later made over the telephone or in person.

We were also required to have interview respondents sign informed-consent forms, indicating that their participation had not been coerced. And these forms, too, were a mixed blessing. One of the institutional review boards even went so far as to ask us to get witnesses to add their signatures to the consent forms along with ours and those of our respondents. We dissuaded them from this by pointing out that it was difficult simultaneously to promise confidentiality and to arrange for someone else to be present for a signing ceremony at the beginning of the interview. Although we also pointed out that we couldn't force anyone to consent to an interview and that we reassured respondents that they could refuse to discuss particular topics (though very few in fact did) or terminate the interview whenever they wished, we nevertheless agreed to have consent forms signed. But it did feel ridiculous asking for the signatures. We knew they had consented; they knew they had consented. It seemed petty to ask them to sign a form—as if we couldn't take them at their word. In some instances, however, the consent procedures ironically became occasions when we could build solidarity with our respondents. Emphasizing that we were required to ask them to sign the form, even though it seemed impossible for us to get an interview with them without their consent, gave us an occasion for alliance against bureaucracy and a point of departure for discussing the ways in which bureaucratic requirements seem either inefficient or counterproductive.

This is not to say that we take either informed consent or providing appropriate introductions to our work lightly. The problem is rather that the routinized forms that seeking consent now takes are insufficiently respectful of the differences among people in what they wish to be told and when they might hesitate to give their consent. We don't have any good solution to this problem. But the arrangements we ended up making with our respondents did vary with their circumstances and their concerns. We have concealed the identities of all of our respondents, even when they initially told us that they wished we would include their real names. But we have taken more pains to conceal the identities of some of our respondents than others. Although we have not altered any essential facts of the cases presented in this book, we have been careful to conceal any identifying information both when a case was more unusual and when the parents expressed more concern about confidentiality. Rather than list the exact occupations of parents, for instance, we have simply referred to their general occupational categories, and rather than list extremely rare medical diagnoses, we have described the child's problems in more general terms.

The problems posed to a researcher by issues of confidentiality vary with the details of the research design. In general, researchers' concerns with protecting anonymity should probably vary directly with the vulnerability of the individual concerned. That means we should probably be more concerned with protecting the identities of parents and children than of hospital staff members. In our case that turns out to be relatively easy. Many of the children whose cases form the core of this book have been patients in more than one medical facility. Their homes are dispersed throughout the Midwest; some live several hundred miles from the facilities where we got their names. We have not identified the years in which we conducted our research, but even in those years, something over nine hundred patients passed through the two units we studied. We thus think it essentially impossible that anyone other than the parents themselves would recognize their case, and even then perhaps only where the case is discussed in some detail.

Some of our initial concerns about protecting the identity of staff members were allayed when one of our NICU informants read an early draft of a paper. She left the paper in her mailbox, intending (with our permission) to share it with a colleague. But before she could pass the draft on, it disappeared from her mailbox. Because we had put in some extended citations to field notes describing particular incidents in the NICU and had been asking for guidance specifically about these passages, we were initially quite concerned about the "theft." But our informant reassured us that only if you knew the location of the NICU and had observed these particular incidents would you be able to identify the location and participants. It was a vivid portrait, but hardly one that revealed the participants' identities. Turnover was high among NICU staff members (because a substantial minority were residents rotating through or fellows in the unit for only a year or two) as well as among parents, so many of the participants we discussed were no longer with the hospital and had only been gathered in the NICU for a very brief period. Further, of course, events that seemed painful or could damage reputations at one point in time are much less capable of doing any damage at a remove of several years.

Locating Mobile and Socially Detached People

Most of our respondents were relatively easy to locate. If they had moved since we copied their address from the medical records, their mail was forwarded and new phone numbers were easy to find. Other parents, however, were exceedingly difficult to contact. But locating people was only the beginning. Getting them to consent to be interviewed and then actually completing the interview were further obstacles.

On a freezing winter day a few years ago, we followed a letter carrier around a ghetto neighborhood asking him if he had any idea where a young woman we were trying to locate lived. We weren't quite dressed for the weather, but figured that he was our last hope. We had devoted the better part of a day to this search. We knocked on the doors of several addresses we had found in the medical record but were often met with wary looks and skeptical, vague responses. People, with good reason, are skeptical of strangers and simply aren't very eager to divulge information about the whereabouts of friends and relatives. In spite of their reluctance, we did manage to convince a few people to give us leads, but they were often quite vague and didn't amount to much: "I don't know, but try that house down the street on the corner," they would say, pointing. With no address and four houses on a corner, we found ourselves knocking on many doors. The letter carrier was also wary, and it took some effort to persuade him that we were not up to anything that would harm the woman in question. But our last-ditch effort paid off, and he directed us to the right house.

Although we had now located our potential respondent, our joy was short-lived. Our work had just begun, because she still had not agreed to an interview. We first had to locate the mother at home to ask her if she would agree to be interviewed. And this was no mean feat. The house where she was living had no telephone, she was unemployed, and she tended to come and go as she pleased. After some weeks, several trips to her home, and at least one occasion where we thought we had an interview scheduled but she was not at home when we arrived, we finally sat down for the interview. It had taken us a great deal of effort to land this interview and get in the door, and when we did, the situation was not one that any treatise on interviewing or field methods would endorse as the way to conduct an interview. Just off the foyer was a living room, and just beyond that a dining room that served as a place to watch television. The front room where we conducted our interview had a couch, some other dilapidated furniture, and a coffee table. During the interview, we could see clearly into the adjoining room where five adults and as many children gathered around the television. Children, especially the respondent's youngest son, wandered freely from one room to the other. Another child came inside with his bicycle and plopped it in front of the door. We had no privacy, but at the same time no one seemed particularly interested in what we were doing. Unfortunately, our respondent sometimes didn't either, perhaps because she wished to rejoin the group in the other room. She alternated between seeming engaged and detached, willing to do the interview but not willing to spend too much time at it. This may have had little to do with us or the content and more to do with our intrusion into their daily life. To us, it may have looked as if they weren't "doing anything," but to her it may have felt as if they were.

But why did it take so long for us to arrange this interview? We stress that this case is not terribly unusual. We had considerable difficulty finding out where the woman lived, to start off with. The medical record contains an address and phone number. But these pieces of information often do not lead directly to the respondent. Young mothers like this one move frequently, often live in someone else's home rather than have their own home, and often have no phone listing of their own. The phone number in the medical record may be for a neighbor's phone, and so of no use if the woman has moved, or it may be for a relative who can be relied on to transmit a message about an emergency but who justifiably may not wish to make a special effort to transmit a message about scheduling an interview appointment. And if the message is transmitted, why should anyone return the call? Typically a message will not supply sufficient context to make it meaningful, and it is nearly impossible to be persuasive about an interview second- or third-hand. Our observations (mainly in chapter 6) about principal/agent relations apply well here—we were the weakest of principals, with little capacity to induce intermediaries to act on our behalf in arranging interviews.

We believe that our difficulties locating people are important data. If we had such great difficulty finding a parent, might not a school teacher or nurse as well? If we had to reschedule our interviews because the respondent did not record appointments on a calendar, might there not be the same difficulties with keeping up on a child's shots? While we may be wrong here, and we were quite sure in a few cases that a scheduled appointment was actually an occasion to be absent from the house (one woman in particular seemed unable to refuse our requests for interviews, but instead refused by repeatedly rescheduling), for the most part the missed appointments seemed to be indicators of disorganization or detachment from a social world that functioned with fixed calendars and timetables. Ironically, it is sometimes more difficult to make appointments with people who are less busy than with those whose lives are very full.

As we have indicated already in the book, we had special difficulties locating fathers who were no longer attached to the mothers of their children. We often could not rely on the medical record to have information about the names and addresses of fathers who were not married to the mothers of their children. And if the parents were no longer involved with each other, mothers were often able to give us only very little to go on in our search. In one instance, the mother had some contact with the father even though they were no longer involved, and she provided his name and a work telephone and address where we could contact him. Unfortunately, the nature of his business required him to be out of the office most of the time, and we never successfully contacted him. We sent a letter to the small shop he owned and left messages on his answering machine, but he never returned our calls. We even drove to his place of business several times hoping to catch him there, but we never did.

Another father was easier to locate, but we were still unsuccessful in getting an interview. Although the mother had no contact with the father of her children, she was able to send us to the family business where she thought we might be able to get some information. After some inquiries, we found him at home. But we couldn't persuade him even to open the door. He peeked at us through the blinds and yelled at us to go away. The mother in this case had told us he was an alcoholic and would be unlikely to agree to be interviewed, and we took his hostile reaction seriously and put his file in the "refused" pile.

Noncustodial fathers were not only more difficult to locate, but they were also considerably less likely to agree to be interviewed even if we did locate them. Because their ties with their children were tenuous at best, we found it very difficult to coax these fathers into talking. Talking about children one doesn't live with and in some cases doesn't even know probably seemed pointless to some and painful to others. And once again, our difficulties in locating fathers and cajoling them into talking with us might be regarded as information about the kinds of troubles teachers and social service workers might encounter in attempting to include fathers in decision making about their children. And in the most extreme cases, our difficulties gave some hints about why couple relationships might have been difficult to sustain.

Despite these and other difficulties, we firmly believe that researchers must be persistent in the pursuit of people who may be hard to locate or reluctant to keep appointments. If we had limited ourselves to those people whose addresses we could easily locate, whom we could contact by telephone, or who honored their appointments with us, we would have eliminated an important part of our sample and shrunk the magnitude of variation we ultimately observed. Of course, there's no magic formula that tells how far to go to contact a respondent. We dedicated ourselves to this venture and would periodically set out with last-known addresses and maps in hand to try to contact those without phones. These people often lived in impoverished and potentially violent neighborhoods, so we would limit our searches to the morning and early afternoon, "before trouble got up," as one social worker advised us. We often had to screw up our courage to knock on a stranger's door inquiring about someone who was also a stranger to us. We were acutely aware that as white women in largely minority neighborhoods, we might be greeted with some skepticism about our intentions. And, indeed, many did seem reluctant as we tried to explain ourselves on the front stoop, speaking quickly before the door was closed in our faces (though we were relieved in one instance when the door closed after a man greeted us with his pants open). And our efforts didn't always pay off. We conducted many searches and pursued many other respondents after they failed to be home for an interview, and came up empty-handed. However, we believe that good social science requires researchers to pursue those people who would be systematically underrepresented if not for the tenacity of the interviewer. Here, even small returns add up to large payoffs.

Interviewing about Painful Subjects and Coding Stream-of-Consciousness Interviews

To some degree our discomfort with the notion of using other people's labor to do interviews or fieldwork stems from the nature of this project. We faced two important difficulties. First, we were trying to measure something that was both morally loaded and difficult to measure. Second, we were working in a setting where people were on an emotional roller coaster (to use a common metaphor). Both of these had profound effects on the way we conducted our research.

Although we knew there was no easy way to measure responsibility, we plunged ahead with our attempt to figure out some realistic way to distinguish more responsible from less responsible behavior in a way that didn't simply reflect common prejudices. Clearly the NICU staff thought they could tell who would be responsible parents, we noted. People who have a strong need to develop a reliable solution to a problem often come up with a fix, and this is often a good place to start in looking for a more general description of a problem and a more generalizable solution.[2] The NICU "solution" is situation specific, of course, and much of this book is an attempt to show how what

2. This is the same strategy that motivated the study of insurance as a starting point for learning about possible solutions to moral hazard and other risk-management problems commonly encountered in everyday life (see Heimer 1985).

happens inside the NICU compares with what happens after families leave the NICU and what might happen in other settings.

But figuring out how to measure something like responsibility is only half the problem. We also needed to convince ourselves and our readers that we were not merely social scientists spouting societal prejudices in dressed-up form. For this reason, we have highlighted the ways in which our findings do not fit with common prejudices. Not all young, unmarried, poor, or minority parents are irresponsible, and not all older, married, middle-class or white parents are responsible. Some of these characteristics are correlated with responsibility, but there are important intervening variables, and these are where our story is focused. We have also tried to provide as much raw data as possible in the text so that readers can assess for themselves the appropriateness of our conclusions.

A second difficulty with studying responsibility (in this setting at least) is that the stories we were asking people to tell were highly emotional, and our respondents often had strong reactions. Our trouble was not, as we had feared, that we had to pull the words out of people—to the contrary, we often had difficulty terminating the interviews. The difficulty was keeping the interview on track. During one of the pilot interviews, for instance, a seemingly innocuous question about whether the family had health insurance led to a twenty-minute discussion about choosing home birth rather than hospital birth, deciding to deliver the baby themselves without professional help, the parents' shock when the baby was stillborn, and more. As it turned out, this was related to the question of insurance—the parents lacked medical insurance and so had chosen home birth to avoid medical expenses they had no way to pay. The point is that in this kind of research, one never really knows where the question is going to lead and what it will be strategic to ask next given the answer that respondents give. For these reasons, the interviewing could not be "farmed out." We had to have a deep understanding of what the research was about to make any sensible judgment about when to probe, when to try to "get back to the subject," and when to let the respondent keep talking.

Further, as it turns out, there is no safe place to start these interviews. We had thought that background information might be a neutral starting point, but, to take one example, the mother's age when the baby was born is not neutral for very young mothers or for women whose conceptions occurred only after they had spent months receiving fertility drugs.

The stream-of-consciousness quality of the interviews made them quite difficult to code. We used an interview guide that would in theory ensure that we always covered certain topics. And while we usually managed to cover those topics, sometimes even heroic efforts and an interview guide didn't help. Sometimes parents had other obligations—they had to go to work, the child had a doctor's appointment. Sometimes, the interview was interrupted so often by children or by the telephone that we were unable to cover much ground. We often scheduled a second session, but were not always able to renew our contact with the family. One family spent a lot of time abroad; other families moved frequently; and, for other families, the obligations of caring for a very sick child simply made it logistically impossible to reschedule. So our data are not fully comparable on every family.

But the situation is worse than that. While it may be a chore to look through fifty to a hundred pages to locate information about the duration of a marriage or to find the ages of siblings, one can at least tell when it has been found. That is not always the case with the more central data. People do not all talk about responsibility in the same way, and often we did not fully understand the significance of some fact until we had reread the interview several times. It is for this reason that on key points (e.g., the coding that underlies the categorization of families in chapter 3), we worked out careful coding instructions and consulted frequently about the appropriate coding of particular statements. In addition, some time after the interviews were complete, transcribed, and the transcriptions corrected, we had research assistants go through the interviews compiling information about key topics. Later we had them sort for information on specific points so that we could check the representativeness of the quotations and examples we had selected for use in the text.

Finally, we should note that conducting the interviews and working with them afterward are a highly emotional enterprise. Our respondents often cried during the interviews. We often cried with them, and we learned to bring tissues, along with tape recorders and spare batteries, to interviews. We are no doubt only faint memories to most of our respondents—although we were astonished and pleased when one family kept us informed of their whereabouts for a few years after the interviews. But to us these people are very much alive, although frozen in time. To the two of us it has been a great comfort to have someone else know who these people are who have so populated our minds and hearts for years. And just as twins experience a special bond with the only other person who shares their invented language, elderly people with the remaining few who remember the era in which they grew up, and survivors of a natural disaster or war with those who experienced the horrors with them, we have been sustained by having someone else who also carries with her vivid mental images of people who are unknown to our friends, colleagues, and families. But, of course, the object here is not to keep these families secret. Although we have worried a great deal about issues of confidentiality, we nevertheless want others to know the essential parts of their stories. We have therefore been gratified when our research assistants commented on the interviews or on parts of the manuscript in ways that suggested that not only did they understand the argument we were making but that they also were moved. If as Zajonc (1980) suggests, feelings typically precede cognitive responses, we hope to grab people's minds by first grabbing their hearts.

Combining Disparate Data

From our point of view, one of the virtues of this project is the diversity of the data it uses. We have collected and analyzed interviews, field notes, and information from medical records. But having collected all these data, we then faced the difficulty of turning thousands of pages of transcriptions and notes into something meaningful. Making the data usable was itself as time consuming an enterprise as collecting them in the first place. One of the main difficulties, we believe, is that there really is no substitute for repeated readings of one's own interviews and field notes. Writing is not a linear process, but an iterative one. We at least cannot think without writing and cannot know how we need to code the data until we have started to write. But writing can't take place without knowing what's in the data, so notes also have to be reread. At most, computerized programs then provide a more sophisticated way of doing the old-fashioned cut and paste, a neater way of keeping track of the myriad files on the topics that become important as writing proceeds. This means that while our earliest coding was a necessary first step that was not in the end very useful, coding done late in the project was quite efficient.

We several times encountered difficulties transforming our data so they spoke to the same questions. Because we could not do all of the work at once, our field observations were done in the units from which our interview samples were drawn, but with a very few exceptions the infants whose parents we interviewed had been discharged a year or so before our observations and interviews began. Thus while we might be able to make statements about how events look to staff members and how they look to parents, we cannot usually say how the exact same events look to the two groups, because the parents we interviewed did not witness the events we witnessed and discussed with staff members. We therefore had to match categories of events rather than actual events, and this adds slippage that we would rather have avoided.

A similar problem occurs with coding information from medical records. Medical records are not produced for sociological research, obviously. Those recording information in the medical record have no reason to be careful about the things we would like them to be careful about. Some of the "errors" are comical. One infant's name was transformed into the name of a central African dictator. We thought it implausible that any parent would give a child that name and were very careful not to use it when we made our first contacts with the parents. And it turned out we were right—the child had an unusual nickname that had, by some weird administrative version of the children's game "telephone," been thoroughly transformed. The records contained errors, certainly, but other information, such as income, education, and other standard demographics, was completely missing. Race was sometimes incorrectly recorded. Occupation, which is hard to code even when one is trained, was haphazardly recorded. At best, intake workers would record the occupation of the parent who carried insurance for the child. But hospitals do care about one indicator of social class—whether the patient is covered by insurance—and that was reliably recorded. We thus ended up with rich, but hardly ideal, data.

The Organization of the Discipline and Funding and Dissemination of Theoretically Oriented Research

Finally, our research has been hampered by the tendency of social scientists to categorize research more by substantive areas than by theoretical questions. What makes our contribution important, we believe, is not so much its substantive focus as the questions it poses in those settings. But that means that at the stage when we needed research support to get the project started, it was hard to find. Sociologists of the family did not always sympathize with our focus. Medical specialists thought we drew too little on the work of medical researchers, and there weren't any researchers who specialized in the study of responsibility. There is no way to state this complaint that doesn't sound like sour grapes, of course, and we do not wish to dwell on this point beyond noting that the organization of the discipline and of research funding may discourage some kinds of work. At some point people have to choose for themselves whether they will do a piece of work even without funding and the legitimacy that funding brings. We ultimately chose to get on with the work rather than to submit more proposals.

As a project nears completion, the balkanization of academic disciplines leads to parallel problems in the dissemination of research results. We are eager for our work to be read by medical sociologists and sociologists of the family, but we believe that our findings are equally important to those interested in questions about the relationship between law and other normative systems, the persistence of gender inequality, incentive systems inside and on the boundaries of organizations, the social psychology of the diffusion of responsibility, and the place of moral discourse in an organizational world. Because we believe that the social organization of responsibility is of fundamental importance to both social theory and social policy, we have tried to pitch our work to a variety of audiences. While we believe that this was the responsible thing to do, we are aware that by attempting to speak to many, we run the risk of speaking to none.

REFERENCES

Abraham, Laurie Kaye. 1993. *Mama Might Be Better Off Dead: The Failure of Health Care in America.* Chicago: University of Chicago Press.

Ahrne, Göran. 1994. *Social Organizations: Interaction Inside, Outside, and between Organizations.* London: Sage Publications.

Aldrich, Howard E. 1979. *Organizations and Environments.* Englewood Cliffs, NJ: Prentice-Hall.

American Academy of Pediatrics Committee on Fetus and Newborn. 1995. "Perinatal Care at the Threshold of Viability." *Pediatrics* 96:974–76.

Anspach, Renée R. 1993. *Deciding Who Lives: Fateful Choices in the Intensive-Care Nursery.* Berkeley: University of California Press.

Arendell, Terry. 1986. *Mothers and Divorce.* Berkeley: University of California Press.

———. 1995. *Fathers and Divorce.* Thousand Oaks, CA: Sage.

Ariès, Philippe. 1962. *Centuries of Childhood.* New York: Vintage.

Arrow, Kenneth J. 1971. *Essays in the Theory of Risk Bearing.* Chicago: Markham.

———. [1985] 1991. "The Economics of Agency." Pp. 37–51 in John W. Pratt and Richard J. Zeckhauser, eds., *Principals and Agents: The Structure of Business.* Boston: Harvard Business School Press.

Barber, Bernard. 1983. *The Logic and Limits of Trust.* New Brunswick, NJ: Rutgers University Press.

Bardach, Eugene, and Robert A. Kagan. 1982. *Going by the Book: The Problem of Regulatory Unreasonableness.* Philadelphia: Temple University Press.

Barnard, Chester I. 1938. *Functions of the Executive.* Cambridge: Harvard University Press.

Becker, Howard S. 1960. "Notes on the Concept of Commitment." *American Sociological Review* 66:32–40.

———. 1963. *Outsiders: Studies in the Sociology of Deviance.* New York: Free Press.

———. 1964. "Personal Changes in Adult Life." *Sociometry* 27 (March):40–53.

Bergen, Mark, Shantanu Dutta, and Orville C. Walker. 1992. "Agency Relationships in Marketing: A Review of the Implications and Applications of Agency and Related Theories." *Journal of Marketing* 56:1–24.

Bielby, Denise D., and William T. Bielby. 1988. "She Works Hard for the Money: Household Responsibilities and the Allocation of Work Effort." *American Journal of Sociology* 93:1031–59.

Blau, Peter M. 1963. *The Dynamics of Bureaucracy.* Rev. ed. Chicago: University of Chicago Press.

Boli-Bennett, John, and John Meyer. 1978. "The Ideology of Childhood and the State:

Rules Distinguishing Children in National Constitutions, 1870–1970." *American Sociological Review* 43:797–812.

Bopp, James, Jr., and Mary Nimz. 1992. "A Legal Analysis of the Child Abuse Amendments of 1984." Pp. 73–104 in A. L. Caplan, R. H. Blank, and J. C. Merrick, eds., *Compelled Compassion: Government Intervention in the Treatment of Critically Ill Newborns.* Totowa, NJ: Humana Press.

Bosk, Charles L. 1979. *Forgive and Remember: Managing Medical Failure.* Chicago: University of Chicago Press.

———. 1992. *All God's Mistakes: Genetic Counseling in a Pediatric Hospital.* Chicago: University of Chicago Press.

Bosk, Charles L., and Joel E. Frader. 1990. "AIDS and Its Impact on Medical Work: The Culture and Politics of the Shop Floor." *Milbank Quarterly* 6:257–79.

Bowditch, Christine. 1993. "Getting Rid of Troublemakers: High School Disciplinary Procedures and the Production of Dropouts." *Social Problems* 40:493–509.

Braithwaite, John B. 1985. *To Punish or Persuade: Enforcement of Coal Mine Safety.* Albany: SUNY Press.

———. 1989. *Crime, Shame, and Reintegration.* Cambridge: Cambridge University Press.

Braithwaite, John B., and Stephen Mugford. 1994. "Conditions of Successful Reintegration Ceremonies: Dealing with Juvenile Offenders." *British Journal of Criminology* 34:139–71.

Brazelton, T. Berry. 1983. *Infants and Mothers: Differences in Development.* Rev. ed. New York: Delta.

Burawoy, Michael. 1979. *Manufacturing Consent.* Chicago: University of Chicago Press.

Campion, Mukti Jain. 1995. *Who's Fit To Be a Parent?* New York: Routledge.

Caplan, Arthur L., Robert H. Blank, and Janna C. Merrick, eds. 1992. *Compelled Compassion: Government Intervention in the Treatment of Critically Ill Newborns.* Totowa, NJ: Humana Press.

Chambliss, Daniel F. 1996. *Beyond Caring: Hospitals, Nurses, and the Social Organization of Ethics.* Chicago: University of Chicago Press.

Chandler, Alfred D., Jr. 1962. *Strategy and Structure.* Cambridge: MIT Press.

Charlton, Joy Carol. 1983. "Secretaries and Bosses." Ph.D. diss., Northwestern University.

Cialdini, Robert B. 1984. *Influence: How and Why People Agree to Things.* New York: Morrow.

Cirillo, Renato. 1979. *The Economics of Vilfredo Pareto.* London: Frank Cass.

Clarke, Lee. 1989. *Acceptable Risk? Making Decisions in a Toxic Environment.* Berkeley: University of California Press.

Cloherty, John P., and Ann R. Stark. 1991. *Manual of Neonatal Care.* 3d ed. Boston: Little, Brown.

Cohen, Michael D., James G. March, and Johan P. Olsen. 1972. "A Garbage Can Model of Organizational Choice." *Administrative Science Quarterly* 17 (March):1–25.

Coleman, James S. 1974. *Power and the Structure of Society.* New York: Norton.

———. 1982. *The Asymmetric Society.* Syracuse, NY: Syracuse University Press.

———. 1990. *Foundations of Social Theory.* Cambridge: Harvard University Press.

Coltrane, Scott. 1996. *Family Man: Fatherhood, Housework, and Gender Equity.* New York: Oxford University Press.

Cook County State's Attorney's Task Force on the Foregoing of Life-Sustaining Treatment. 1990. *Report of the Cook County State's Attorney's Task Force on the Foregoing of Life-Sustaining Treatment.* Cook County, IL: Cook County State's Attorney's Office.

Cornblath, Marvin, and Russell L. Clark. 1984. "Neonatal 'Brain Damage': An Analysis of 250 Claims." *Western Journal of Medicine* 140:298–302.

Coser, Lewis A. 1974. *Greedy Institutions.* New York: Free Press.

Cotton, Robert B. 1994. "A Model of the Effect of Surfactant Treatment on Gas Exchange in Hyaline Membrane Disease." *Seminars in Perinatology* 18:19–22.

Darling, Rosalyn Benjamin. 1979. *Families against Society: A Study of Reactions to Children with Birth Defects.* Beverly Hills, CA: Sage.

Devers, Kelly J. 1994. "Triage in Adult Intensive Care Units: How Organizations Allocate Resources." Ph.D. diss., Northwestern University.

DiLeonardo, Micaela. 1987. "The Female World of Cards and Holidays: Women, Families, and the Work of Kinship." *Signs* 12:440–53.

Dilley, Becki, and Keith Dilley, with Sam Stall. 1995. *Special Delivery: How We Are Raising America's Only Sextuplets. . .and Loving It.* New York: Random House.

Dingwall, Robert, John Eekelaar, and Topsy Murray. 1983. *The Protection of Children: State Intervention and Family Life.* Oxford: Basil Blackwell.

Douglas, Mary, and Baron Isherwood. 1978. *The World of Goods.* New York: Basic.

Durkheim, Emile. [1895] 1982. *The Rules of Sociological Method.* Trans. W. D. Halls. New York: Free Press.

Economist. 1996. "Sex and Drugs and Nutty Schools," 341 (October 12–18):31.

Edin, Kathryn, and Laura Lein. 1996. "Work, Welfare, and Single Mothers' Economic Survival Strategies." *American Sociological Review* 61:253–66.

Eisenberg, Arlene, Heidi E. Murkoff, and Sandee E. Hathaway. 1989. *What to Expect the First Year.* New York: Workman.

Emerson, Robert M. 1969. *Judging Delinquents: Context and Process in Juvenile Court.* Chicago: Aldine.

———. 1981. "On Last Resorts." *American Journal of Sociology* 87:1–22.

———. 1983. "Holistic Effects in Social Control Decision-Making." *Law and Society Review* 17:425–55.

———. 1991. "Case Processing and Interorganizational Knowledge: Detecting the 'Real' Reasons for Referrals." *Social Problems* 38 (2):198–212.

———. 1992. "Disputes in Public Bureaucracies." *Studies in Law, Politics, and Society* 12:3–29.

Emerson, Robert M., and Sheldon L. Messinger. 1977. "The Micro-Politics of Trouble." *Social Problems* 25:121–34.

Erikson, Kai T. 1966. *Wayward Puritans: A Study in the Sociology of Deviance.* New York: Wiley.

Espeland, Wendy Nelson. 1992. "Contested Rationalities: Commensuration and the Representation of Value in Public Choice." Ph.D. diss., University of Chicago. [Revised as *The Struggle for Water: Politics, Rationality, and Identity in the American Southwest,* Chicago: University of Chicago Press, 1998.]

Faden, Ruth R., and Tom L. Beauchamp, with Nancy M. P. King. 1986. *A History and Theory of Informed Consent.* New York: Oxford University Press.

Fama, Eugene F. 1980. "Agency Problems and the Theory of the Firm." *Journal of Political Economy* 88:288–307.

Fama, Eugene F., and Michael C. Jensen. 1983. "Agency Problems and Residual Claims." *Journal of Law and Economics* 26:327–49.

Faulkner, Robert R. 1983. *Music on Demand.* New Brunswick, NJ: Transaction.
Fineman, Martha Albertson. 1995. *The Neutered Mother, the Sexual Family, and Other Twentieth Century Tragedies.* New York: Routledge.
Fost, Norman. 1989. "Do the Right Thing: Samuel Linares and Defensive Law." *Law, Medicine and Health Care* 17:330–34.
———. 1992. "Infant Care Review Committees in the Aftermath of Baby Doe." Pp. 285–98 in A. L. Caplan, R. H. Blank, and J. C. Merrick, eds., *Compelled Compassion: Government Intervention in the Treatment of Critically Ill Newborns.* Totowa, NJ: Humana Press.
Freeman, Caroline. 1982. "The 'Understanding Employer.'" Pp. 135–53 in Jackie West, ed., *Women, Work, and the Labour Market.* London: Routledge and Kegan Paul.
Freidson, Eliot. 1970. *Professional Dominance: The Social Structure of Medical Care.* New York: Atherton.
———. [1970] 1988. *Profession of Medicine: A Study in the Sociology of Applied Knowledge.* Chicago: University of Chicago Press.
———. 1989. *Medical Work in America: Essays on Healthcare.* New Haven, CT: Yale University Press.
Frey, Darcy. 1995. "Does Anyone Here Think This Baby Can Live?" *New York Times Magazine* (July 9, section 6): 22–31, 36, 44–45.
Friedman, Debra. 1995. *Towards a Structure of Indifference: The Social Origins of Maternal Custody.* New York: Aldine de Gruyter.
Frohock, Fred M. 1986. *Special Care: Medical Decisions at the Beginning of Life.* Chicago: University of Chicago Press.
———. 1992. *Healing Powers: Alternative Medicine, Spiritual Communities, and the State.* Chicago: University of Chicago Press.
Garfinkel, Harold. 1967. *Studies in Ethnomethodology.* Englewood Cliffs, NJ: Prentice-Hall.
Gerry, Martin H., and Mary Nimz. 1987. "Federal Role in Protecting Babies Doe." *Issues in Law and Medicine* 2:339–77.
Gerson, Kathleen. 1985. *Hard Choices: How Women Decide about Work, Career, and Motherhood.* Berkeley: University of California Press.
———. 1993. *No Man's Land: Men's Changing Commitments to Family and Work.* New York: Basic.
Gibbs, Jack P., and Maynard L. Erickson. 1975. "Major Developments in the Sociological Study of Deviance." *Annual Review of Sociology* 1:21–42.
Giddens, Anthony. 1979. *Central Problems in Social Theory: Action, Structure, and Contradictions in Social Analysis.* Berkeley: University of California Press.
Gilboy, Janet A. 1991. "Deciding Who Gets In: Decisionmaking by Immigration Inspectors." *Law and Society Review* 25 (3):571–99.
———. 1992. "Penetrability of Administrative Systems: Political 'Casework' and Immigration Inspections." *Law and Society Review* 26 (2):273–314.
Gilligan, Carol. 1982. *In a Different Voice.* Cambridge: Harvard University Press.
Goffman, Erving. 1967. "Where the Action Is." Pp. 149–270 in *Interaction Ritual: Essays on Face-to-Face Behavior.* Garden City, NY: Doubleday.
———. 1971. "The Insanity of Place." Pp. 35–90 in *Relations in Public: Microstudies of the Public Order.* New York: Basic.
Goldman, Gilbert M., Karen M. Stratton, and Max Douglas Brown. 1989. "What Actu-

ally Happened: An Informed Review of the Linares Incident." *Law, Medicine and Health Care* 17:298–307.

Gostin, Larry. 1989. "Editor's Introduction: Family Privacy and Persistent Vegetative State." *Law, Medicine and Health Care* 17:295–97.

Guillemin, Jeanne Harley, and Lynda Lytle Holmstrom. 1986. *Mixed Blessings: Intensive Care for Newborns.* New York: Oxford University Press.

Halpern, Sydney A. 1988. *American Pediatrics.* Berkeley: University of California Press.

Haralambie, Ann M. 1987. *Family Law Series.* Vols. 1–2. Colorado Springs, CO: Shepard's McGraw-Hill.

Harrison, Helen. 1986. "Neonatal Intensive Care: Parents' Role in Ethical Decision Making." *Birth* 13:165–75.

Harrison, Helen, with Ann Kositsky. 1983. *The Premature Baby Book.* New York: St. Martin's.

Hawkins, Keith. 1983. "Assessing Evil." *British Journal of Criminology* 23 (2):101–27.

———, ed. 1992. *The Uses of Discretion.* Oxford: Clarendon Press.

Hays, Sharon. 1996. *The Cultural Contradictions of Motherhood.* New Haven, CT: Yale University Press.

Heimer, Carol A. 1984. "Organizational and Individual Control of Career Development in Engineering Project Work." *Acta Sociologica* 27 (4):283–310.

———. 1985. *Reactive Risk and Rational Action: Managing Moral Hazard in Insurance Contracts.* Berkeley: University of California Press.

———. 1986. "Producing Responsible Behavior in Order to Produce Oil: Bringing Obligations, Rights, Incentives, and Resources Together in the Norwegian State Oil Company." Report #76, Institute of Industrial Economics, Bergen, Norway. Also issued as a working paper at Center for Urban Affairs and Policy Research, Northwestern University.

———. 1988. "Social Structure, Psychology, and the Estimation of Risk." *Annual Review of Sociology* 14:491–519.

———. 1990. "Dimensions of the Agency Relationship." Northwestern University. Unpublished paper.

———. 1992a. "Doing Your Job *and* Helping Your Friends: Universalistic Norms about Obligations to Particular Others in Networks." Pp. 143–64 in Nitin Nohria and Robert G. Eccles, eds., *Networks and Organizations: Structure, Form, and Action.* Boston: Harvard Business School Press.

———.1992b. "Your Baby's Fine, Just Fine: Certification Procedures, Meetings, and the Supply of Information in Neonatal Intensive Care Units." Pp. 161–88 in James F. Short, Jr. and Lee Clarke, eds., *Organizations, Uncertainties, and Risk.* Boulder, CO: Westview Press.

———. 1993. "Competing Institutions: Law, Medicine, and Family in Neonatal Intensive Care." American Bar Foundation Working Paper #9308.

———. 1996a. "Explaining Variation in the Impact of Law: Organizations, Institutions, and Professions." *Studies in Law, Politics and Society* 15:29–59.

———. 1996b. "Gender Inequalities in the Distribution of Responsibility." Pp. 241–73 in James Baron, David Grusky, and Donald Treiman, eds., *Social Differentiation and Social Inequality: Essays in Honor of John Pock.* Boulder, CO: Westview Press.

Heimer, Carol A., and Lisa R. Staffen. 1995. "Interdependence and Reintegrative Social

Control: Labeling and Reforming 'Inappropriate' Parents in Neonatal Intensive Care Units." *American Sociological Review* 60 (October):635–54.

Heimer, Carol A., and Mitchell L. Stevens. 1997. "Caring for the Organization: Social Workers as Frontline Risk Managers in Neonatal Intensive Care Units." *Work and Occupations* 24 (2):133–63.

Heimer, Carol A., and Arthur L. Stinchcombe. 1980. "Love and Irrationality: It's Got to Be Rational to Love You because It Makes Me So Happy." *Social Science Information* 19 (4/5):697–754.

Hertz, Rosanna. 1986. *More Equal than Others.* Berkeley: University of California Press.

Hirschman, Albert O. 1970. *Exit, Voice, and Loyalty: Responses to Decline in Firms, Organizations, and States.* Cambridge: Harvard University Press.

Hochschild, Arlie Russell. 1997. *The Time Bind: When Work Becomes Home and Home Becomes Work.* New York: Metropolitan.

———, with Anne Machung. 1989. *The Second Shift.* New York: Viking.

Hodgman, Joan E. 1990. "Neonatology." *Journal of the American Medical Association* 263 (19):2656–57.

Holmstrøm, Bengt. 1979. "Moral Hazard and Observability." *Bell Journal of Economics* 10:74–91.

———. 1982. "Moral Hazard in Teams." *Bell Journal of Economics* 13:324–40.

Hughes, Everett C. (1958) 1981. *Men and Their Work.* Westport, CT: Greenwood Press.

———. 1971. *The Sociological Eye.* Chicago: Aldine-Atherton.

Jaques, Elliott. 1972. *Measurement of Responsibility.* New York: Wiley.

Jencks, Christopher, Lauri Perman, and Lee Rainwater. 1988. "What Is a Good Job? A New Measure of Labor Market Success." *American Journal of Sociology* 93:1322–57.

Kant, Immanuel. [1785] 1949. *Fundamental Principles of the Metaphysic of Morals.* Trans. Thomas K. Abbott. Indianapolis: Bobbs-Merrill.

———. [1781] 1965a. *Critique of Pure Reason.* Trans. Norman Kemp Smith. New York: St. Martin's.

———. [1797] 1965b. *The Metaphysical Elements of Justice.* Trans. John Ladd. Indianapolis: Bobbs-Merrill.

Kaplan, Elaine Bell. 1996. "Black Teenage Mothers and Their Mothers: The Impact of Adolescent Childbearing on Daughters' Relations with Mothers." *Social Problems* 43:427–43.

Katz, Jay. 1984. *The Silent World of Doctor and Patient.* New York: Free Press.

Kidder, Tracy. 1981. *The Soul of a New Machine.* New York: Avon.

Kitsuse, John I. 1972. "Deviance, Deviant Behavior, and Deviants: Some Conceptual Problems." Pp. 233–43 in W. J. Filstead, ed., *An Introduction to Deviance.* Chicago: Markham.

Kliegman, R. M. 1995. "Neonatal Technology, Perinatal Survival, Social Consequences, and the Perinatal Paradox." *American Journal of Public Health* 85:909–13.

Kohlberg, Lawrence. 1981. *Essays on Moral Development.* New York: Harper and Row.

Kopelman, Loretta M., Arthur E. Kopelman, and Thomas G. Irons. 1992. "Neonatologists, Pediatricians, and the Supreme Court Criticize the 'Baby Doe' Regulations." Pp. 237–66 in A. L. Caplan, R. H. Blank, and J. C. Merrick, eds., *Compelled Compassion: Government Intervention in the Treatment of Critically Ill Newborns.* Totowa, NJ: Humana Press.

Lantos, John D., Steven H. Miles, and Christine K. Cassel. 1989. "The Linares Affair." *Law, Medicine and Health Care* 17:308–15.

LaRossa, Ralph, and Maureen Mulligan LaRossa. 1981. *Transition to Parenthood.* Beverley Hills, CA: Sage.

Latané, Bibb, and John M. Darley. 1970. *The Unresponsive Bystander.* New York: Meredith Corporation.

Layne, Linda L. 1990. "Motherhood Lost: Cultural Dimensions of Miscarriage and Stillbirth in America." *Women and Health* 16 (3/4):69–89.

Leach, Penelope. 1983. *Babyhood.* 2d ed. New York: Knopf.

Leidner, Robin L. 1993. *Fast Food, Fast Talk.* Berkeley: University of California Press.

Lempert, Richard. 1972. "Norm-Making in Social Exchange: A Contract Law Model." *Law and Society Review* 7 (1):1–32.

Lempert, Richard, and Joseph Sanders. 1986. *An Invitation to Law and Social Science: Deserts, Disputes, and Distribution.* Philadelphia: University of Pennsylvania Press.

Letherby, Gayle. 1993. "The Meanings of Miscarriage." *Women's Studies International Forum* 16:165–85.

Levine, Judith A. 1996. "Policy Incentives Confront Everyday Realities: Integrating Economic and Sociological Perspectives on the Welfare-to-Work Transition." Institute for Policy Research Working Paper Series #WP-96–3, Northwestern University.

Lieberman, Adrienne B., and Thomas G. Sheagren. 1984. *The Premie Parents' Handbook.* New York: E. P. Dutton.

Lieberman, Jethro K. 1981. *The Litigious Society.* New York: Basic.

Loewenstein, George, and Jon Elster. 1992. *Choice over Time.* New York: Russell Sage Foundation.

Luker, Kristin. 1996. *Dubious Conceptions: The Politics of Teenage Pregnancy.* Cambridge: Harvard University Press.

Lyon, Jeff. 1985. *Playing God in the Nursery.* New York: Norton.

Macaulay, Stewart. 1963. "Non-contractual Relations in Business: A Preliminary Study." *American Sociological Review* 28:55–66.

Maccoby, Eleanor E., and Robert H. Mnookin. 1992. *Dividing the Child: Social and Legal Dilemmas of Custody.* Cambridge: Harvard University Press.

McCarthy, John D., and Dean R. Hoge. 1987. "The Social Construction of School Punishment: Racial Disadvantage out of Universalistic Process." *Social Forces* 65: 1101–20.

McCormick, Marie C. 1989. "Long-term Follow-up of Infants Discharged from Neonatal Intensive Care Units." *Journal of the American Medical Association* 261 (12): 1767–72.

McKeon, Richard. [1957] 1990. "The Development and Significance of the Concept of Responsibility." Pp. 62–87 in *Freedom and History and Other Essays.* Chicago: University of Chicago Press.

———. 1957. "Responsibility as Sign and as Instrumentality." Paper, Institute on Ethics of the Institute for Religious and Social Studies, Jewish Theological Seminary of America.

McMahon, Martha. 1995. *Engendering Motherhood: Identity and Self-Transformation in Women's Lives.* New York: Guilford Press.

Mansbridge, Jane J. 1990. "On the Relation of Altruism and Self-Interest." Pp. 133–43 in J. Mansbridge, ed., *Beyond Self-Interest.* Chicago: University of Chicago Press.

March, James G., and Johan P. Olsen, eds. 1976. *Ambiguity and Choice in Organizations.* Bergen: Norwegian University Press.

Matsueda, Ross L. 1992. "Reflected Appraisals, Parental Labeling, and Delinquency:

Specifying a Symbolic Interactionist Theory." *American Journal of Sociology* 97: 1577–1611.

Maynard, Douglas W. 1996. "The Forecasting of Bad News as a Social Relation." *American Sociological Review* 61 (1):109–31.

Mehren, Elizabeth. 1991. *Born Too Soon.* New York: Doubleday.

Meisel, Alan, and Lisa D. Kabnick. 1980. "Informed Consent to Medical Treatment: An Analysis of Recent Legislation." *University of Pittsburgh Law Review* 41:407–564.

Menkel-Meadow, Carrie. 1996. "What's Gender Got to Do with It? The Politics and Morality of an Ethic of Care." *New York University Review of Law and Social Change* 22 (1):265–93.

Merton, Robert K. [1949] 1968. *Social Theory and Social Structure.* Enl. ed. New York: Free Press.

———. 1987. "Three Fragments from a Sociologist's Notebook: Establishing the Phenomenon, Specified Ignorance, and Strategic Research Material." *Annual Review of Sociology* 13:1–28.

Merton, Robert K., David Sills, and Stephen Stigler. 1984. "The Kelvin Dictum and Social Science: An Excursion into the History of an Idea." *Journal of the History of the Behavioral Sciences* 20:319–31.

Mnookin, Robert H., and Lewis Kornhauser. 1979. "Bargaining in the Shadow of the Law: The Case of Divorce." *Yale Law Journal* 88:950–97.

Monsma, Karl. 1993. "Contracts or Exchange? Principals and Agents on a 19th-Century Ranching Frontier." Paper presented at Social Science History Association Annual Meetings, Baltimore.

Mynatt, Clifford, and Steven J. Sherman. 1975. "Responsibility Attribution in Groups and Individuals: A Direct Test of the Diffusion of Responsibility Hypothesis." *Journal of Personality and Social Psychology* 32:1111–18.

Nelson, Lawrence J., and Ronald E. Cranford. 1989. "Legal Advice, Moral Paralysis and the Death of Samuel Linares." *Law, Medicine and Health Care* 17:316–24.

New, Caroline, and Miriam David. 1985. *For the Children's Sake: Making Childcare More than Women's Business.* Harmondsworth: Penguin.

Newman, Stephen A. 1989. "Baby Doe, Congress and the States: Challenging the Federal Treatment Standard for Impaired Infants." *American Journal of Law and Medicine* 15:1–60.

New York Times. 1995. "Father Acquitted in Death of His Premature Baby," February 3 (late ed.), section A, p. 15.

Nocon, James J., and David A. Coolman. 1987. "Perinatal Malpractice: Risks and Prevention." *Journal of Reproductive Medicine* 32:83–90.

Nussbaum, Martha C. 1986. *The Fragility of Goodness: Luck and Ethics in Greek Tragedy and Philosophy.* Cambridge: Cambridge University Press.

O'Connell, Jeffrey. 1979. *The Lawsuit Lottery.* New York: Free Press.

Padgett, John F., and Christopher K. Ansell. 1993. "Robust Action and the Rise of the Medici, 1400–1434." *American Journal of Sociology* 98:1259–1319.

Page, Clarence. 1996. "Calm the Chaos over Kissing Kids." *Chicago Tribune,* October 9, p. 15.

Paneth, Nigel. 1990. "Technology at Birth." *American Journal of Public Health* 80 (7):791–92.

Parsons, Talcott. 1956. "A Sociological Approach to the Theory of Organizations." *Administrative Science Quarterly* 1:63–85, 225–39.

———. 1968. "Professions." Pp. 536–47 in *International Encyclopedia of the Social Sciences.* New York: Macmillan.

Parsons, Talcott, and Edward A. Shils. 1951. "Categories of the Orientation and Organization of Action." Pp. 53–109 in T. Parsons and E. A. Shils, eds., *Towards a General Theory of Action.* New York: Harper and Row.

Paternoster, Raymond, and Leeann Iovanni. 1989. "The Labeling Perspective and Delinquency: An Elaboration of the Theory and an Assessment of the Evidence." *Justice Quarterly* 6 (3):359–94.

Pegalis, Steven E., and Harvey F. Wachsman. 1992. *American Law of Medical Malpractice 2nd,* vol 1. Deerfield, IL: Clark Boardman Callaghan.

———. 1993. *American Law of Medical Malpractice 2nd,* vol. 2. Deerfield, IL: Clark Boardman Callaghan.

Petersen, Trond. 1993. "Recent Developments in the Economics of Organizations: The Principal-Agent Relationship." *Acta Sociologica* 36 (3):277–93.

Pleck, Joseph H. 1977. "The Work-Family System." *Social Problems* 26:417–27.

Pollock, Linda A. 1983. *Forgotten Children: Parent-Child Relations from 1500 to 1900.* Cambridge: Cambridge University Press.

Popenoe, David. 1996. *Life without Father: Compelling New Evidence that Fatherhood and Marriage Are Indispensable for the Good of Children and Society.* New York: Martin Kessler.

Pratt, John W., and Richard J. Zeckhauser, eds. [1985] 1991. *Principals and Agents: The Structure of Business.* Boston: Harvard Business School Press.

Raab, Francis. 1968. "History, Freedom and Responsibility." Pp. 694–704 in May Brodbeck, ed., *Readings in the Philosophy of the Social Sciences.* New York: Macmillan.

Rathi, Manohar, ed. 1989. *Current Perinatology.* New York: Springer-Verlag.

Rawls, John. 1971. *A Theory of Justice.* Cambridge: Harvard University Press.

Raz, Joseph. 1986. *The Morality of Freedom.* Oxford: Clarendon Press.

Reinharz, Shulamit. 1988. "Controlling Women's Lives: A Cross-Cultural Interpretation of Pregnancy Accounts." *Research in the Sociology of Health Care.* 7:3–37.

Ribbens, Jane. 1994. *Mothers and Their Children: A Feminist Sociology of Childrearing.* Thousand Oaks, CA: Sage.

Robinson, J. P. 1977. *How Americans Use Time.* New York: Praeger Press.

Rosenbaum, James E., and Takehiko Kariya. 1989. "From High School to Work: Market and Institutional Mechanisms in Japan." *American Journal of Sociology* 94:1334–65.

Rossi, Alice S. 1968. "Transition to Parenthood." *Journal of Marriage and the Family* 30:26–39.

———. 1977. "A Biosocial Perspective on Parenting." *Daedalus* 106 (2):1–31.

———. 1985. "Gender and Parenthood." Pp. 161–91 in Alice S. Rossi, ed., *Gender and the Life Course.* New York: Aldine.

Rossi, Alice S., and Peter H. Rossi. 1990. *Of Human Bonding.* New York: Aldine de Gruyter.

Roth, Julius A. 1972. "Some Contingencies of the Moral Evaluation and Control of Clientele: The Case of the Hospital Emergency Service." *American Journal of Sociology* 77:836–49.

Rothman, Barbara Katz. 1986. *The Tentative Pregnancy: Prenatal Diagnosis and the Future of Motherhood.* New York: Viking Penguin.

Rothman, David J. 1991. *Strangers at the Bedside: A History of How Law and Bioethics Transformed Medical Decision Making.* New York: Basic.

Rutkowski, G. K., C. L. Gruder, and D. Romer. 1983. "Group Cohesion, Social Norms, and Bystander Intervention." *Journal of Personality and Social Psychology* 44:545–52.

Sanchez, Lisa E. 1997. "Boundaries of Legitimacy: Sex, Violence, Citizenship and Community in a Local Sexual Economy." *Law and Social Inquiry* 22:543–80.

Schelling, Thomas C. 1960. *The Strategy of Conflict.* Cambridge: Harvard University Press.

Scheppele, Kim Lane. 1991. "Law without Accidents." Pp. 267–93 in Pierre Bourdieu and James S. Coleman, eds., *Social Theory for a Changing Society.* Boulder, CO: Westview Press.

Schuck, Peter H. 1994. "Rethinking Informed Consent." *Yale Law Journal* 103:899–959.

Schutz, Alfred. 1962. *Collected Papers.* Vol. I: *The Problem of Social Reality.* Ed. M. Natanson. The Hague: Martinus Nijhoff.

Scott, James C. 1985. *Weapons of the Weak: Everyday Forms of Peasant Resistance.* New Haven, CT: Yale University Press.

Scott, Marvin B., and Stanford M. Lyman. 1968. "Accounts." *American Sociological Review* 33:46–62.

Seligman, Milton, and Roslyn Benjamin Darling. 1989. *Ordinary Families, Special Children: A Systems Approach to Childhood Disability.* New York: Guilford Press.

Selznick, Philip. 1992. *The Moral Commonwealth: Social Theory and the Promise of Community.* Berkeley: University of California Press.

Sewell, William H., Jr. 1992. "A Theory of Structure: Duality, Agency, and Transformation." *American Journal of Sociology* 98:1–29.

Shapiro, Robyn S., and Richard Barthel. 1986. "Infant Care Review Committees: An Effective Approach to Baby Doe's Dilemma?" *Hastings Law Journal* 37:827–62.

Shapiro, Susan P. 1987. "The Social Control of Impersonal Trust." *American Journal of Sociology* 93:623–58.

Silverman, William A. 1980. *Retrolental Fibroplasia: A Modern Parable.* New York: Grune and Stratton.

Simmons, Roberta G., Susan D. Klein, and Richard L. Simmons. 1977. *Gift of Life.* New York: Wiley.

Sobel, Joel. 1993. "Information Control in the Principal-Agent Problem." *International Economic Review* 34:259–69.

Soltan, Karol E. 1987. *The Causal Theory of Justice.* Berkeley: University of California Press.

Spitze, Glenna, and John R. Logan. 1990. "Sons, Daughters, and Intergenerational Social Support." *Journal of Marriage and the Family* 52:420–30.

Spock, Benjamin. 1976. *Baby and Child Care.* New York: Simon and Schuster.

Stacey, Judith. 1996. *In the Name of the Family: Rethinking Family Values in the Postmodern Age.* Boston: Beacon Press.

Staffen, Lisa R. 1994. "Heroic Medicine, Physician Autonomy, and Patient Rights." *Law and Social Inquiry* 19:753–73.

Starr, Paul. 1982. *The Social Transformation of American Medicine.* New York: Basic.

Stevens, Mitchell L. 1996. "Kingdom and Coalition: Hierarchy and Autonomy in the Home Education Movement." Ph.D. diss., Northwestern University.

Stinchcombe, Arthur L. 1990. *Information and Organizations.* Berkeley: University of California Press.

Stinson, Robert, and Peggy Stinson. 1979. "On the Death of a Baby." *Atlantic Monthly* 244 (July):64–72.

———. 1983. *The Long Dying of Baby Andrew.* Boston: Little, Brown.

Stone, Christopher D. 1975. *Where the Law Ends: The Social Control of Corporate Behavior.* New York: Harper and Row.

Strandjord, Thomas P., and W. Alan Hodson. 1992. "Neonatology." *Journal of the American Medical Association* 268 (3):377–78.

Stubblefield, Phillip G. 1984. "Causes and Prevention of Preterm Birth: An Overview." Pp. 3–20 in Fritz Fuchs and Phillip G. Stubblefield, eds., *Preterm Birth: Causes, Prevention and Management.* New York: Macmillan.

Sudnow, David. 1965. "Normal Crimes: Sociological Features of the Penal Code in a Public Defender Office." *Social Problems* 12:255–76.

Szalai, Alexander, ed. 1972. *The Use of Time.* The Hague: Mouton.

Taylor, Verta. 1996. *Rock-a-by Baby: Feminism, Self-Help, and Postpartum Depression.* New York: Routledge.

Thompson, James D. 1967. *Organizations in Action.* New York: McGraw-Hill.

Tronto, Joan C. 1993. *Moral Boundaries: A Political Argument for an Ethic of Care.* New York: Routledge.

Tversky, Amos, and Daniel Kahneman. 1974. "Judgment under Uncertainty: Heuristics and Biases." *Science* 185:1124–31.

U.S. Bureau of the Census. 1996. *Statistical Abstract of the United States: 1993.* 116th ed. Washington, DC: Government Printing Office.

Van Maanen, John. 1978. "The Asshole." Pp. 221–38 in P. K. Manning and J. Van Mannen, eds., *Policing: A View from the Street.* Santa Monica, CA: Goodyear.

Vaughan, Diane. 1996. *The Challenger Launch Decision: Risky Technology, Culture, and Deviance at NASA.* Chicago: University of Chicago Press.

Waegel, William B. 1981. "Case Routinization in Investigative Police Work." *Social Problems* 28:263–75.

Walman, Terry. 1992. "Decision Making in the Neonatal Intensive Care Unit: The Impact of the 1984 Child Abuse Amendments." Pp. 299–316 in A. L. Caplan, R. H. Blank, and J. C. Merrick, eds., *Compelled Compassion: Government Intervention in the Treatment of Critically Ill Newborns.* Totowa, NJ: Humana Press.

Walzer, Susan. 1996. "Thinking about the Baby: Gender and Divisions of Infant Care." *Social Problems* 43:219–34.

Weir, Robert F. 1984. *Selective Nontreatment of Handicapped Newborns.* New York: Oxford University Press.

White, Martha S. 1970. "Psychological and Social Barriers to Women in Science." *Science* 170:413–16.

Whyte, William Foote. 1993. *Street Corner Society: The Social Structure of an Italian Slum.* 4th ed. Chicago: University of Chicago Press.

Whyte, William H. 1956. *The Organization Man.* New York: Simon and Schuster.

Wieder, D. Lawrence. 1983. "Telling the Convict Code." Pp. 78–90 in Robert M. Emerson, ed., *Contemporary Field Research: A Collection of Readings.* Prospect Heights, IL: Waveland Press.

Wrong, Dennis. 1961. "The Oversocialized Conception of Man in Modern Sociology." *American Sociological Review* 26:183–93.

Wuthnow, Robert. 1991. *Acts of Compassion.* Princeton, NJ: Princeton University Press.

———. 1994. *Sharing the Journey: Support Groups and America's New Quest for Community.* New York: Free Press.

Zajonc, Robert B. 1980. "Feeling and Thinking: Preferences Need No Inferences." *American Psychologist* 35 (2):151–75.
Zelizer, Viviana A. Rotman. 1985. *Pricing the Priceless Child: The Changing Social Values of Money.* New York: Basic.
Zey, Mary. 1993. *Banking on Fraud.* New York: Aldine de Gruyter.
Zussman, Robert. 1992. *Intensive Care: Medical Ethics and the Medical Profession.* Chicago: University of Chicago Press.
Zylke, Jody W. 1990. "Individualized Care, as well as Intensive Care, May Reduce Morbidity among Premature Infants." *Journal of the American Medical Association* 264 (20):2611–12.

Cases Cited

Canterbury v. Spence, 464 F.2d 772, 787 (D.C. Cir. 1972)
Helling v. Carey, 83 Wash. 2d 514, 519 P.2d 981 (1974)
Jehovah's Witnesses in the State of Washington v. King County Hospital Unit 1 (Harborview) 390 U.S. 598 (1967)

INDEX OF INTERVIEWS

This index includes interviews that are cited individually in the book. Additional, uncited interviews were used in making the computations reported in tables and contribute in a more general way to our conclusions. An explanation of the interview code numbers can be found in footnote 1 on page 1.

Family Interviews

GENERAL INDEX